MW01253793

Immunology of Oral Diseases

TO
MARGARET
AND
GRETA

Immunology of Oral Diseases

IVAN M. ROITT MA, DSc(Oxon),
FRCPath, FRS, *Professor and Head of Department of
Immunology, Middlesex Hospital Medical School, London W1*

THOMAS LEHNER MD, BDS,
FDS, FRCPath, *Professor of Oral Immunology,
Head of Department of Oral Immunology and Microbiology,
United Medical Schools of Guy's and
St Thomas's Hospitals, London SE1*

SECOND EDITION

BLACKWELL SCIENTIFIC PUBLICATIONS

OXFORD LONDON
EDINBURGH BOSTON MELBOURNE

First published 1980
Second edition 1983

Japanese edition 1982

Photoset by Enset Ltd
Midsomer Norton, Bath, Avon
and printed and bound
in Great Britain by
Butler & Tanner Ltd
Frome, Somerset

DISTRIBUTORS

USA
  Blackwell Mosby Book
  Distributors
  11830 Westline Industrial Drive
  St Louis, Missouri 63141

Canada
  Blackwell Mosby Book
  Distributors
  120 Melford Drive, Scarborough
  Ontario, M1B 2X4

Australia
  Blackwell Scientific Book
  Distributors
  214 Berkeley Street, Carlton
  Victoria 3053

British Library
Cataloguing in Publication Data

Roitt, Ivan M
    Immunology of oral diseases.—
    2nd ed.
    1. Mouth—Diseases—Immuno-
    logical aspects
    I. Title   II. Lehner, T.
    616.3'1079   RC815

ISBN 0–632–01079–7

Contents

Preface to second edition

Within about a year of launching the first textbook of *Immunology of Oral Diseases* in this country and probably in the world, the necessity for the second edition became evident. A great deal of feedback and helpful advice from students and colleagues alike persuaded us to revise and expand the section on applied oral immunology at the expense of the section on basic immunology. Elective surgery was performed on some of the more theoretical and less essential concepts of basic immunology, bearing in mind the requirements of dental students. However, immunology will not stay still and new sections have been introduced dealing particularly with monoclonal antibodies, the diotypic network and certain technological advances.

The section on immunology of oral diseases has been extensively revised to bring it up-to-date. This applies particularly to the chapter dealing with periodontal disease in which there have been important advances in the immune responses to newly discovered micro-organisms. Recent views on the role of helper and suppressor cells in the regulation of the immune responses involved in both caries and periodontal disease have been included in the corresponding chapters. Overall, the number of pages has been reduced from 464 to 448 which will decrease the pain and, we hope, increase the pleasure of the reader.

Ivan Roitt
Thomas Lehner

Preface to first edition

It is becoming increasingly clear that immunological processes are involved in the pathogenesis of many oral diseases. All the microbial diseases affecting the mouth have an immunological component and this applies particularly to the two principal diseases—caries and periodontal disease. Immunological factors are also implicated in the pathogenesis of oral ulcers, tumours and mucosal lesions, and sytemic immunological abnormalities may have oral manifestations.

We felt that there was now a need for a book on this subject which would enable dental students, postgraduates, oral biologists, teachers of dentistry and practitioners to make an appraisal of the current situation. The section on basic immunology represents a modified and revised version of *Essential Immunology* by I. M. Roitt; It covers much of the ground required by dental students in their general course of pathology and should also be suitable for postgraduate dental students during the basic medical sciences course. The section dealing with immunology of oral diseases, written by T. Lehner, has been aimed to cover the requirements of dental students in their applied pathology course. The latter section is also suitable for postgraduate students and for this reason a large number of references have been included to encourage the student to consult the original literature.

The authors wish to acknowledge the long, pleasant and fruitful exchange of ideas with Drs Mark Wilton, Lida Ivanyi, Steve Challacombe and Mike Russell which have led to many of the concepts of the immunology of oral diseases expressed in this book.

Ivan Roitt
Thomas Lehner

1 Basic immunology

1 Introduction

The essential function of the immune system is defence against infection. Babies born with a defect in a critical part of this system suffer continued infections and in many cases may die if recourse to advanced medical technology is not available. Lower animal forms possess so-called *innate* or *non-specific* immune mechanisms such as phagocytosis of bacteria by specialized cells, which afford them protection against infecting organisms. Additionally, higher animals have evolved an *adaptive* or *acquired immune response* which provides a flexible, *specific* and more effective reaction to different infections.

At the heart of the adaptive immune response lie three important features, memory, specificity and the recognition of 'non-self'. Our experience of the subsequent protection (*immunity*) afforded by exposure to many infectious illnesses can in fact lead us to this view.

We rarely suffer twice from such diseases as measles, mumps, chicken-pox, whooping cough and so forth. The first contact with an infectious organism clearly imprints some information, imparts some *memory*, so that the body is effectively prepared to repel any later invasion by that organism. This protection is provided by the adaptive immune response evoked as a reaction to the infectious agent behaving as an antigen (figure 1.1). One of the agents of the immune response is antibody which combines with antigen to cause its elimination.

By following the production of antibody on the first and second contacts with antigen we can see the basis for the development of immunity. For example, when we inject a bacterial product such as staphylococcal toxoid into a rabbit, several days elapse before antibodies can be detected in the blood; these reach a peak and then fall (figure 1.2). If we now allow the animal to rest and then give a second injection of toxoid, the course of events is dramatically altered. Within two to three days the antibody level in the blood rises steeply to reach much higher values than were observed in the *primary response*. This *secondary response* then is characterized by a more rapid and more abundant production of antibody resulting from the 'tuning up' or priming of the antibody-forming system

3

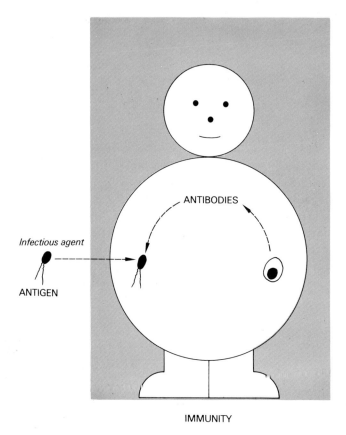

Infectious agent

ANTIGEN

ANTIBODIES

IMMUNITY

FIGURE 1.1. Antibodies (*anti*-foreign *bodies*) are produced by host white cells on contact with the invading micro-organism which is acting as an antigen (i.e. *gene*rates antibodies). The individual may then be immune to further attacks.

to provide a population of memory cells after first exposure to antigen.

Vaccination utilizes this principle by employing a relatively harmless form of the antigen (e.g. a killed virus) as the primary stimulus to imprint 'memory'. The body's defences are thereby alerted and any subsequent contact with the virulent form of the organism will lead to a secondary response with an early and explosive production of antibody which will usually prevent the infection from taking hold.

Specificity was mentioned earlier as a fundamental feature of the adaptive immunological response. The establishment of memory or immunity by one organism does not confer protection against another unrelated organism. After an attack of measles we are immune to further infection but are susceptible to other agents such as the polio or mumps viruses. The body

4

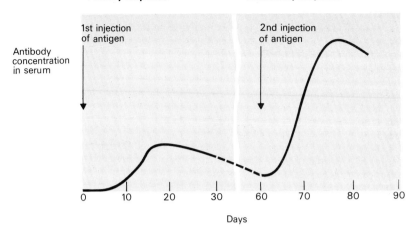

Primary response   **Secondary response**

FIGURE 1.2. Primary and secondary response. A rabbit is injected on two separate occasions with staphylococcal toxoid. The antibody response on the second contact with antigen is more rapid and more intense.

can, in fact, differentiate specifically between the two organisms.

This ability to recognize one antigen and distinguish it from another goes even further. The individual must also recognize what is foreign, i.e. what is *non-self*. The failure to discriminate between 'self' and 'non-self' could lead to the synthesis of antibodies directed against components of the subject's own body (*autoantibodies*) which in principle could prove to be highly embarrassing. On purely theoretical grounds it seemed to Burnet and Fenner that the body must develop some mechanism whereby 'self' and 'non-self' could be distinguished, and they postulated that those circulating body components which were able to reach the developing lymphoid system in the perinatal period could in some way be 'learnt' as 'self'. A permanent unresponsiveness or tolerance would then be created so that as immunological maturity was reached there would normally be an inability to respond to 'self' components. As we shall see later, these predictions have been amply verified.

The non-specific immunity mechanisms, such as the uptake of bacteria by phagocytic cells which we mentioned earlier, are not heightened by subsequent infections and in this respect differ fundamentally from the adaptive immune response. Clearly this has evolved to provide more effective defence in that the small fraction of immunological cells which are capable of recognizing the particular agents infecting the body at any one time increase in number and synthesize antibodies which greatly speed up the disposal of these organisms by facilitating their adherence to phagocytic cells (see chapter 7). In other words the specific adaptive immune response operates to a considerable extent by increasing the efficiency of the non-specific immunity systems.

Some historical perspectives

Space does not allow more than a cursory survey of some of the outstanding contributions to the early development of immunology.

India and China (ancient times)—Practice of 'variolation' in which protection against smallpox was obtained by inoculating live organisms from disease pustules (dangerous!).

Jenner (1798)—Protection effect of vaccination with non-virulent cowpox against smallpox infection (noting the pretty pox-free skin of the milkmaids).

Pasteur (1881)—Vaccine for anthrax using attenuated organisms.

Metchnikoff (1883)—Role of phagocytes in immunity.

Von Behring (1890)—Recognized antibodies in serum to diphtheria toxin.

Denys & Leclef (1895)—Phagocytosis greatly enhanced by immunization—innate response amplified by adaptive.

Ehrlich (1897)—Side-chain receptor of antibody synthesis.

Bordet (1899)—Lysis of cells by antibody requires co-operation of serum factors now collectively termed complement.

Landsteiner (1900)—Human ABO groups and natural iso-haemagglutinins.

Richet & Portier (1902)—Anaphylaxis (opposite of prophylaxis).

Wright (1903)—Relation of opsonic activity to phagocytosis. (Basis for Sir Colenso Ridgeon's assertion in Shaw's *The Doctor's Dilemma* that vaccines stimulate antibodies (opsonins) which 'butter' the germs for ingestion by phagocytes, in contrast with 'B.B.'s' resonant belief that any anti-toxin would non-specifically 'stimulate the phagocytes'.)

von Pirquet & Schick (1905)—Description of serum sickness following injection of foreign serum.

von Pirquet (1906)—Relation of immunity and hypersensitivity.

Fleming (1922)—Lysozyme.

Zinsser (1925)—Contrast between immediate and delayed-type hypersensitivity.

Heidelberger & Kendall (1930–35) Quantitative precipitin studies on antigen–antibody interactions.

Let us examine the work of Heidelberger and Kendall and its implications in more detail and with some benefit.

The classical precipitin reaction

When an antigen solution is mixed in correct proportions with a potent antiserum, a precipitate is formed. Quantitative analysis of this interaction by the method shown in figure 1.3 gives both the antibody content of the immune serum and also an indication of the valency of the antigen, i.e. the effective number of combining sites. This can vary enormously depending on the antigen, its size, and the species making the antibody. With rabbit antisera, ovalbumin may have a valency of 10 and human thyroglobulin as many as 40 combining sites on its surface. By splitting antigens into large fragments with proteolytic enzymes it has become clear that the separate combining areas on the surface of a given protein (called antigenic *determinants* or *epitopes*) are by no means identical.

It will be noted from the precipitin curve in figure 1.3 that as more and more antigen is added, an optimum is reached after which consistently less precipitate is formed. At this stage the supernatant can be shown to contain soluble complexes of antigen (Ag) and antibody (Ab), many of composition Ag_4Ab_3, Ag_3Ab_2 and Ag_2Ab. In extreme antigen excess (AgXS, figure 1.3) ultracentrifugal analysis reveals the complexes to be mainly of the form Ag_2Ab, suggesting that the rabbit antibodies studied are bivalent (figure 1.4; see also figures 2.5 and 2.6). Between these extremes the cross-linking of antigen and antibody will generally give rise to three-dimensional lattice structures, as suggested by Marrack, which coalesce to form large precipitating aggregates.

The basis of specificity

Much of our understanding of the factors governing antigen specificity has come from the studies of Landsteiner and of Pauling and their colleagues on the interaction of antibody with small chemically defined groupings termed *haptens*, a typical example being *m*-aminobenzene sulphonate (figure 1.5). Whereas an antigen will both evoke antibody formation and combine with the resulting antibody, *a hapten is defined as a small molecule which by itself cannot stimulate antibody synthesis but will combine with antibody once formed.*

7

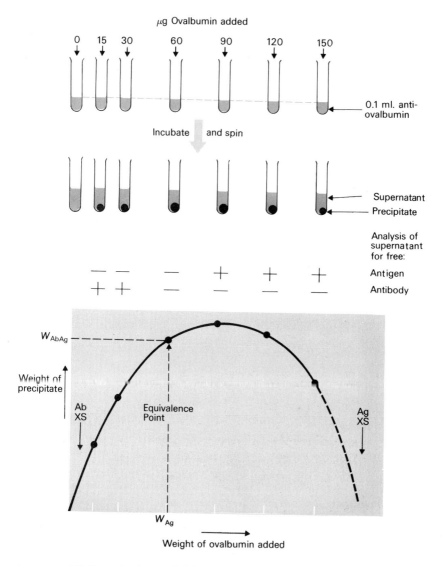

FIGURE 1.3. Quantitative precipitin reaction between rabbit anti-ovalbumin and ovalbumin (after Heidelberger & Kendall). Increasing amounts of ovalbumin are added to a constant volume of the antiserum placed in a number of tubes. After incubation the precipitates formed are spun down and weighed. Each supernatant is split into two halves: by adding antigen to one and antibody to the other, the presence of reactive antibody or antigen respectively can be demonstrated. The antibody content of the serum can be calculated from the equivalence point where no antigen or antibody is present in the supernatant. All the antigen added is therefore complexed in the precipitate with all the antibody available and the antibody content in 0.1 ml of serum would therefore be given by $(W_{AgAb}-W_{Ag})$. Analysis of the precipitate formed in antibody excess (AbXS), where the antigen-combining sites are largely saturated, gives a measure of the molar ratio of antibody to antigen in the complex and hence an estimate of the antigen valency.

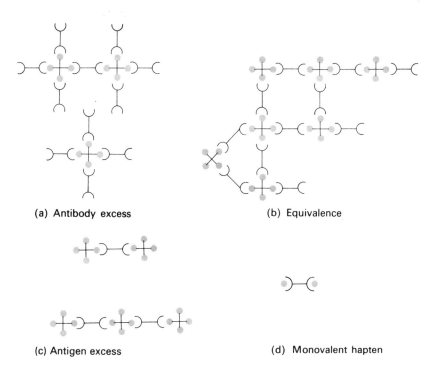

(a) Antibody excess

(b) Equivalence

(c) Antigen excess

(d) Monovalent hapten

FIGURE 1.4. Diagrammatic representation of complexes formed between a hypothetical tetravalent antigen (-+-) and bivalent antibody (>-<) mixed in different proportions. In practice, the antigen valencies are unlikely to lie in the same plane or to be formed by identical determinants as suggested in the figure.

(a) In extreme antibody excess, the antigen valencies are saturated and the molar ratio Ab:Ag approximates to the valency of the antigen.

(b) At equivalence, large lattices are formed which aggregate to form a typical immune precipitate. This secondary aggregation, and hence precipitation, tends to be inhibited by high salt concentration.

(c) In extreme antigen excess where the two valencies of each antibody molecule become rapidly saturated, the complex Ag_2Ab tends to predominate.

(d) A monovalent hapten binds but is unable to cross-link antibody molecules.

The problem of how to produce these antibodies was solved by injecting the haptens coupled to proteins which acted as 'carriers'. It then became possible to relate variations in the chemical structure of a hapten to its ability to bind to a given antibody. It would appear that the overall *configuration* of the hapten is even more important than its *chemical* nature, i.e. the hapten is recognized by the overall three-dimensional shape of its outer electron cloud as distinct from its chemical reactivity. The production of antibodies against such strange moieties as benzene sulphonate and arsonate becomes more comprehen-

9

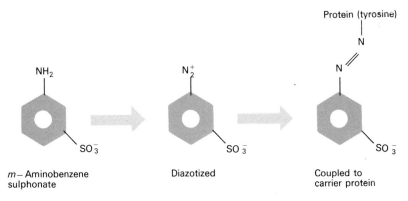

FIGURE 1.5. Coupling of hapten to carrier protein by diazotization.

sible if they are thought to be directed against a particular electron-cloud shape rather than a specific chemical structure. This view is consistent with the nature of antigen–antibody binding which is known not to involve covalent linkages.

THE FORCES BINDING ANTIGEN TO ANTIBODY

It should be stressed immediately that the forces which hold antigen and antibody together are in essence no different from the so-called 'non-specific' protein–protein interactions which occur between any two unrelated proteins (or other macro-molecules) as, for example, human serum albumin and human transferrin. These intermolecular forces may be classified under four headings:

(1) *Electrostatic*

These are due to the attraction between oppositely charged ionic groups on the two protein side chains as, for example, an *ionized amino group* (NH_3^+) on a lysine of one protein and an ionized carboxyl group ($-COO^-$) of, say, aspartate on the other (figure 1.6a).

(2) *Hydrogen bonding*

The formation of the relatively weak and reversible hydrogen bridges between hydrophilic groups such as .OH, .NH₂ and COOH depends very much upon the close approach of the two molecules carrying these groups (figure 1.6b).

10

(3) *Hydrophobic*

In the same way that oil droplets in water merge to form a single large drop, so non-polar, hydrophobic groups such as the side chains of valine, leucine and phenylalanine, tend to associate in an aqueous environment (figure 1.6c).

(4) *Van der Waals*

These are the forces between molecules which depend upon interaction between the external 'electron clouds'. The deviation of gaseous molecules of say nitrogen or hydrogen from 'ideal' behaviour according to the kinetic theory is attributable to the Van der Waals attractions between them.

There is one essential feature common to all four types of force—they depend upon the close approach of both molecules before the forces become of significant magnitude. This is at the heart of the combination of antigen and antibody. By having *complementary* electron-cloud shapes on the combining site of the antibody and the surface determinant of the antigen, the two molecules can fit snugly together like a lock and key (figure 1.8a). The intermolecular distance becomes very small and the non-specific protein interaction forces are considerably increased; the greater the areas of antigen and antibody which fit together, the greater the force of attraction, particularly if there is apposition of opposite charges and hydrophobic groupings.

ANTIBODY AFFINITY

The combination of antibody with the surface determinant of an antigen or a monovalent hapten molecule (cf. figure 1.4d) is reversible and the complex may readily dissociate, depending upon the strength of binding. This can be defined through the equilibrium constant (K) of the reaction:

$$Ab + Hp \rightleftharpoons AbHp$$

$$(\supset\!\!-\!\!c) \quad (\,\bullet\,) \quad (\supset\!\!-\!\!-\!\!-\!\!\bullet)$$

given by the mass action equation,

$$K = \frac{[AbHp]}{[Ab][Hp]}$$

where [Ab] is the concentration of free antibody combining sites

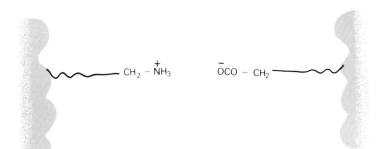

Lysine
side – chain

Aspartate
side – chain

(a)

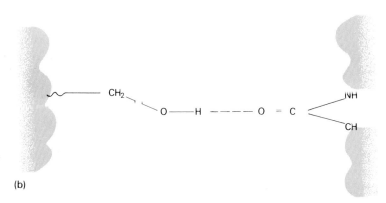

(b)

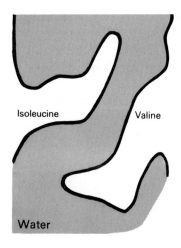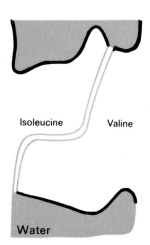

Isoleucine

Valine

Water

Isoleucine

Valine

Water

(c)

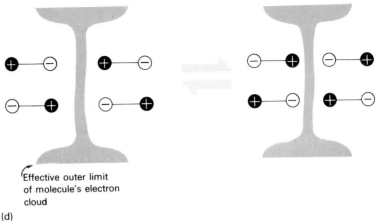

Effective outer limit
of molecule's electron
cloud

(d)

FIGURE 1.6. Protein–protein interactions.

(a) Coulombic attraction between oppositely charged ionic groupings.

(b) Hydrogen bonding between two proteins: the example shows an H-bond between a serine or threonine side-chain on one protein and a peptide carbonyl group on the other.

(c) Hydrophobic bonding: the region in which the water molecules are in contact with the hydrophobic groups (indicated by the thickened line) is considerably reduced when the hydrophobic groups on two proteins are in contact with each other and the lower free-energy of this system makes this a more probable state than separation of the hydrophobic groups.

(d) Van der Waals forces: the interaction between the electrons in the external orbitals of two different macromolecules may be envisaged (for simplicity!) as the attraction between induced oscillating dipoles in the two electron clouds.

and [Hp] the concentration of free hapten. If the antibody and hapten fit together very closely, the equilibrium will lie well over to the right; we refer to such antibodies which bind strongly to the hapten as *high affinity antibodies*. At a certain *free* hapten concentration $[Hp_c]$ where half of the antibody sites are bound, $[AbHp] = [Ab]$ and $K = 1/[Hp_c]$, i.e. K is equal to the reciprocal of the concentration of free hapten at the equilibrium point where half the antibody sites are in the bound form. In other words, when an antibody has a high affinity constant and binds hapten strongly, it only needs a low hapten concentration to half-saturate the antibody. Affinity constants, which can be determined by methods such as that shown in figure 1.7, may reach values as high as 10^{11} l/mol.

Analysis of the binding at different hapten concentrations generally shows a heterogeneity which indicates that most antisera, even those raised against antigens with a simple structure, contain a variety of different antibodies with a range of binding affinities which depend upon the area of contact between the antibody and the antigenic determinant, the

13

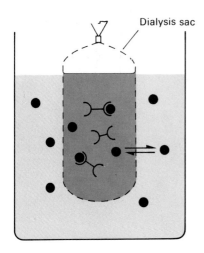

FIGURE 1.7. Antibody affinity determined by studying the equilibrium between antibody (✕) and hapten (●). Within the dialysis sac the hapten is partly in the free form and partly bound to antibody according to the affinity of the antibody. Only hapten can diffuse through the dialysis membrane and the external concentration then will equal the concentration of unbound hapten within the sac. Measurement of total hapten in the dialysis sac then enables the amount bound to antibody to be calculated. By repeating this at different concentrations of hapten, one can calculate the average affinity constant (K) as described in the text. Constant renewal of the external buffer will lead to total dissociation and loss of hapten from inside the dialysis sac showing the reversible nature of the antigen–antibody bond.

closeness of fit (figure 1.8) and the distribution of charged and hydrophobic groups. If we bear in mind that antigen determinants are not two-dimensional as represented in the figures, but have a three-dimensional electron-cloud shape, one can realize that antibodies are confronted with very many different configurations even in a single determinant, depending upon the direction from which the antibody molecule approaches.

AVIDITY AND THE BONUS EFFECT OF
MULTIVALENT BINDING

The strength of the interaction of antibody with a monovalent hapten or a single antigen determinant we have labelled antibody affinity. In most practical situations we are concerned with the interaction of an antiserum with a multivalent antigen molecule and the term employed to express this binding,

$$n\mathrm{Ab} + m\mathrm{Ag} \rightleftharpoons \mathrm{Ab}_n\mathrm{Ag}_m$$

is *avidity*. The factors which contribute to avidity are complicated. Not only must we contend with the heterogeneity of

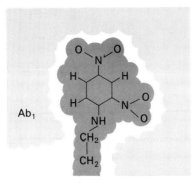

(a) High affinity

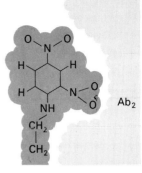

(b) Moderate affinity

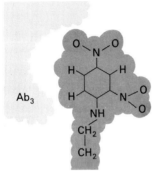

(c) Low affinity

FIGURE 1.8. Binding of antibodies present in the same antiserum with different affinities to the same hapten (dinitrobenzene linked to the amino group of lysine). (a) Antibody₁ fits with nearly the whole of the hapten and is thus of high affinity. (b) Antibody₂ fits with less of the molecule and not so closely, and has a moderate binding affinity while (c) the low affinity antibody₃ is complementary in shape to so little of the hapten surface that its binding energy is very little above that occurring between completely unrelated proteins. Only a portion of the antibody combining site is shown.

antibodies in a given serum which are directed against each determinant on the antigen, but we must also recognize that the differing amino acid sequences on different parts of a protein surface, for example, lead to the formation of a number of antigenic patches or determinants on a single molecule, each with its distinct shape and specificity.

The multivalence of most antigens leads to an interesting 'bonus' effect in which the binding of two antigen molecules by antibody is always greater than the arithmetic sum of the individual antibody links. This is illustrated in figure 1.9. The mechanism of this effect may be interpreted by considering an analogy. Let us fabricate an unheard of disease in which we cannot stop our hands opening and closing continuously. If we

15

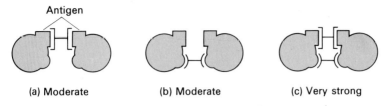

Antigen

(a) Moderate   (b) Moderate   (c) Very strong

FIGURE 1.9. The 'bonus' effect of multivalent attachment on binding strength. The force binding the two antigen molecules in (c) with two antibody bridges is often at least ten times greater than (a+b) where only single antibody molecules provide the link. The effect varies with K values; the weaker the affinity the more the bonus.

now try to hold an object in *one* hand it will fall the moment we open that hand. However, if we use *both* hands to hold the object, provided we open and close our hands at different times, there is much less chance of the object falling. The reversible combination of antigen and antibody is like the opening and closing of the hand; the more valencies holding the antigen the less likely it is to be lost when the complex dissociates at any one binding site (figure 1.10).

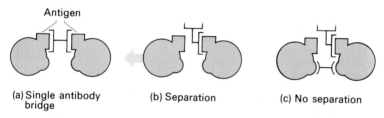

Antigen

(a) Single antibody bridge   (b) Separation   (c) No separation

FIGURE 1.10. The mechanism of the bonus effect. Each antigen–antibody bond is reversible and with a single antibody bridge between two antigen molecules (a), dissociation of either bond could enable an antigen molecule to 'escape' as in (b). If there are two antibody bridges, even when one dissociates the other prevents the antigen molecule from escaping and holds it in position ready to reform the broken bond.

SPECIFICITY AND CROSS-REACTIONS

An antiserum raised against a given antigen can cross-react with a partially related antigen which bears one or more identical or similar determinants. In figure 1.11 it can be seen that an antiserum to antigen₁ will react less strongly with antigen₂ which bears just one identical determinant because only certain of the antibodies in the serum can bind. Antigen₃ which possesses a similar but not identical determinant will not fit as well with the antibody and the binding is even weaker. Antigen₄ which has no structural similarity at all will not react significantly with the antibody.* Thus, based upon stereochemical considerations, we can see why the avidity of the antiserum for antigens$_{2+3}$ is less than for the homologous antigen, while for the unrelated antigen$_4$ it is negligible. It is in this way that the *specificity* of an antiserum is expressed.

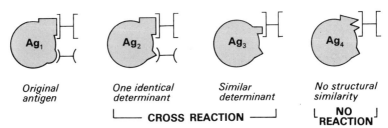

| Original antigen | One identical determinant | Similar determinant | No structural similarity |

CROSS REACTION — NO REACTION

FIGURE 1.11. Specificity and cross-reaction. The avidity of the serum (antibodies ⊣, ⊁) for Ag$_1$ > Ag$_2$ > Ag$_3$ ≫ Ag$_4$ so that the serum shows specificity.

THE ANTIBODY SITE AND ANTIGEN DETERMINANTS

The forces which bind antigen to antibody are largely similar to those binding enzyme to substrate. The elucidation of the three-dimensional structures of certain enzymes such as lysozyme by X-ray cyrstallography has shown that the substrate lies within a long cleft in the surface of the molecule. Similar studies on homogeneous antibody preparations indicate that the combining site is approximately 1.5–2.0 nm long, 1.5 nm wide and 0.5–1.2 nm deep (Poljak and colleagues).

These dimensions are consistent with studies using *linear* haptens formed from repeating units of sugar molecules (Kabat) or amino acids (Sela) which have indicated that the site probably accommodates roughly six such units. Of these units, the terminal one usually shows the highest binding energy to the antibody and may be termed the 'immunodominant' group; successive units contribute progressively less to the overall binding.

It is worth emphasizing that our analysis has been concerned with the interaction of an antigenic determinant or a hapten with antibody but several further factors govern the ability of a given substance to act as an *antigen*, i.e. to stimulate the antigen-reactive cells in the host animal to produce antibody. These include the content of polymeric repeating structures, the rate

*If the antigenic determinant is appreciably smaller than the antibody site, there could be a cross-reaction with an unrelated antigen which bound fortuitously to the remainder of the site.

17

of catabolism, the size, the degree of 'foreignness'—i.e. dissimilarity from self—and the ability of the body to recognize the substance.

Summary

The purpose of the immune response is to defend the host against infection. 'Non-specific' immune mechanisms (e.g. phagocytosis) are enhanced by the development of *adaptive* immunity characterized by memory, specificity and the recognition of non-self. The more rapid and intense antibody response which occurs on the second contact with antigen explains the protection afforded by a primary infection against subsequent disease and provides the rationale for the immunological education of the body by vaccination.

Antigens bind to antibodies reversibly by non-covalent molecular interactions including electrostatic, hydrogen-bonding, hydrophobic and Van der Waals forces which become significant when complementarity of shape between antigen and antibody allows them to approach each other closely ('lock and key' fit like enzymes and substrate).

The binding strength of an antibody for a single determinant or hapten is measured by *affinity*. The term *avidity* describes the binding of an antiserum for the whole antigen molecule, this being influenced relative to affinity, by the bonus effect of multivalency. Antibodies discriminate between two antigens, i.e. show *specificity*, by their greater avidity for one rather than the other. Where some determinants (epitopes) on two antigens are identical or similar, they will give cross-reactions directly dependent upon their relative binding strengths to the antibodies.

The antigenic determinant must be capable of lying within the groove forming the antibody combining site. With linear antigens, primary structure is crucially important for the formation of a determinant but in the case of globular molecules, tertiary conformation is usually of even greater significance.

Further reading

Cunningham A.J. (1978) *Understanding Immunology*. Academic Press, New York.

Davis B.D., Dulbecco R., Eisen H.N., Ginsberg H.S. & Wood W.B. (1973) *Microbiology* (Including Immunology), 2nd edn. Harper International Edition.

Fougerean M. & Dausset J. (eds) (1980) *Progress in Immunology IV*. Academic Press, London. (Papers from the 4th Int. Congress of Immunology.)

Fudenberg H.H., Stites D.P., Caldwell J.L. & Wells J.V. (1978) *Basic and Clinical Immunology*, 2nd edn. Lange Medical Publications, Los Altos, California.

Glynn L.E. & Steward M.W. (eds) (1977) *Immunochemistry: an Advanced Textbook*. John Wiley & Sons, Chichester.

Humphrey J.H. & White R.G. (1970) *Immunology for Students of Medicine*, 3rd edn. Blackwell Scientific Publications, Oxford. (Dated but scholarly.)

Kabat E.A. (1976) *Structural Concepts in Immunology and Immunochemistry*. Holt, Rinehart & Winston, New York.

McConnell I., Munro A. & Waldmann H. (1980) *The Immune System: a Course on the Molecular and Cellular Basis of Immunity*, 2nd edn. Blackwell Scientific Publications, Oxford.

Richards F.F., Konisberg W.H. & Rosenstein R.W. (1975) On the specificity of antibodies: Biochemical and biophysical evidence indicates the existence of polyfunctional antibody combining regions. *Science*, **187**, 130.

Sela M. (ed.) (1974) *The Antigens*. Academic Press, New York.

Thaler M.S., Klausner R.D. & Cohen H.J. (1977) *Medical Immunology*. J.B. Lippincott, Philadelphia.

Historical

Landsteiner K. (1946) *The Specificity of Serological Reactions*. Harvard University Press, Cambridge, Massachusetts. (Reprinted 1962 by Dover Publications, New York.)

Metchnikoff E. (1893) *Comparative Pathology of Inflammation*. Transl. F.A. and E.H. Starling. Kegan Paul, Trench, Trubner & Co., London.

Parish H.J. (1968) *Victory with Vaccines*. Churchill Livingstone, Edinburgh.

Series for the advanced student

*Advances in Immunology (annual). Academic Press, London.
Progress in Allergy. Karger, Basle.
Modern Trends in Immunology. Butterworth, London.
*Immunological Reviews (ed. G. Moller). Munksgaard, Copenhagen.
Essays in Fundamental Immunology. Blackwell Scientific Publications, Oxford.
Contemporary Topics in Molecular Immunology. Plenum Press, New York.
Contemporary Topics in Immunobiology. Plenum Press, New York.
Protides of the Biological Fluids. Pergamon Press, Oxford.

*In depth treatment.

Current information

Current Titles in Immunology, Transplantation and Allergy. MSK Books, London.
Immunology Today. North-Holland, Amsterdam.

Major journals

Nature, Lancet, Science, J.exp.Med., Immunology, J.Immunol., Clin.exp.Immunol., Mol. Immunol., Immunopharmacology, Infect Immunity, Int.Arch.Allergy, Cell.Immunol., Eur.J.Immunol., Scand.J.Immunol., Clin.Immunol.Immunopath., J.Immunogenetics, J.Immunol.Methods, J.Reticuloendoth.Soc., Tissue Antigens, Immunogenetics, Transplantation, Ann.d'Immunologie, Cancer Immunol. Immunotherapy, J.AllergyClin.Immunol., Clin.Allergy, Ann.Allergy, J.Clin.Lab.Immunol., ParasiticImmunol.

2

The immunoglobulins

The association of antibody activity with the classical γ-globulin fraction of serum was shown many years ago by Tiselius and Kabat. They hyperimmunized rabbits with pneumococcal polysaccharide to produce a high concentration of circulating antibody and then examined the effect of absorbing the serum with antigen on the electrophoretic profile. Only the γ-globulin fraction was significantly reduced after removal of antibody (figure 2.1). With the recognition of heterogeneity in the types of molecules which can function as antibodies, it has now become customary to use the general term 'immunoglobulin'. In each species, the immunoglobulin molecules can be subdivided into different classes on the basis of the structure of their 'backbone' (rather than on their specificity for given antigens). Thus, in the human for example, five major structural types or classes can be distinguished: immunoglobulin G (abbreviated to IgG), IgM, IgA, IgD and IgE.

The basic structure of the immunoglobulins

The antibody fraction of serum consists predominantly of one group of proteins with molecular weight around

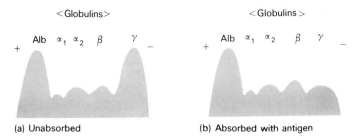

FIGURE 2.1. Association of antibody activity with γ-globulin serum fraction. Hyperimmune serum is separated into major fractions by electrophoresis before (a) and after (b) absorption with antigen. Only the γ-globulin fraction is reduced.

150,000 (sedimentation coefficient 7S) of which the major component is IgG, and another of molecular weight 900,000 (19S IgM). The IgG antibodies can be split by papain into three fragments (R.R. Porter). Two of these are identical and are able to combine with antigen to form a soluble complex which will not precipitate; these are therefore univalent antibody fragments and are given the nomenclature Fab ('fragment antigen binding'). The third fragment has no power to combine with antigen and is termed Fc ('fragment crystallizable' obtainable in crystalline form). Another proteolytic enzyme, pepsin, cleaves the Fc part from the remainder of the antibody molecule, leaving a large fragment (5S) which can still precipitate with antigen and is formulated as $F(ab')_2$ since it is clearly still divalent.

Antibodies can also be broken down into their constituent peptide chains. First the disulphide bonds linking different chains must be broken by reduction with *excess* of a sulphydryl reagent. The reduced molecule still has a sedimentation coefficient of 7S because the chains are held together by non-covalent forces but they can be separated by lowering the pH into two sizes of peptide chain termed *light* and *heavy chains* (G. Edelman).

On the basis of these findings Porter put forward a symmetrical four-peptide model for antibody consisting of two heavy and two light chains linked together by interchain

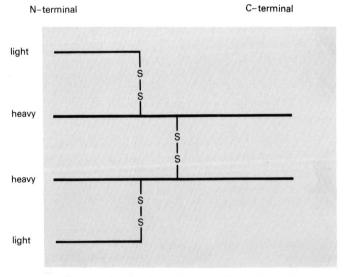

FIGURE 2.2. Antibody model proposed by R.R. Porter with two heavy and two light polypeptide chains held by interchain disulphide bonds. In the diagram the amino-terminal residue is on the left for each chain.

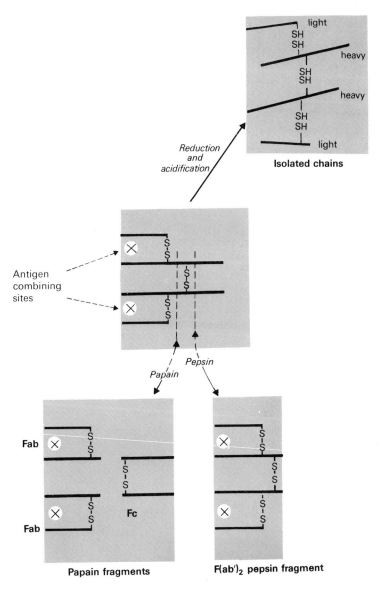

FIGURE 2.3. Degradation of immunoglobulin to constituent peptide chains and to proteolytic fragments showing divalence of pepsin F(ab')₂ and univalence of the papain Fab. After pepsin digestion the pFc' fragment representing the C-terminal half of the Fc region is formed. The portion of the heavy chain in the Fab fragment is given the symbol Fd.

disulphide bonds (figure 2.2). The formation of the various fragments by proteolysis and reduction is represented in figure 2.3.

Purified IgG antibodies when visualized in the electron microscope by negative staining can be seen to be Y-shaped molecules whose arms can swing out to an angle of 180°

23

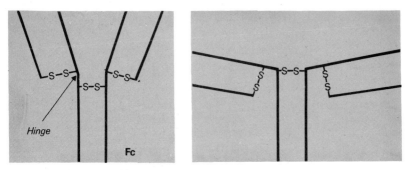

FIGURE 2.4. Illustrating the flexibility of the immunoglobulin molecule at the hinge region. Compare with the conformation of immunoglobulin molecules in figure 2.5.

through the papain and pepsin sensitive region acting as a hinge (figure 2.4). Amino acid analysis of the hinge region has revealed an unusual feature—a large number of proline residues; because of its structure, proline prevents the peptide chain assuming α-helix conformation, and so this stretch of the chain is extended and accessible to proteolytic enzymes.

Elegant confirmation of the correctness of these general views on the structure of the antibody molecule has come from studies using a divalent hapten, bis-N-dinitrophenyl (DNP)-octamethylene-diamine:

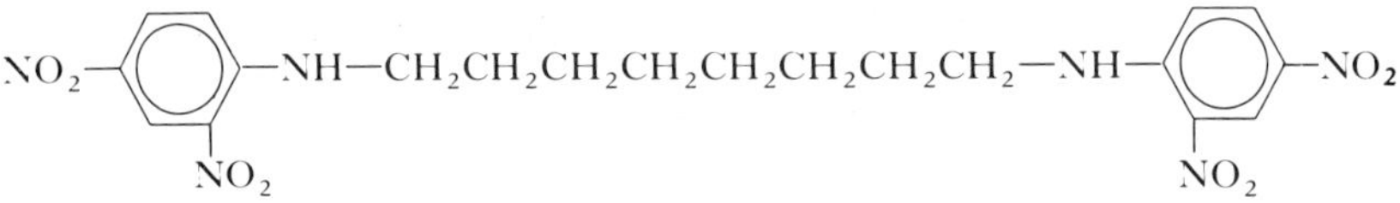

$$NO_2 - \bigcirc - NH - CH_2CH_2CH_2CH_2CH_2CH_2CH_2CH_2 - NH - \bigcirc - NO_2$$

where the two haptenic DNP groups are far enough apart not to interfere with each other's combination with antibody. When mixed with purified IgG antibody to DNP, the divalent hapten brings the antigen-combining sites on two different antibodies together end to end; when viewed by negative staining in the electron microscope a series of geometric forms are observed which represent the different structures to be expected if a Y-shaped hinged molecule with a combining site at the end of each of the two arms of the Y were to complex with this divalent hapten. Triangular

FIGURE 2.5. (a)–(d) Electron micrograph ($\times 1,000,000$) of complexes formed on mixing the divalent DNP hapten with rabbit anti-DNP antibodies. The 'negative stain' phosphotungstic acid is an electron-dense solution which penetrates in the spaces between the protein molecules. Thus the protein stands out as a 'light' structure in the

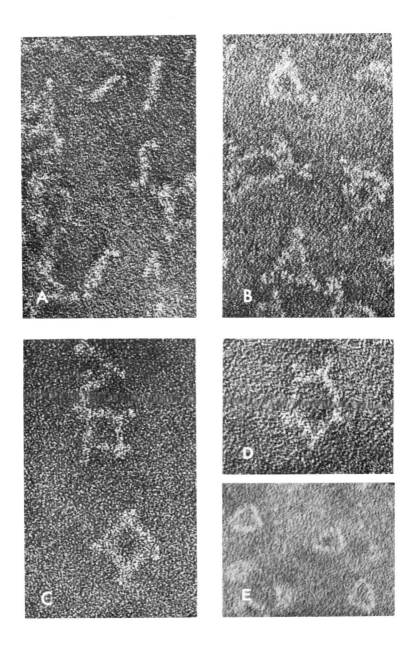

electron beam. The hapten links together the Y-shaped antibody molecules to form (a) dimers, (b) trimers, (c) tetramers and (d) pentamers (cf. figure 2.6). The flexibility of the molecule at the hinge region is evident from the variation in angle of the arms of the 'Y'.

(e) As in (b), trimers formed using the F(ab')$_2$ antibody fragment from which the Fe structures have been digested by pepsin ($\times 500,000$). The trimers can be seen to lack the Fc projections at each corner evident in (b). (After Valentine R.C. & Green N.M. (1967) *J. mol. Biol.* **27,** 615; courtesy of Dr Green and with the permission of Academic Press, New York.)

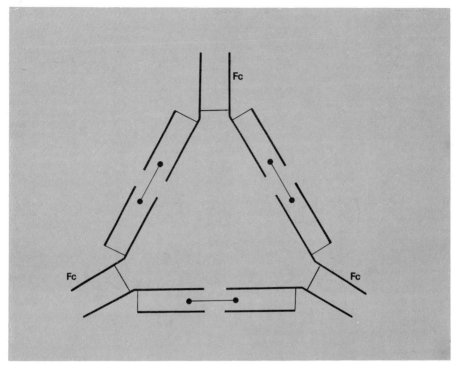

FIGURE 2.6. Three DNP antibody molecules held together as a trimer by the divalent hapten (●———●). Compare figure 2.5b. When the Fc fragments are first removed by pepsin, the corner pieces are no longer visible (figure 2.5e).

trimers, square tetramers and pentagonal pentamers may be readily discerned (figure 2.5). The way in which these polymetric forms arise is indicated in figure 2.6. The position of the Fc fragments and its lack of involvement in the combination with antigen are apparent from the shape of the polymers formed using the pepsin $F(ab')_2$ fragment (figure 2.5e).

Variations in structure of the immunoglobulins

Any attempt to analyse the amino acid structure of the immunoglobulins in normal serum is bedevilled by the incredible number of different molecules present. This heterogeneity may be inferred from analysis by immuno-electrophoresis, the principle of which is explained in figure 2.7. It is evident that the immunoglobulins occur in different classes of molecules and also that they have a very wide range of electrophoretic mobilities within each class, ranging in the case of IgG, from slow γ- to α_2-globulin

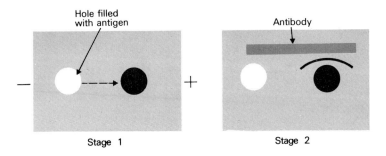

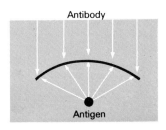

FIGURE 2.7. The principle of immunoelectrophoresis. Stage 1: Electrophoresis of antigen in agar gel. Antigen migrates to the hypothetical position shown. Stage 2: The current is stopped and a trough cut in agar and filled with antibody. A precipitin arc is formed.

Because antigen theoretically at a point source diffuses radially and antibody from the trough diffuses with a plane front, they meet in optimal proportions for precipitation along an arc. The arc is closest to the trough at the point where antigen is in highest concentration.

(figure 2.8). This range of mobilities is due to different net charges on the different immunoglobulin molecules and is indicative of variations in amino acid structure (e.g. replacement of a neutral residue such as valine with a basic amino acid like lysine will tend to increase the net charge by $+1$). Even 'purified' antibodies directed against a simple hapten may show a wide spectrum of electrophoretic mobilities since, as mentioned in the previous chapter, they represent a variety of antibodies of varying degrees of fit for various shapes on the hapten surface.

The answer to this seemingly insoluble problem of analysing amino acid structure has come from study of the *myeloma proteins*. In the human disease known as multiple myeloma, one cell making one particular individual immunoglobulin divides over and over again in the uncontrolled way a cancer cell does, without regard for the overall requirement of the host. The patient then possesses enormous numbers of identical cells derived as a clone from

27

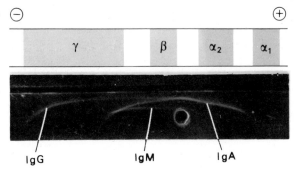

FIGURE 2.8. Major human immunoglobulin classes demonstrated by immunoelectrophoretic analysis of human serum using a rabbit antiserum in the trough. The position of the main electrophoretic globulin fractions are indicated. Three of the five major immunoglobulin classes can be recognized: immunoglobulin G (IgG), immunoglobulin A (IgA) and immunoglobulin M (IgM). The IgG precipitin arc extends from the γ region well into the α_2-globulin mobility range. (Photograph provided by Dr F.C. May.)

the original cell and they all synthesize the same immunoglobulin—the myeloma or M-protein—which appears in the serum, sometimes in very high concentrations. By purification of the myeloma protein we can obtain a preparation of an immunoglobulin having a unique structure. These myeloma proteins have been studied in two ways: amino acid analysis and the recognition of major characteristic groups on the molecules using specific antibodies produced in experimental animals.

STRUCTURAL VARIATION IN RELATION
TO ANTIBODY SPECIFICITY

Amino acid analysis of a number of purified myeloma proteins has revealed that, within a given major immunoglobulin class such as IgG, the N-terminal portions of both heavy and light chains show quite considerable variations whereas the remaining parts of the chains are relatively constant in structure (figure 2.9). Each variable region has a basic overall amino acid structure which is common to a number of antibodies with differing specificities. They are said to belong to the same *subgroup* and to give an example, the heavy chain variable regions in a normal individual form three such subgroups (table 2.3, p. 42). This subgroup 'framework' structure cannot be related to antibody specificity since so many different antibodies belong to the same subgroup. What is striking, however, is the hypervariability in amino acid residues at certain positions in the

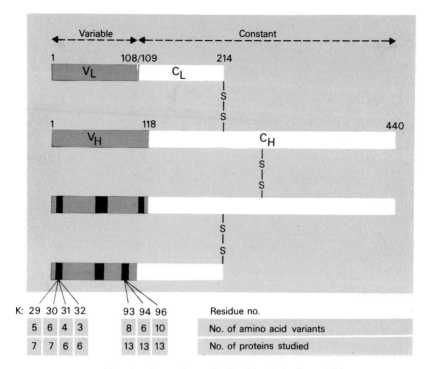

K: 29 30 31 32	93 94 96	Residue no.
5 6 4 3	8 6 10	No. of amino acid variants
7 7 6 6	13 13 13	No. of proteins studied

FIGURE 2.9. Showing the regions of IgG with relatively variable (▬) and constant (▭) amino acid composition. The terms 'V region' and 'C region' are used to designate the variable and constant regions respectively. 'V_L' and 'C_L' are generic terms for these regions on the light chain and 'V_H' and 'C_H' specify variable and constant regions on the heavy chain. The amino acid residues are numbered starting from the N-terminal end. C_L starts at residue 108 for κ-types and 109 for λ (see also figure 2.12). Examples are given of the degree of variation in amino acid residues seen in the hypervariable regions (▬).

peptide chain. For example, when 13 myeloma light chains were sequenced, eight different amino acids were found at residue number 93, six at residue 94 and ten and residue 96 (figure 2.9). The most attractive view, supported by the latest X-ray analysis, is that these 'hot spots', three on the light and three on the heavy chain, lie relatively close to each other to form the antigen binding site (figures 2.10, 2.14), their heterogeneity ensuring diversity in combining specificities through variation in the shape and nature of the surface they create (cf. p. 15). Thus each hypervariable region may be looked upon as an independent structure contributing to the complementarity of the binding site for antigen and perhaps one can speak of complementarity determinants.

That these variable regions on heavy and light chains

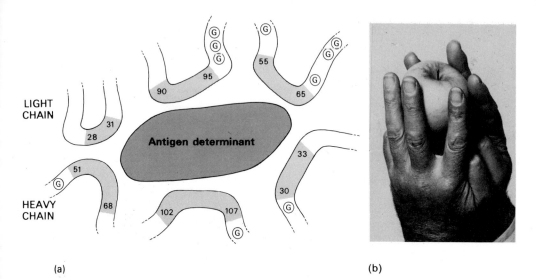

(a)   (b)

FIGURE 2.10. (a) Two-dimensional representation of an antigen binding
site formed by spatial apposition of peptide loops containing the
hypervariable regions (hot spots: ▬) on light and heavy chains.
The numbers refer to amino acid residues. Glycine residues (Ⓖ) are
invariably present at the positions indicated whatever the specificity or
animal species of the immunoglobulin. They are of importance in
enabling peptide chains to fold back and form β-pleated sheet structures
which enable the hypervariable regions to lie close to each other (figure
2.14). Wu and Kabat have suggested that the flexibility of bond angle in
this amino acid is essential for the effective formation of a binding site.
On this basis the greater frequency of invariant glycines on the light chain
might indicate that coarse specificity for antigen binding was provided by
the heavy chain and 'fine tuning' by the light chain. Through binding to
different combinations of hypervariable regions and to different residues
within each of these regions, each antibody molecule can form a complex
with a variety of antigenic determinants (with a comparable variety of
affinities).
    (b) A simulated combining site formed by apposing the three middle
fingers of each hand, each finger representing a hypervariable loop.
(Photograph by B.N.A. Rice.)

both contribute to antibody specificity is suggested by
experiments in which isolated chains were examined for
their antigen combining power. In general, varying degrees
of residual activity were associated with the heavy chains
but relatively little with the light chains; on recombination,
however, there was always a significant increase in antigen-
binding capacity.

Even the 'constant' portions of the immunoglobulin peptide chains which are not directly concerned in antigen binding show considerable heterogeneity. This has largely been analysed through the recognition of characteristic groupings on the molecules by use of specific antisera raised usually in other species. Let us consider, for example, studies on human immunoglobulin light chains.

Light chains

A convenient source of human material is the urinary Bence-Jones' protein which is found in a proportion of patients with myeloma. The Bence-Jones' protein represents a dimer of light chains derived from the pool used in the synthesis of the myeloma protein. By raising antisera in rabbits to a number of Bence-Jones' proteins it was found that light chains could be divided into two groups (called *kappa* (κ) and *lambda* (λ)) depending upon their reactions with the antisera. The Bence-Jones' light chains of the κ-group all gave precipitin reactions with anti-κ sera but no reaction with anti-λ sera. Parallel reactions were always obtained with the parent myeloma protein as would be

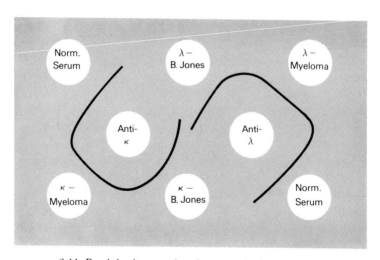

FIGURE 2.11. Precipitation reactions in agar-gel using antisera prepared against κ and λ Bence-Jones' proteins (urinary light chain dimers). The anti-κ reacted with κ but not λ light chains and gave reactions of 'identity' with the related myeloma protein and with normal serum. Parallel results were obtained with the anti-λ serum.

expected if they were derived from light chains produced by one clone of myeloma plasma cells (figure 2.11). The reactions with normal serum show that molecules with κ- and λ-chains are present. They occur on different molecules and approximately 65% of the immunoglobulin molecules in normal serum are of κ-type, the remainder being λ-type. It is of interest that myeloma proteins of type κ occur with nearly twice the frequency of type λ, suggesting that cells synthesizing molecules with λ-chains carry the same risk of becoming malignant as those making κ-chains. The $\kappa:\lambda$ ratio varies in different species.

Heavy chains

Similar studies using antisera prepared against normal and myeloma proteins have established the existence of *five* major types of heavy chain in the human, each of which gives rise to a distinct immunoglobulin class. As mentioned earlier these are IgG, IgA, IgM, IgD and IgE. But whereas each immunoglobulin class is associated with a particular type of heavy chain, they all have κ- and λ-light chains; thus each myeloma protein so far studied, whatever its class, has possessed light chains of either κ- or λ-specificity (but never of both together).

We have already considered the view that the variable portion of the immunoglobulin molecule is bound up with antibody specificity and all classes have been shown to have binding affinity for antigen associated with the Fab regions. What of the constant region, particularly the Fc part of the heavy chain backbone which makes no contribution to specificity? Almost certainly the Fc structure directs the *biological activity* of the antibody molecule. As will be seen below, it determines to some extent the distribution of the immunoglobulin throughout the body, e.g. the selective passage of IgG across the placenta and the secretion of IgA into the external body fluids. But also after combination with antigen a new or enhanced activity such as the ability to fix complement, or to bind effectively to macrophages may arise. It has been suggested that this occurs through an allosteric change in Fc conformation due to the opening of the 'hinge' Fc. However, the flexibility of the hinge makes this rather unlikely and physical measurements with nuclear magnetic resonance and electron spin probes only detect conformational changes in the Fab not the Fc region after complexing with antigen. The complement system (cf.

32

p. 134) may be activated if the combination of antibody with antigen causes a shift in the relative spatial orientation of Fab and Fc fragments and permits access of the initiating complement component (C1) to the appropriate site in the Fc region; this contention is strengthened by the finding that IgG4 (a *sub*class variant of IgG, see below) with a very short hinge can only activate complement when the Fc is cleaved from the Fab. Secondary biological properties of

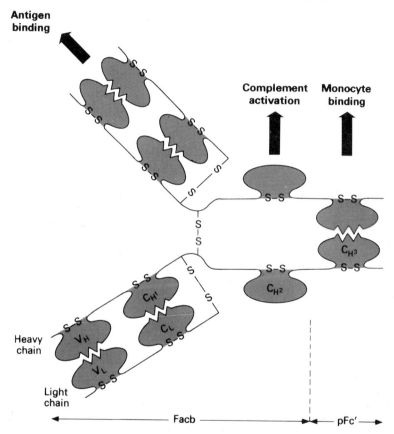

FIGURE 2.12. Immunoglobulin domains in IgG. Each loop in the peptide chain formed by an *intrachain* disulphide bond represents a single domain (shaded) and these are labelled V_H, C_H1, etc. as indicated. They show considerable homology (i.e. similarities in amino acid structure) but each domain appears to be specialized for a specific function as shown. The involvement of the C_H2 region in complement activation is indicated by the activity of the plasmin Facb fragment which contains the C_H2 domain, and the inactivity of the $F(ab')_2$ fragment which lacks it. The active site is a hydrophobic region near the hinge. The pepsin pFc′ fragment which bears the C_H3 domain can bind directly to the monocyte surface and inhibit the formation of Fc rosettes with antibody-coated red cells. Staphylococcal protein-A reacts at the interface between C_H2 and C_H3.

antibodies which are mediated through interaction with cell surface receptors for the immunoglobulin Fc may depend upon greatly increased binding to the cell due to the multivalent Fc sites present in an immune complex (cf. bonus effect of multivalency, p. 14) or the cross-linking of Fc receptors by the complex, or both mechanisms. Each of these biological functions may require a different type of Fc structure and hence amino acid sequence. Thus the multiplicity of Fc structures as expressed in the different immunoglobulin classes and subclasses may be looked upon as a system which has evolved to provide antibodies with different biological capabilities in relation to antigens.

In summary, the variable part provides specificity for binding antigen; the constant part is associated with different biological properties which vary from one immunoglobulin class to another, depending upon the primary structure, and which may require combination with antigen for their activation.

Immunoglobulin domains

In addition to the *interchain* disulphide bonds which bridge heavy and light chains, there are internal, *interchain* disulphide links which form loops in the peptide chain (figure 2.12) As Edelman predicted, the loops are compactly folded to form globular domains (figure 2.14). These interact spatially through their hydrophobic regions (figure 2.13) and individual domains subserve separate functions.

Thus the variable region domains (V_L and V_H) are responsible for the formation of a specific antigen-binding site. The C_H2 region in IgG binds C1q to initiate the classical complement sequence (cf. p. 137) while adherence to the monocyte surface is mediated largely through the terminal C_H3 domain (figure 2.12).

Comparison of immunoglobulin classes

The physical and biological characteristics of the five major immunoglobulin classes in the human are summarized in tables 2.1 and 2.2. The following comments are intended to supplement this information.

Immunoglobulin G

During the secondary response IgG is probably the major immunoglobulin to be synthesized. Through its ability to cross

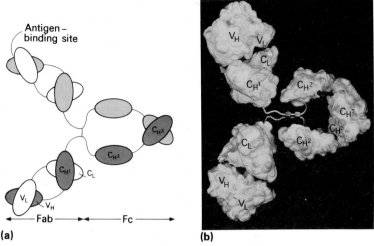

Antigen–
binding site

C_H3
C_H2
C_H1
C_L
V_L
V_H

Fab

Fc

(a)

(b)

FIGURE 2.13. The disposition and interaction of Ig domains in IgG.
(a) Diagram showing apposing domains making contact through
hydrophobic regions (after Dr A. Feinstein). These regions on the two
complement fixing C_{H2} domains are partly masked by carbohydrate and
remain independent. This separation allows the formation of a hinge region
which is extremely flexible both with respect to variation in the angle of the
Fab fragments and their rotation about the hinge peptide chain. Thus
combining sites in IgG can be readily adapted to spatial variations in the
presentation of the antigenic epitopes. (b) Space filling model (courtesy of Dr
A. Feinstein).

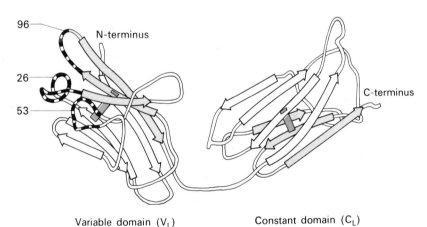

96
N-terminus
26
53
C-terminus

Variable domain (V_L)   Constant domain (C_L)

FIGURE 2.14. Structure of the globular domains of a light chain (from X-ray
crystallographic studies of a Bence-Jones' protein by Schiffler *et al.*, (1973)
Biochemistry, **12**, 4620). One surface of each domain is composed essentially of
four chains arranged in an anti-parallel β-pleated structure (white arrows)
and the other of three such chains (grey arrows): the dark bar represents the
intra-chain disulphide bond. This structure is characteristic of all
immunoglobulin domains. Of particular interest is the location of the
hypervariable regions (■━■━■━■) in three separate loops which are
closely disposed relative to each other and form the light chain contribution to
the antigen binding site (cf. figure 2.10). One numbered residue from each
complementarity determinant is identified.

35

TABLE 2.1. Physical properties of major human immunoglobulin classes

WHO designation	IgG	IgA	IgM	IgD	IgE
Sedimentation coefficient	$7S$	$7S, 9S, 11S$*	$19S$	$7S$	$8S$
Molecular weight	150,000	160,000 and dimer	900,000	185,000	200,000
Number of basic 4-peptide units	1	1, 2*	5	1	1
Heavy chains	γ	α	μ	δ	ϵ
Light chains $\kappa+\lambda$	$\kappa+\lambda$	$\kappa+\lambda$	$\kappa+\lambda$	$\kappa+\lambda$	$\kappa+\lambda$
Molecular formula†	$\gamma_2\kappa_2, \gamma_2\lambda_2$	$(\alpha_2\kappa_2)_{1-2}$ $(\alpha_2\lambda_2)_{1-2}$ $(\alpha_2\kappa_2)_2S$* $(\alpha_2\lambda_2)_2S$*	$(\mu_2\kappa_2)_5$ $(\mu_2\lambda_2)_5$	$\delta_2\kappa_2(\delta_2\lambda_2?)$	$\epsilon_2\kappa_2\epsilon_2\lambda_2$
Valency for antigen binding	2	2, 4	5(10)	2	2
Concentration range in normal serum	8–16 mg/ml	1.4–4 mg/ml	0.5–2 mg/ml	0–0.4 mg/ml	17–450 ng/ml‡
% total immunoglobulin	80	13	6	0–1	0.002
Carbohydrate content %	3	8	12	13	12

*Dimer in external secretions carries secretory component–S.
†IgA dimer and IgM contain J chain.
‡ng = 10^{-9} g.

the placenta it provides a major line of defence against infection for the first few weeks of a baby's life which may be further reinforced by the transfer of colostral IgG across the gut mucosa in the neonate. IgG diffuses more readily than the other immunoglobulins into the extravascular body spaces where as the predominant species it carries the major burden of neutralizing bacterial toxins and of binding to micro-organisms to enhance their phagocytosis. The complexes of bacteria with IgG antibody activate complement, thereby chemotactically attracting polymorphonuclear phagocytic cells (cf. p. 138) which adhere to the bacteria through surface receptors for complement and the Fc portion of IgG (Fcγ); binding to the Fc receptor then stimulates ingestion of micro-organisms through phagocytosis. In a similar way, the extracellular killing of target cells coated with IgG antibody is mediated through recognition of the surface Fcγ by K cells bearing the appropriate receptors (cf. p. 194). The interaction of IgG complexes with platelet Fc receptors presumably leads to aggregation and vasoactive

TABLE 2.2. Biological properties of major immunoglobulin classes in the human

	IgG	IgA	IgM	IgD	IgE
Major charac-teristics	Most abundant Ig of internal body fluids particularly extra-vascular where it combats micro-organisms and their toxins	Major Ig in sero-mucous secretions where it defends external body surfaces	Very effective agglutinator; produced early in immune re-sponse—effective first line defence vs. bacteraemia	Most, if not all, present on lympho-cyte surface	Protection of external body surfaces Recruits anti-microbial agents Raised in parasitic infections Responsible for symptoms of atopic allergy
Complement fixation					
Classical	++	−	+++	−	
Alternative	−	±	−	−	
Cross placenta	+	−	−	−	−
Fix to homo-logous mast cells and basophils	−	−	−	−	+
Binding to macrophages and poly-morphs	+	±	−	−	−

amine release but the physiological significance of Fcγ binding sites on other cell types, particularly lymphocytes, has not yet been clarified. Although unable to bind firmly to mast cells in human skin, IgG alone among the human immunoglobulins has the somewhat useless property of fixing to guinea pig skin. The thesis that the biological individuality of different immuno-globulin classes is dependent on the heavy chain constant regions, particularly the Fc, is amply borne out in relation to the activities we have discussed such as transplacental passage, complement fixation and binding to various cell types, where function has been shown to be mediated by the Fc part of the molecule.

With respect to overall regulation of IgG levels in the body, the catabolic rate appears to depend directly upon the total IgG concentration whereas synthesis is largely governed by antigen stimulation so that in germ-free animals, for example, IgG levels are extremely low but rise rapidly on transfer to a normal environment.

Immunoglobulin A

IgA appears selectively in the sero-mucous secretions such as saliva, tears, nasal fluids, sweat, colostrum and secretions of the lung, genito-urinary and gastro-intestinal tracts where it clearly has the job of defending the exposed external surfaces of the body against attack by micro-organisms. It is present in these fluids as a dimer stabilized against proteolysis by combination with another protein—the secretory component which is synthesized by local epithelial cells and has a single peptide chain of molecular weight 60,000. The IgA is synthesized locally by plasma cells and dimerized intracellularly together with a cysteine-rich polypeptide called J-chain of molecular weight 15,000. If dimerization occurred randomly *after* secretion, dimers of mixed specificity would be formed which would not be as effective in combining with antigen as those of single specificity which would have a higher effective valency. The dimeric IgA binds strongly to secretory component present on the surface of the cell in which it was produced and the complex is then actively endocytosed, transported across the cytoplasm and secreted into the external body fluids (figure 2.15).

IgA antibodies function by inhibiting the adherence of coated micro-organisms to the surface of mucosal cells thereby preventing entry into the body tissues. Aggregated IgA binds to polymorphs and can also activate the alternative (p. 139) as distinct from the classical complement pathway which

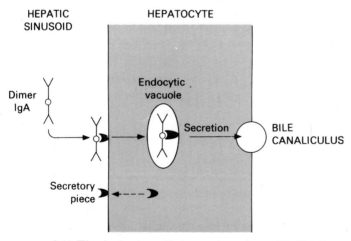

FIGURE 2.15. The mechanism of IgA secretion as exemplified by the transfer of circulating IgA into the bile. Dimeric IgA in the sinusoid binds to a surface secretory piece thereby activating the uptake and secretion of the immunoglobulin. There is perhaps an analogy with the uptake of IgG into macrophages through stimulation of the surface IgG receptors.

probably accounts for reports of a synergism between IgA, complement and lysozyme in the killing of certain coliform organisms. Human plasma contains relatively high concentrations of monomeric IgA and its role is still something of a mystery.

Immunoglobulin M

Often referred to as the macroglobulin antibodies because of their high molecular weight, IgM molecules are polymers of five 4-peptide subunits each bearing an extra C_H domain. As with IgA, polymerization of the subunits depends upon the presence of J-chain whose function may be to stabilize the Fc sulphydryl groups during Ig synthesis so that they remain available for cross-linking the subunits to give the structure shown in figure 2.16a. Under negative staining in the electron microscope, the free molecule in solution assumes a 'star' shape but when combined as an antibody with an antigenic surface membrane it can adopt a 'crab-like' configuration (figures 2.16b and c). The theoretical combining valency is of course 10 but this is only observed on interaction with small haptens; with larger antigens the effective valency falls to 5 and this must be attributed to some form of steric restriction due to lack of flexibility in the molecule. IgM antibodies tend to be of relatively low affinity as measured against single determinants (haptens) but, because of their high valency, they bind with quite respectable avidity to antigens with multiple epitopes (bonus effect of multivalency p. 14).

For the same reason, these antibodies are extremely efficient agglutinating and cytolytic agents and since they appear early in the response to infection and are largely confined to the blood stream, it is likely that they play a role of particular importance in cases of bacteraemia. The isohaemagglutinins (anti-A, anti-B) and many of the 'natural' antibodies to micro-organisms are usually IgM; antibodies to the typhoid 'O' antigen (endotoxin) and the 'WR' antibodies in syphilis also tend to be found in this class. IgM would appear to precede IgG in the phylogeny of the immune response in vertebrates.

Immunoglobulin D

This class was recognized through the discovery of a myeloma protein which did not have the antigenic specificity of IgG, A or M, although it reacted with antibodies to immunoglobulin light chains and had the basic four-peptide structure. Among the

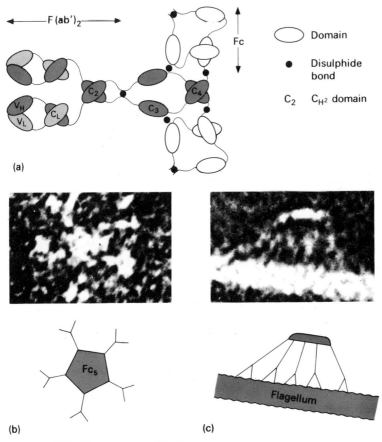

FIGURE 2.16. The structure of IgM.

(a) The arrangements of domains in one of the five subunits showing how the pentamer is built up through the disulphide linkages between $C_{H}3$ and C terminal regions (after Hilschman & Feinstein). Without too much aggravation, I hope the reader will appreciate that the hinge region in IgG (cf. fig. 2.13) is replaced by a rigid pair of extra domains ($C_{H}2$), while $C_{H}3$ and $C_{H}4$ domains in IgM are structurally equivalent to the $C_{H}2$ and $C_{H}3$ regions respectively in IgG.

(b) As shown by electron microscopy of a human Waldenström's macroglobulin in free solution adopting a 'star'-shaped configuration.

(c) As revealed in an E.M. preparation of specific sheep IgM antibody bound to *Salmonella paratyphi* flagellum where the immunoglobulin has assumed a 'crab-like' conformation in establishing its links with antigen. With the $F(ab')_{2}$ arms bent out of the plane of the central Fc_{5} region, the $C_{H}3$ complement binding domains are now readily accessible to the first component of complement (cf. p. 136). The Fc_{5} constellation obtained by papain cleavage can activate complement directly.

(Electron micrographs—kindly provided by Dr Feinstein and Dr E.A Munn—are negatively stained preparations of magnification ×2,000,000, i.e. 1 mm represents 5 Å.)

different immunoglobulin classes it is uniquely susceptible to proteolytic degradation, and this may account for its short half-life in plasma (2.8 days). An exciting development has been the demonstration that nearly all the IgD is present on the surface of a proportion of blood lymphocytes together with IgM, and it seems likely that they may function as mutually interacting antigen receptors for the control of lymphocyte activation and suppression.

Immunoglobulin E

Only very low concentrations of IgE are present in serum and only a very small proportion of the plasma cells in the body are synthesizing this immunoglobulin. It is not surprising, therefore, that so far only six cases of IgE myeloma have been recognized compared with tens of thousands of IgG para-proteinaemias. IgE antibodies remain firmly fixed for an extended period when injected into human skin where they are probably bound to mast cells. Contact with antigen leads to degranulation of the mast cells with release of vasoactive amines. This process is responsible for the symptoms of hay fever and of extrinsic asthma when patients with atopic allergy come into contact with the allergen, e.g. grass pollen.

The main *physiological* role of IgE would appear to be protection of the external mucosal surfaces of the body by local recruitment of plasma factors and effector cells. Infectious agents penetrating the IgA defences would combine with specific IgE on the mast cell surface and trigger the release of vasoactive agents and factors chemotactic for granulocytes so leading to an influx of plasma IgG, complement, polymorphs and eosinophils (cf. p. 157). In such a context, the ability of eosinophils to damage IgG-coated helminths and the generous IgE response to such parasites would constitute an effective defence.

IMMUNOGLOBULIN SUBCLASSES

Antigenic analysis of IgG myelomas revealed further variation and showed that they could be grouped into four *subclasses* now termed IgG1, IgG2, IgG3 and IgG4. The differences all lie in the heavy chains which have been labelled $\gamma 1$, $\gamma 2$, $\gamma 3$ and $\gamma 4$ respectively. These heavy chains show considerable homology and have certain structures in common with each other—the ones which react with specific anti-IgG antisera—but each has one or more additional structures characteristic of its own subclass arising from differences in primary amino acid composition and in disulphide bridging. These give rise to differences in biological behaviour.

Two subclasses of IgA have also been found. The IgA2 subclass is unusual in that it lacks interchain disulphide bonds between heavy and light chains. Class and subclass variation is not restricted to human immunoglobulins but is a feature of all the higher mammals so far studied: monkey, sheep, rabbit, guinea-pig, rat and mouse.

OTHER IMMUNOGLOBULIN VARIANTS

Isotypes

The heavy chain constant region structures associated with the different classes and subclasses are termed isotypic variants, i.e. they are all present together in the serum of a normal subject. Other examples are provided by the types and subtypes of the

TABLE 2.3. Summary of immunoglobulin variants

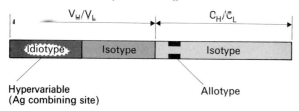

Type of variation	Distribution	Variant	Location	Examples
ISOTYPIC	All variants present in serum of a normal individual	Classes	C_H	IgM, IgE
		Subclasses	C_H	IgA1, IgA2
		Types	C_L	κ, λ
		Subtypes	C_L	$\lambda Oz^+, \lambda Oz^-$
		Subgroups	V_H/V_L	$V_{\kappa I}, V_{\kappa II}, V_{\kappa III}$ $V_{HI}, V_{HIII}, V_{HIII}$
ALLOTYPIC	Alternative forms: genetically controlled so not present in all individuals	Allotypes	Mainly C_H/C_L sometimes V_H/V_L	Gm groups (human) b4, b5, b6, b9 (rabbit light chains)
IDIOTYPIC	Individually specific to each immunoglobulin molecule	Idiotypes	Variable regions	Probably one or more hypervariable regions forming the antigen-combining site

42

C_L domain and by the subgroups of the light and heavy chain variable regions (table 2.3).

Allotypes

These represent yet a further type of variation which depends upon the existence of allelic forms (encoded by alleles or alternative genes at a single locus). In somewhat the same way as the red cells in genetically different individuals can differ in terms of the blood group antigen system A, B, O, so the Ig heavy chains differ in the expression of their allotypic groups. Typical allotypes are the Gm specificities on IgG (Gm = *marker* on Ig*G*) which are recognizable by the ability of the individual's IgG to block agglutination of red cells coated with anti-rhesus D bearing the Gm allotype by sera from patients with rheumatoid arthritis containing the appropriate anti-Gm rheumatoid factors.

Idiotypes

We have seen that it is possible to obtain antibodies that recognize isotypic and allotypic variants; it is also possible to raise antisera which are specific for individual antibody molecules and discriminate between one monoclonal antibody and another or one myeloma protein and another independently of isotypic or allotypic structures. These individual or idiotypic determinants (Kunkel, Oudin) are located in the variable part of the antibody, almost certainly in the combining site, and it seems likely that each hypervariable region could contribute to an idiotype. Thus in many cases, an anti-idiotypic serum directed against an anti-hapten antibody can block the binding of hapten. Anti-idiotypic sera which do not block are presumably directed to hyper-variable regions not concerned in the binding of that hapten (we know that small haptens do not fill the whole of the potential combining site of the antibody molecule). The existence of anti-idiotypes provides further support for the idea that each antibody has a unique structure. These antisera provide useful reagents, e.g. for demonstrating the same V region on different heavy chains and on different cells, for identification of specific immune complexes in patients' sera, for recognition of V_L type amyloid in subjects excreting Bence-Jones proteins, for detection of residual monoclonal protein after therapy and perhaps for selecting lymphocytes with certain surface receptors.

Summary

Immunoglobulins (Ig) have a basic 4 peptide structure of two identical heavy and two identical light chains joined by interchain disulphide links. Papain splits the molecule at the exposed flexible hinge region to give two identical univalent antigen binding fragments (Fab) and a further fragment (Fc). Pepsin proteolysis gives a divalent Ag binding fragment $F(ab')_2$ lacking the Fc.

There are perhaps 10^8 or more different Ig molecules in normal serum. Analysis of myeloma proteins which are homogeneous Ig produced by single clones of malignant plasma cells has shown the N terminal region of heavy and light chains to have a variable amino acid structure and the remainder to be relatively constant in structure. Each chain is folded into globular domains. The variable region domains bind Ag and three *hypervariable* loops on the heavy and three on the light chain form the Ag binding site. The constant region domains of the heavy chain (particularly the Fc) carry out a secondary biological function after the binding of Ag, e.g. complement fixation and macrophage binding.

In the human there are five major types of heavy chain giving five classes of Ig. IgG is the most abundant Ig particularly in the extravascular fluids where it combats micro-organisms and toxins; it fixes complement, binds to phagocytic cells and crosses the placenta. IgA exists mainly as a monomer (basic 4 peptide unit) in plasma, but in the seromucous secretions where it is the major Ig concerned in the defence of the external body surfaces, it is present as dimer linked to a secretory component. IgM is a pentameric molecule, essentially intravascular, produced early in the immune response. Because of its high valency it is a very effective bacterial agglutinator and mediator of complement dependent cytolysis and is therefore a powerful · first line defence against bacteraemia. IgD is largely present on the lymphocyte and probably functions as an Ag receptor. IgE binds firmly to mast cells and contact with antigen leads to local recruitment of anti-microbial agents through degranulation of the mast cells and release of inflammatory mediators. IgE is of importance in certain parasitic infections and is responsible for the symptoms of atopic allergy. Further diversity of function is possible through subdivision of classes into subclasses based on structural differences in heavy chains present in each normal individual.

Allotypic structural variations are controlled by allelic genes and provide genetic markers. Idiotypic determinants unique to a given immunoglobulin are recognizable by anti-idiotypic antibodies and are associated with the hypervariable regions forming the Ag binding site.

Further reading

Benacerraf B. (ed.) (1975) *Immunogenetics and Immunodeficiency*. (Articles by B. Frangione on Ig structure and by H.G. Kunkel & T. Kindt on allotypes and idiotypes.) MTP, Lancaster.

Edelman G.M. *et al.* (1969) Complete sequence of human IgG1. *Proc. Nat. Acad.Sci.*, **63**, 78.

Fougerean M. & Dausset J. (eds) (1980) *Progress in Immunology IV*. Academic Press, London.

Givol D. (1974) Affinity labelling and topology of the antibody combining site. In *Essays in Biochemistry*, 10. p. 73. Campbell P.N. & Dickens F. (eds). Biochemistry Society, London.

Glynn L.E. & Steward M.W. (eds) (1977) *Immunochemistry: an Advanced Textbook*, John Wiley & Sons, Chichester.

Leslie R.G.Q. & Cohen S. (1973) The active sites of immunoglobulin molecules. In *Essays in Fundamental Immunology 1*. p. 1. Roitt I.M. (ed.). Blackwell Scientific Publications, Oxford.

Moller G. (ed.) (1978) Immunoglobulin E. *Immunol. Rev.*, **41**.

Poljak R.J. (1973) Three-dimensional structure, function and genetic control of immunoglobulin. *Nature*, **256**, 373.

3

The immune response
I—Fundamentals

Two types of immune response

When antigen enters the body, two different types of adaptive immunological action may occur:

(1)   The synthesis and release of free antibody into the blood and other body fluids (*humoral immunity*). This antibody acts, for example, by coating bacteria to enhance their phagocytosis and by combination with and neutralization of bacterial toxins.

(2)   The production of 'sensitized' lymphocytes which are themselves the effectors of *cell-mediated immunity*. This confers protection against organisms such as the tubercle bacillus and viruses which are characterized by an ability to live and replicate *within* the cells of the host. In individuals immune to tubercle infection, the 'sensitized' lymphocytes interact with injected tuberculin antigen to produce the delayed type hyper sensitivity skin response, well known as the Mantoux reaction. Cells of this type are also involved in the rejection of skin grafts.

Role of the small lymphocyte

The central importance of the lymphocyte for both types of immune response was established largely by the work of Gowans. By labelling the lymphocytes with radioisotope and following their fate in the body it could be shown that there is a pool of recirculating lymphocytes which pass from the blood into the lymph nodes, spleen and other tissues and back to the blood by the major lymphatic channels such as the thoracic duct (figure 3.1).

PRIMARY RESPONSE

When rats are depleted of their lymphocytes by chronic drainage of lymph from the thoracic duct by an indwelling cannula, they have a grossly impaired ability to mount a primary antibody response to antigens such as tetanus toxoid and sheep red blood cells, or to reject a skin graft. Immunological reactivity can be restored by injecting thoracic duct

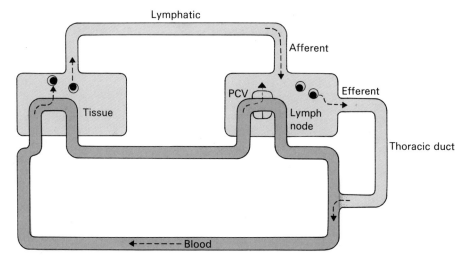

FIGURE 3.1. Traffic and recirculation of lymphocytes. Blood-borne lymphocytes enter the tissues and lymph nodes passing between the high cuboidal cells of the post-capillary venules (PCV) and leave via the draining lymphatics. The efferent lymphatics finally emerging from the last node in each chain join to form the thoracic duct which returns the lymphocytes to the blood stream where it empties into the left subclavian vein (in the human). In the spleen, lymphocytes enter the lymphoid area (white pulp) from the arterioles, pass to the sinusoids of the erythroid area (red pulp) and leave by the splenic vein.

lymphocytes obtained from another rat. The same effects can be obtained if, before injection, the thoracic duct cells are first incubated at 37°C for 24 hours under conditions which kill off large and medium-sized cells and leave only the small lymphocytes. Thus the small lymphocyte is necessary for the primary response to antigen.

Transfer experiments have also shown that small lymphocytes can become antibody synthesizing cells (plasma cells) and effector cells in cell-mediated immunity transplantation reactions.

SECONDARY RESPONSE—MEMORY

An immunologically 'virgin' rat, i.e. one which has had no previous contact with a specific antigen, may be inoculated with small lymphocytes from a rat which has already given a primary response to that antigen. Challenge of the recipient rat with antigen leads to a secondary type response with the rapid production of high-titre antibodies. If the recipient had not been injected with small lymphocytes from the 'primed' donor, a primary response with the relatively slow development of

48

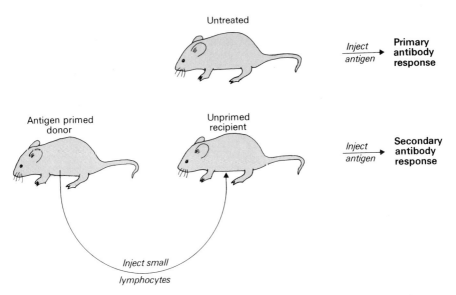

Untreated

Inject antigen → **Primary antibody response**

Antigen primed donor

Unprimed recipient

Inject antigen → **Secondary antibody response**

Inject small lymphocytes

FIGURE 3.2. Transfer of immunological memory by small lymphocytes from a primed donor rat. In these transfer experiments, genetically identical animals of the same strain are used to prevent complications arising from transplantation reactions between the transferred lymphocytes and the host.

lower-titre antibodies would have been seen (figure 3.2). Thus the small lymphocytes carry the *memory* of the first contact with antigen.

In the primary response, the relatively small number of virgin cells specific for the antigen are induced to *proliferate*; some go on to produce antibody- or cell-mediated immunity while others form an expanded population of antigen-sensitive memory cells which are capable of a faster response to antigen (figure 3.3). This combination of increase in cell number and more rapid maturation after antigen triggering is responsible for the characteristically brisk and heightened course of the secondary antibody response.

The thymus

This gland is organized into a series of lobules made up essentially of a meshwork of epithelial cells within which are packed aggregates of lymphocytes. The outer cortical area is densely populated with actively mitotic and some dying lymphoid cells and surrounds an inner medullary zone of prominent reticular dendritic and epithelioid cells with considerably fewer lymphocytes and isolated Hassall's corpuscles (figure 3.4). The occurrence of frequent thymic abnormalities in children with immunological deficiency disorders led to the

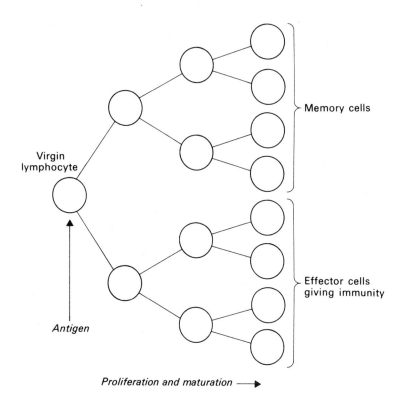

Virgin
lymphocyte

Antigen

Memory cells

Effector cells
giving immunity

Proliferation and maturation ⟶

FIGURE 3.3 The cellular basis of the primary response. After stimulation by antigen the previously resting virgin lymphocyte proliferates and during these divisions the cells mature. Some become non-dividing memory cells and others the effector cells of humoral or cell-mediated immunity. Memory cells require fewer cycles before they develop into effectors and this shortens the reaction time for the secondary response. The expanded clone of cells with memory for the original antigen provides the basis for the greater secondary relative to the primary immune response. Priming with low doses of antigen can often stimulate effective memory without producing very adequate antibody synthesis.

suggestion that the thymus was related in some way to the development of immune responses (Good and colleagues). The relationship was clarified by Miller's demonstration that removal of the thymus gland in mice at birth led to:

(1) decrease in circulating lymphocytes;

(2) severe impairment of graft rejection;

(3) reduced humoral antibody response to some but not all antigens;

(4) wasting after 1–3 months—probably a result of inability to combat infection effectively since neonatally thymectomized mice reared under germ-free conditions did not waste.

X-irradiation of adult mice destroys the ability of their

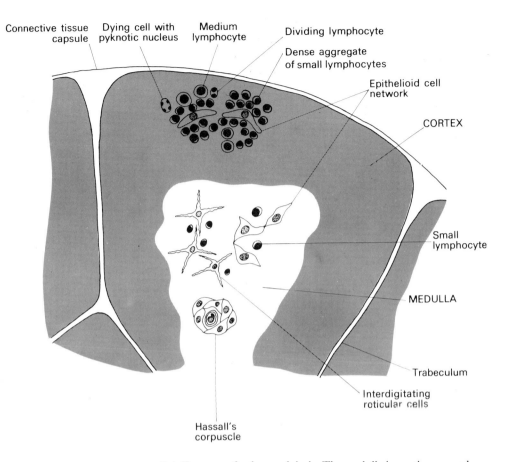

Connective tissue capsule

Dying cell with pyknotic nucleus

Medium lymphocyte

Dividing lymphocyte

Dense aggregate of small lymphocytes

Epithelioid cell network

CORTEX

Small lymphocyte

MEDULLA

Trabeculum

Interdigitating roticular cells

Hassall's corpuscle

FIGURE 3.4. Features of a thymus lobule. The medulla is continuous and sends finger-like processes into each lobule. The meshwork of epithelioid cells forms an almost continuous cytoplasmic barrier around the blood vessels ('blood-thymus barrier'). Whorled, possibly degenerate aggregates of epithelial cells appear as the characteristic Hassall's corpuscles. Reticular dendritic cells are prominent in the medulla. The densely packed, rapidly dividing lymphocytes in the cortex are mostly immunologically immature and readily destroyed by cortisone; 90% are small, 1% large and the remainder are medium-sized. Lymphocytes in the medulla are more sparse and more cortisone resistant.

lymphocytes to divide and hence their immunological responsiveness. This can be restored by injection of bone marrow cells. However, bone marrow cells fail to restore X-irradiated adult mice which have been thymectomized; on the other hand, mature cells from adult spleens or lymph node were effective. It is thus concluded that the thymus acts on primitive cells coming from the bone marrow to make them immunologically competent.

The Bursa of Fabricius

In chickens, another lymphoid organ termed the Bursa of Fabricius can be recognized. It is similar to the thymus and also embryologically derived from gut epithelium. Just as the thymus appears to act as a central lymphoid organ controlling the maturation of lymphocytes concerned largely with cell-mediated immunity, so the Bursa of Fabricius is responsible for the development of immunocompetence in cells destined to make humoral antibody. This differentiation of function may be readily seen from the results of the experiments documented in table 3.1: the thymus or bursa was removed from newborn chicks which were then irradiated to inactivate any competent lymphocytes which had already reached the peripheral tissues. After several weeks the chickens were tested and it was found that bursectomy had a profound effect on humoral antibody synthesis but did not unduly influence the cell mediated reactions responsible for tuberculin skin reactivity and graft rejection. On the other hand, as in the mice, thymectomy grossly impaired cell-mediated reactions and had some effect on antibody production.

TABLE 3.1. Effect of neonatal bursectomy and thymectomy on the development of immunological competence in the chicken. (From Cooper M.D., Peterson R.D.A., South M.A. & Good R.A. (1966) *J.exp.Med.*, **123**, 75, with permission of the editors.)

All X-irradiated after birth	Peripheral blood lymphocyte count	Ig concn.	Antibody	Delayed skin reaction to tuberculin	Graft rejection
Intact	14,800	++	+++	++	++
Thymectom-ized	9000	++	+	−	−
Bursectomized	13,200	−	−	+	+

Two populations of lymphocytes:
T- and B-cells

Thus primitive lymphoid cells from the bone marrow appear to differentiate into two small lymphocyte populations:

(1) *T-lymphocytes*, processed by or in some way dependent on the thymus, and responsible for cell-mediated immunity;

(2) *B-lymphocytes*, bursa-dependent, and concerned in the synthesis of circulating antibody.

Both populations on appropriate stimulation by antigen

proliferate and undergo morphological changes (figure 3.5). The B-lymphocytes develop into the plasma cell series. The mature plasma cell (figure 3.6 d & h) is actively synthesizing and secreting antibody and has a well-developed rough surfaced endoplasmic reticulum (figure 3.7c) characteristic of a cell producing protein for 'export'. T-lymphocytes transform to lymphoblasts (figure 3.6c) which in the electron microscope are seen to have virtually no rough-surfaced endoplasmic reticulum although there are abundant free ribosomes, either single or as polysomes (figure 3.7d). This high ribosome content makes them basophilic so that they show superficial resemblance to plasmablasts in the light microscope but no antibody can be detected in their cytoplasm nor in their secretions. However, they do elaborate a series of soluble factors which act largely through the macrophage in establishing cell-mediated immunity, the other arm of this response being provided by a

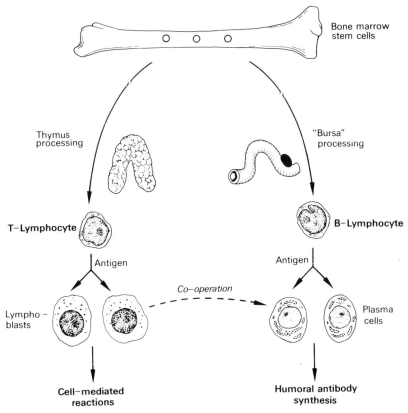

FIGURE 3.5. Processing of bone marrow cells by thymus and gut-associated central lymphoid tissue to become immunocompetent T- and B-lymphocytes respectively. Proliferation and transformation to cells of the lymphoblast and plasma cell series occurs on antigenic stimulation.

53

sub-population of activated T-lymphocytes which are cytotoxic for virus-infected cells (cf. p. 71).

The equivalent of the bursa in man and other mammals has not yet been clearly defined but experiments involving the culture of bone marrow or fetal liver *in vitro* make it seem likely that haemopoietic tissue itself provides the appropriate micro-environment for maturation of B-lymphocytes from precursor stem cells.

IDENTIFICATION OF B- AND T-LYMPHOCYTES

From the morphological standpoint it is difficult to differentiate T and B small lymphocytes at the light microscope level with conventional histological stains although some differences are now becoming apparent in their enzyme content and their ultrastructure (figures 3.6 a & b, 3.7 a & b). Fortunately the two populations differ strikingly in their surface markers (table 3.2) and these have been widely exploited.

Immunoglobulins are readily demonstrable on the surface of B- but not T-lymphocytes using an immunofluorescent technique with reagents such as fluorescein-labelled anti-immunoglobulin light chain (cf. figure 3.9b); this has also been shown in the electron microscope using peroxidase coupled (figure 6.11) or ^{125}I-labelled anti-Ig. Nearly all B-cells bear surface IgM, probably as monomer, but a proportion also stain with antisera directed against the Fc portion of other Ig classes, particularly IgD. Antisera specific for the terminal heavy chain domain (pFc' cf. p.33) stain more weakly suggesting attachment to the membrane through this region. The heavy chain of the surface IgM, which is present as a monomer, has an extra hydrophobic sequence relative to secreted pentameric IgM as revealed by its ability to bind detergent in the Fc region, to be labelled by lipophilic reagents and to insert itself into artificial membrane vesicles (liposomes). It must be supposed that the hydrophobic sequence anchors the molecule to the surface membrane and that removal of this sequence by mRNA splicing can be suitably arranged should the cell be turned on for Ig secretion as an antibody forming cell. I would like now to make an exceedingly important point. As we will see later, *each lymphocyte is programmed to make Ig of only one specificity and it is this Ig, placed on the B-lymphocyte surface, which is used as a specific receptor for antigen.*

In some circumstances, a proportion of T-cells do stain for surface immunoglobulin. This is not a product of the T-cell itself but is acquired by adsorption and probably represents immune complexes binding to receptors for Ig Fc region which are displayed by some T-cells. These can be demonstrated by the formation of rosettes with red cells coated with IgG antibody; clusters of red cells surround the lymphocyte to which they bind through the Fc of the coating IgG. Other T-cells have Fcμ receptors (i.e. binding sites for the Fc region of IgM heavy chains) and some features of these two sub-populations are contrasted in figures 3.6 and 3.7. Most if not all B-cells carry Fc receptors and form 'Fcγ rosettes' (figure 3.8a). In addition, approximately one half of the B-lymphocytes and perhaps some T-cells form clusters with red cells coated with the third component of complement (C3; cf. p.138) (figure 3.8b).

TABLE 3.2. Tests for surface markers on B- and T-cells

Lymphocytes	Immunofluorescent staining for:		Rosette formation using sheep r.b.c. coated with:				Virus receptors	Approx. % of human blood lymphocytes
	Ig	Thy 1 (θ)	Nothing	IgG	IgM	C$_3$		
T		+ +	+ +*	+	+ +	±	Measles	70
B	+ +	−	−	+ +	±	+ +	EB	10–20

*Human T-cells.

Interestingly, human T-cells can be persuaded to form so-called 'spontaneous' rosettes with uncoated sheep erythrocytes, a useful if fortuitous reaction without any immunological foundation. The T-lymphocyte membrane also possesses a specific discriminating antigen which is shared by the brain. In the mouse this is recognized as the Thy1 isoantigenic system (watch for the old nomenclature—θ) which is acquired as the cells differentiate within the milieu of the thymus gland.

At the time of writing, the most popular means of enumerating lymphocyte populations in human blood is to use fluorescent anti-immunoglobulin for B-cells and spontaneous rosette formation with neuraminidase-treated sheep erythrocytes for T-cells. Values given by these two tests usually add up to a few per cent short of 100%; without giving anything away, the remaining lymphocyte-like cells, negative on both counts, are termed 'null-cells'.

FIGURE 3.6. Light microscopy of cells involved in immune responses.

(a) Small lymphocytes. Condensed chromatin gives rise to heavy staining of the nucleus. The cell on the left is a typical T-cell with receptors for IgM with a thin rim of cytoplasm. The other cell has more cytoplasm and azurophilic granules are evident; it bears receptors for IgG and sheep red cells and has therefore been defined as a T_G lymphocyte. Isolated platelets are visible. B-lymphocytes have a similar appearance. Giemsa stain ×2500.

(b) T_M lymphocytes. Acid esterase staining giving the characteristic 'dot'-like appearance ×2500.

(c) Transformed lymphocyte (lymphoblast) following stimulation of lymphocytes in culture with a polyclonal activator. The large lymphoblasts with their relatively high ratio of cytoplasm to nucleus may be compared in size with the isolated small lymphocyte. One cell is in mitosis. May–Grünewald–Giemsa stain ×2500.

(d) Plasma cells. The nucleus is eccentric. The cytoplasm is strongly basophilic due to high RNA content. The juxta-nuclear lightly-stained zone corresponds with the Golgi region. May–Grünewald–Giemsa stain ×2500.

(e) Monocyte, showing 'horseshoe-shaped' nucleus and moderately abundant pale cytoplasm with well defined granules. A small lymphocyte with a more strongly stained nucleus is shown for comparison. Staining for peroxidase is frequently positive. Giemsa stain ×5000.

(f) Four polymorphonuclear leucocytes (neutrophils) and one eosinophil. The multi-lobed nuclei and the cytoplasmic granules are clearly shown, those of the eosinophil being heavily stained. Leishman stain ×2000.

(g) Macrophages in monolayer cultures after phagocytosis of mycobacteria (stained red). Carbol–Fuchsin counterstained with Malachite Green ×1000.

(h) Plasma cells stained to show intracellular immunoglobulin using a fluorescein-labelled anti-IgG (green) and a rhodamine-conjugated anti-IgM (red) ×2500.

(a), (b), (c) and (g) were photographed by Dr P.M. Lydyard. The material for (a) was supplied by Dr K. McLennan and (g) by Dr G. Rooke. (d) and (h) were given by Professor C. Grossi, (e) by Professor J. Stewart and (f) by Professor J.J. Owen.

FIGURE 3.7. (pp. 58–61). Electron microscopy of cells involved in immune responses (most cells may be seen in figure 8.6).

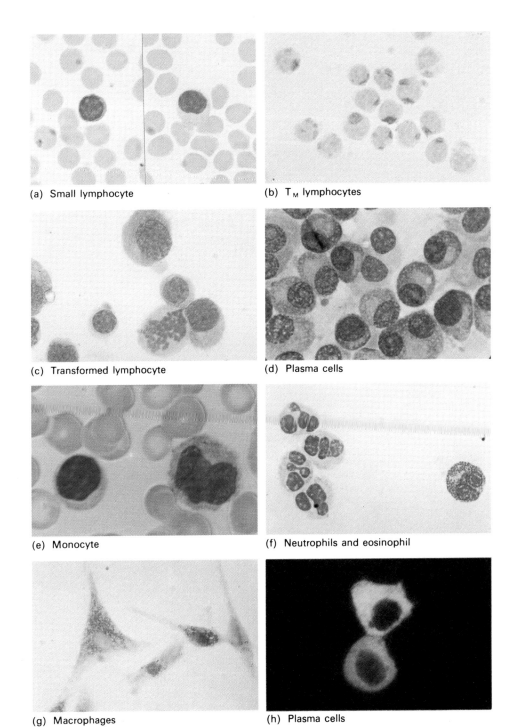

(a) Small lymphocyte

(b) T$_M$ lymphocytes

(c) Transformed lymphocyte

(d) Plasma cells

(e) Monocyte

(f) Neutrophils and eosinophil

(g) Macrophages

(h) Plasma cells

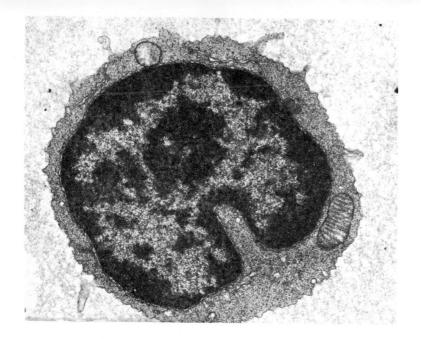

FIGURE 3.7. (a) Small T-lymphocyte with receptors for IgM. Indented nucleus with condensed chromatin and sparse cytoplasm: a single mitochondrion is shown and many free ribosomes but otherwise few organelles (×13,000). B-lymphocytes are essentially similar with slightly more cytoplasm and occasional elements of rough-surfaced endoplasmic reticulum.

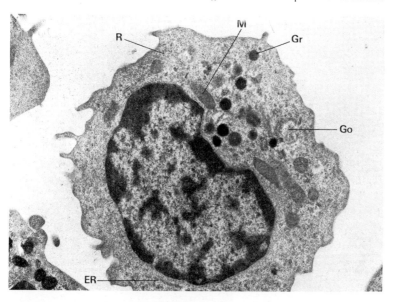

(b) T-lymphocyte with receptors for IgG (×7500). The more abundant cytoplasm contains several mitochondria (M), free ribosomes (R) with some elements of rough-surfaced endoplasmic reticulum (ER), prominent Golgi apparatus (Go) and characteristic membrane-bound electron-dense granules (Gr). The nuclear chromatin is less condensed than that of the T_M cell. (Courtesy of Drs A. Zicca & C.E. Grossi.)

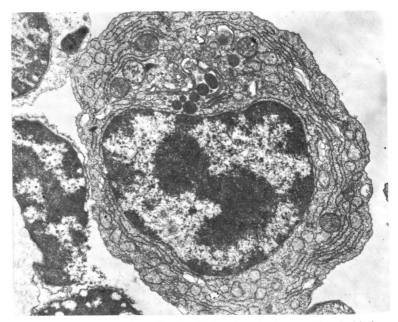

(c) Plasma cell (×10,000). Prominent rough-surfaced endoplasmic reticulum associated with the synthesis and secretion of Ig.

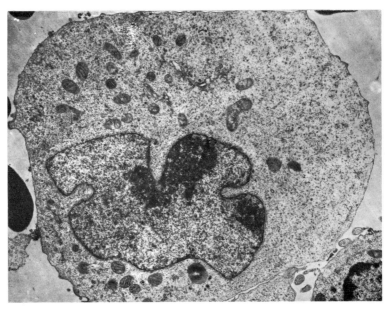

(d) Transformed lymphocyte (lymphoblast) (×7000). The nuclear chromatin is less condensed than in the small lymphocyte (a). The more extensive cytoplasm shows numerous mitochondria and free polyribosomes. (Courtesy of Miss V. Petts.)

59

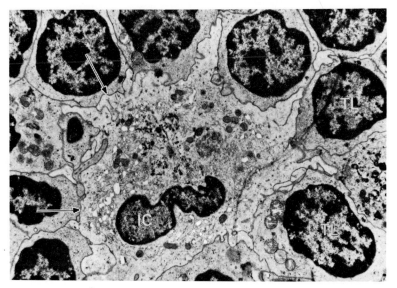

(e) Interdigitating cell (IC) in the thymus dependent area of the rat lymph node. This is thought to be an antigen-presenting cell derived from the Langerhans' cell in the skin which travels to the node in the afferent lymph as a 'veiled' cell bearing antigen on its profuse surface processes. Intimate contacts are made with the surface membranes (arrows) of the surrounding T-lymphocytes (TL). The cytoplasm of the IC contains relatively few organelles and does not show Birbeck granules (racket-shaped cytoplasmic organelles, characteristic of the Langerhans' cell), but these granules appear after antigenic stimulation. (×2000) (From Kamperdijk E.W.A., Hoefsmit E.Ch.H., Drexhage H.A. & Balfour B.II. (1980) In *Mononuclear Phagocytes*. Furth R.v. III (ed.). Rijhoff, The Hague, courtesy of authors and publishers.)

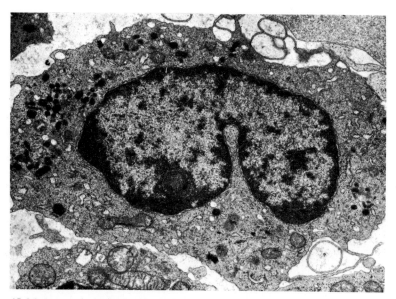

(f) Monocyte (×10,000). 'Horseshoe' nucleus. Phagocytic and pinocytic vesicles, lysosomal granules, mitochondria and isolated profiles of rough-surfaced endoplasmic reticulum are evident.

60

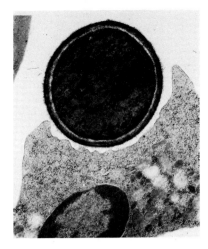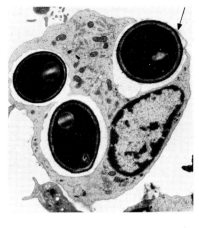

(g) (Left) Phagocytosis of *Candida albicans* by a polymorphonuclear leucocyte (Neutrophil). Adherence to the surface initiates enclosure of the fungal particle within arms of cytoplasm. Lysosomal granules are abundant but mitochondria are rare. (×15,000)

(h) (Right) Phagocytosis of *C. albicans* by a monocyte showing near completion of phagosome formation (arrowed) around one organism and complete ingestion of two others. (×5000)

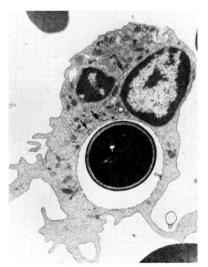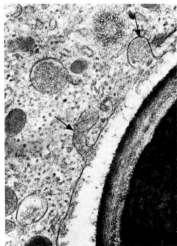

(i) (Left) Neutrophil 30 minutes after ingestion of *C. albicans*. The cytoplasm is already partly degranulated and two lysosomal granules (arrowed) are fusing with the phagocytic vacuole. Two lobes of the nucleus are evident. (×5000)

(j) (Right) Higher magnification of (i) showing fusing granules discharging their contents into the phagocytic vacuole (arrowed). (×33,000) (Figs 3.7 g–j courtesy of Dr H. Valdimarsson.)

61

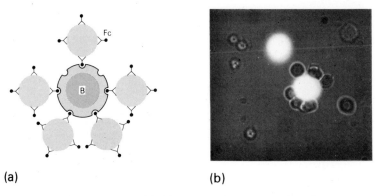

(a)   (b)

FIGURE 3.8. B-cell rosettes. (a) Diagrammatic representation of rosette formed with IgG (Y) coated erythrocytes binding to the receptor for Fcγ. (b) Cluster of C₃ coated red cells around B-lymphocyte (visualized in u.v. light after staining with acridine orange). (Courtesy of Dr A. Arnaiz-Villena.)

LYMPHOCYTE SURFACE PHENOMENA

When viable B-lymphocytes are stained in the cold with a fluorescein-conjugated anti-Ig, the fluorescence is seen as patches on the cell surface (figure 3.9b). However, if the experiment is repeated using monovalent (Fab) anti-Ig, a smooth ring of surface fluorescence is observed (figure 3.9a). The interpretation of these findings is that the lymphocyte surface immunoglobulins are floating freely in the plasma membrane (like icebergs in a sea of lipid) and are agglutinated into little patches by the divalent anti-Ig (figure 3.9d and e). If the lymphocytes are now allowed to warm up, the patches coalesce to form a cap over one pole of the cell (figure 3.9c) and the complexes are taken into the cytoplasm by endocytosis leaving the surface free of immunoglobulin. The cell will resynthesize its surface immunoglobulin within a few hours if washed and incubated at 37° in fresh medium.

When rabbit lymphocytes are cultured in the presence of anti-Ig for a minimum of 16–20 hours, they go on to transform into blast-like cells (cf. figure 3.6c) and divide. Activation also occurs with the divalent F(ab')₂ pepsin fragment derived from the anti-Ig but not the monovalent Fab, with the strong implication that cross-linking and aggregation of surface Ig is an important step in B-lymphocyte stimulation which would normally be brought about by antigen combining with complementary surface Ig receptors on those lymphocytes capable of synthesizing the appropriate antibody. However the blast cells induced by such activation do not make antibody and current thinking is that in most circumstances an additional non-specific or 'second' signal (Bretscher & Cohn) is required

62

particularly for the triggering of antibody production by thymus-dependent antigens (i.e. those antigens which provoke a grossly depressed response in animals deprived of T-lymphocytes by neonatal thymectomy or other means: cf. p. 50).

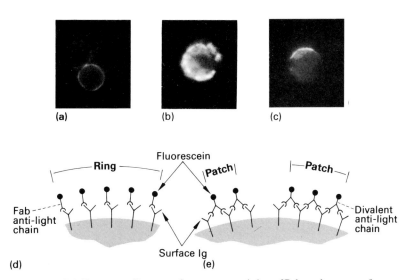

FIGURE 3.9. Patterns of immunofluorescent staining of B-lymphocyte surface immunoglobin using fluorescein-conjugated anti-Ig (cf. p. 127 for discussion of technique). Provided the reaction is carried out in the cold to prevent pinocytosis, the labelled antibody cannot penetrate to the interior of the viable lymphocytes and reacts only with surface components. (a) Ring staining with monovalent (Fab) anti-Ig; (b) patch formation with whole anti-Ig; (c) cap formation on warming the cells in (b); (d) diagram of ring staining by monovalent anti-Ig; (e) diagram of patch formation by divalent anti-Ig. During cap formation, submembraneous myosin becomes redistributed in association with the surface Ig and induces locomotion of the previously sessile cell in a direction away from the cap. (Photographs kindly provided by Drs A. Arnaiz-Villena & L. Hudson.)

Cellular co-operation in the antibody response

THE ROLE OF MACROPHAGES

The mononuclear cells of the monocyte-macrophage series play a central role in the induction of the immune response with respect to the presentation of antigen to lymphocytes. Intimate cytoplasmic contacts between macrophages and lymphocytes have been observed (cf. figure 3.7e) and co-operative effects of macrophages for antibody production are clearly revealed by tissue culture studies showing that the antibody response to most antigens is largely abrogated when glass-adherent cells are first removed from the responding lymphoid cell population, and that this defect can be overcome by the addition of macrophages. Furthermore, antigens such as bovine serum albumin provoke a vastly superior antibody response when injected together with macrophages rather than as a free solution; interestingly the more thymus-dependent the response to a given antigen, the greater the enhancing effect due to macrophages. Antigen trapping and concentration of antigen at the cell surface for effective presentation to the lymphocyte seems to be important. Antigen-antibody complexes formed in antigen excess and containing the third component of complement (C3b, p. 138) localize efficiently in lymphoid follicles where they persist on the surface of dendritic cells and trap antigen-specific B-cells to generate B-cell memory. In general, when antigen is taken up by macrophages, a proportion is degraded by phagocytic digestion while part is fixed to the cell surface where it is thought to be in a strongly immunogenic state in some form of association with the Ia antigens of the major histocompatibility complex (p. 88). Cells of the macrophage series adopt many morphological forms which vary greatly in their expression of these two mechanisms for handling antigens. Some, like the Kupffer cells of the liver, the alveolar macrophages or the lining cells of splenic cords, have well-developed lysosomal granules and are actively phagocytic. We may look upon them as 'professional phagocytes' destined for a life of microbe-crunching. In contrast with these men of violence, the dendritic macrophages of the lymph node cortex and skin (Langerhans' cells) are far more genteel; largely eschewing the degrading process of phagocytosis, they prefer to incorporate antigen into their surface membranes for the more aristocratic purpose of presentation to and activation of lymphocytes. Even the dendritic macrophages are specialized depending upon the particular lymphocyte sub-population they serve.

CO-OPERATION BETWEEN T- AND B-CELLS

Attention has already been drawn to the fact that the antibody response to certain antigens is considerably depressed following neonatal thymectomy. However, we know from the work of Davies with chromosome (T6) marked thymus cells, that the T-lymphocytes do not themselves secrete antibody even though they actively divide after contact with antigen. This involvement of the T-lymphocyte in antibody synthesis without itself producing antibody is now seen to be due to a form of *co-operation* by the T-cell which helps the antigenic stimulation of B-lymphocytes to be more effective (figure 3.5). Using an irradiated mouse (which cannot itself make an immune response) as a 'living test-tube', Claman and his colleagues showed that thymocytes or bone marrow cells (containing B-cell precursors) injected together with sheep red cells gave only poor or modest antibody production. When T- and B-cells were injected together, there was a very marked increase in the number of cells engaged in antibody synthesis (table 3.3).

TABLE 3.3. Co-operation of bone marrow and thymus cells in production of antibody to sheep red cells in irradiated recipient

Irradiated recipient given antigen plus:	Antibody response
Spleen cells	+++
Thymocytes (T-cells)	±
Bone marrow (B-cells)	+
Thymocytes and bone marrow	+++

The cellular origin of the antibody-forming cells was elegantly demonstrated by Miller and his colleagues in co-operation experiments involving transfer of T-cells and bone marrow from genetically different mouse strains. The antibody-forming cells in the recipient spleen were studied *in vitro* by the Jerne plaque technique (p. 79) and could be inhibited only by an antiserum to the transplantation antigens of the strain providing the bone marrow *not* the thymus cells (figure 3.10).

At the molecular level, further light on the nature of co-operation has been shed by the experiments with carrier-hapten conjugates. The reader may recall that haptens are small groups which can combine with preformed antibody but fail to stimulate antibody synthesis unless coupled with an antigenic carrier (usually a protein; cf. p. 9). Both Mitchison and Rajewsky have shown that primed B-cells make a secondary antibody response to a hapten bound to protein carrier only when T-cells primed to the carrier ('helper cells') are also present. In other words, when T-cells recognize and respond to carrier determinants, they help B-lymphocytes specific for the hapten to develop into antibody-forming cells, presumably by providing the required second or accessory signal(s) discussed earlier (figure 3.11).

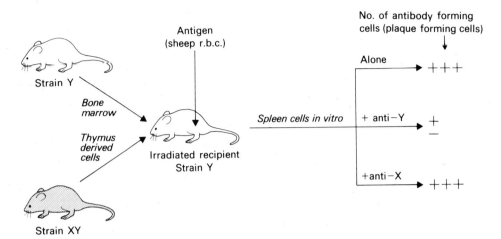

FIGURE 3.10. Bone marrow origin of antibody-forming cells. Antibody-forming cells were studied in the antigen stimulated recipient of a bone marrow/thymus mixture. Antibodies to the transplantation antigens of the strain providing bone marrow inhibited the plaque-forming cells whereas antibodies to the thymocyte donor were ineffective. (Based on Miller J.F.A.P. & Mitchell G.F. (1968) *J.exp.Med.*, **128,** 821: in these studies thymus derived cells from the thoracic duct were used).

The mechanisms underlying co-operation are not yet clearly defined. They involve complex interactions between macrophages, T-cells and B-cells in which association of the carrier determinants with Ia antigens of the major histocompatibility complex is crucial (p. 88) and in which various soluble growth factors are implicated. Activated B-blasts produced during the limited antigen-specific first phase are driven by non-antigen specific growth factors (usually resulting from a specific antigenic stimulus; cf. p. 161) to divide extensively and mature to form an expanded clone of plasma cells (figure 3.12).

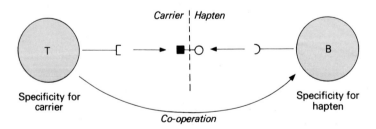

FIGURE 3.11. T-B *co-operation*. The T-cells on recognizing carrier determinants on the antigen provide a co-operative signal which enables B-cells that recognize hapten to mature into antibody-secreting plasma cells.

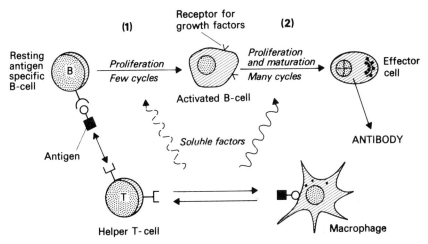

FIGURE 3.12. T-B co-operation in the response to a carrier (■)—hapten (●).

Stage 1—*Antigen-specific:* helper T-cells activated by macrophage processed antigen stimulate the resting B-cell, which has bound antigen through its hapten-specific Ig receptors, to transform after a small number of divisions to a blast cell with receptors for soluble growth factors.

Stage 2—*Non-antigen specific:* these soluble growth factors produced by interactions between the T-cell and macrophages (possibly different from the original type initially presenting the antigen) stimulate the blast cells to repeated division and maturation to become antibody-producing effector cells.

The cell-mediated immune response

Immunity to those infectious organisms which have developed the capacity for living and multiplying *within* the cells of the host is masterminded by the T-lymphocytes independently of the B-cells. Thus infections with intracellular facultative parasites such as tubercle and leprosy bacilli, budding viruses like smallpox and parasites such as toxoplasma, pose serious problems for children with thymic insufficiency in contrast to infants with primary immunoglobulin deficiency who cope relatively well with these organisms. Support for this view is also afforded by studies on thymectomized and bursectomized chicks and by the demonstration that T-cells from mice which had recovered from infection with TB could passively confer immunity on previously uninfected animals into which they had been injected (cf. figure 7.7).

The T-cells are antigen-sensitive in that they show specificity for antigen in their response to carriers in delayed hypersensitivity reactions and in their cytotoxicity for virally infected cells or allogeneic (cf. p. 71) targets. The fact that such cytotoxic cells can be specifically adsorbed onto fibroblasts bearing the transplantation antigens to which the animal was initially sensitized clearly indicates that T-cells do have surface receptors which recognize antigen although it must be said that the nature of these receptors is still hotly debated. The presence of binding sites on different T-lymphocytes for Fcγ and Fcμ led to the inevitable suggestion that the antigen receptors were nothing more than exogenously acquired cytophilic antibody and in some instances (e.g. the Thy1 positive cells from immunized mice which form rosettes with sheep erythrocytes) this is undoubtedly the case. Nonetheless, the ability of neonatally bursectomized chickens and of a-γ-globulinaemic children to mount specific cell-mediated hypersensitivity responses is powerful evidence that T-cells possess their own endogenous receptors independently of B-cells and their products, a view reinforced by the phenomena of selective T-cell tolerance (p. 96) and the deletion of specific T-helpers by 'suicide' with radioactive antigen.

The receptors are not conventional Ig molecules. Very sensitive techniques have failed to detect light chain determinants on the surface of T-cells from bursectomized chickens and so far, with the exception of anti-idiotypic sera, which are probably directed against the antigen-combining site, no anti-Ig serum has been able to block the killing of allogeneic targets by cytotoxic T-cells. These anti-idiotypic sera have provided evidence for common or closely similar combining sites on cytotoxic T-cells and antibodies directed against the same major histocompatibility (transplantation) antigen, and for shared idiotypes on helper T-cells and antibodies with specificity for a given bacterial antigen determinant. In the latter case, the gene encoding the helper T-cell idiotype is found to be on the same chromosome and close to the cluster of genes for the Ig heavy chains. The present tentative view is that the receptor has a molecular weight of 150,000 daltons and consists of two chains, each of which uses an Ig heavy chain variable region gene (cf. p. 115) linked to a constant region gene different from those coding for conventional heavy chain peptides. A curious feature of the receptor is its ability to recognize antigen in association with a constituent of the major histocompatibility complex (pp. 88 and 234).

The T-cell receptor is triggered by antigen on the surface of an appropriate macrophage where it may be present in a special 'processed' form in association with Ia. The cell membrane becomes activated and the signal is transmitted to the interior of the cell where the nucleus of the small lymphocyte with its compact chromatin becomes derepressed; the cell transforms into a large blast cell and proliferates in response to macrophage

—derived growth factors rather like the later stages of B-cell differentiation (figure 3.12). One sub-population of the stimulated T-cells releases a number of soluble factors, another develops cytotoxic powers, while a further proportion become memory cells; together, these phenomena form the basis of cell-mediated immunity.

THE TWO ARMS OF THE CELL-MEDIATED RESPONSE

Proliferation of the stimulated T-cells provides the mechanism for amplification of the cell-mediated immune response which depends upon these two major effector mechanisms—the generation of cytotoxic cells and the release of biologically active soluble factors (termed 'lymphokines' by Dumonde)

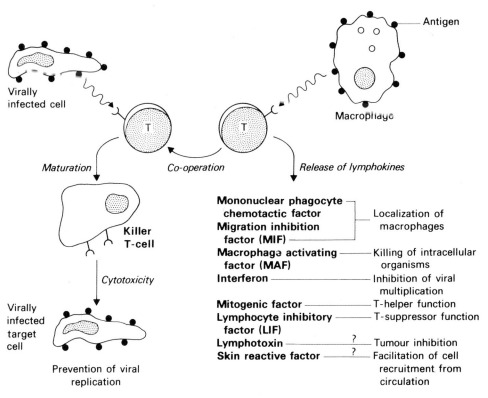

FIGURE 3.13. The cell-mediated immune response. This operates through the generation of cytotoxic T-cells and the release of lymphokines through the stimulation of two distinct T-sub-populations. Different lymphokines may be produced by different lymphocyte subsets. The intense proliferation induced by antigenic stimulation has not been shown but is an essential factor in the amplification of the response.

which modulate the behaviour of other cells, particularly the mononuclear phagocytes (monocytes and macrophages) (figure 3.13).

Lymphokines

The supernatant fluid recovered after stimulating sensitized lymphocytes with antigen possesses several biological activities, some of which have been ascribed to different molecular species. These lymphokines have molecular weights of the order of 20,000–80,000. Among them is a group which directly influence the movement and activity of macrophages. *Macrophage chemotactic factor* causes an accumulation of mononuclear phagocytes at the site of antigen-mediated lymphokine release; this can be demonstrated in Boyden chambers where monocytes or macrophages move across Millipore membranes into the chamber containing higher concentrations of factor. Once attracted, the cells are discouraged from leaving by macrophage *migration inhibition factor* (MIF); interaction with the cells appears to involve a fucose residue on MIF and a useful control for its assay is abrogation of a positive test by added fucose. Stimulation by *macrophage activating factor* (MAF) produces significant morphological changes with a ruffling of the surface membrane which gives the cell an 'angry' appearance, and leads to an increase in lysosomal enzyme content and a heightened ability to kill off ingested intracellular organisms. The movement of monocytes from blood vessels into the extravascular spaces is facilitated by another lymphokine, the *skin reactive factor* which also increases capillary permeability. *Immune interferon*, which inhibits intracellular viral replication, is present in lymphokine supernatants but it is not clear whether it is synthesized by T-cells or is secondarily released from activated macrophages.

Two lymphokines, *mitogenic factor* and *lymphocyte inhibitory factor* (LIF), with opposite effects on the proliferation of lymphocytes could well be related to T-helper and suppressor effects respectively. *Lymphotoxin*, although only mildly cytolytic for certain cultured cell lines, showed quite marked cytostatic activity and one is tempted to postulate a role in the constraint of tumour growth. Other biological activities which have been ascribed to lymphokines include effects on the migration and adhesiveness of polymorphs and eosinophils and on the aggregation of platelets.

Cytotoxic T-cells

Viral infection can generate a population of killer T-cells which are specifically cytotoxic for host cells infected with that virus. Similarly, a graft from a genetically dissimilar member of the same species (allogenic graft) provokes the formation of cytotoxic T-cells directed against target cells bearing the major histocompatibility antigens of the donor. The first stage in this interaction, which may be followed *in vitro,* involves intimate binding of effector to target through recognition of the transplantation antigens by surface receptors; this stage is Ca^{2+} independent and cytochalasin B sensitive. Within a matter of minutes, a change occurs in the target cell, a 'kiss of death' so to speak, which leads irrevocably to cytolysis; this phase is Ca^{2+} dependent and cytochalasin insensitive. Thus by carrying out the binding step in the absence of Ca^{2+} and then allowing cytolysis to proceed by adding Ca^{2+} and cytochalasin (which inhibits cell movement and prevents binding to further target cells), each cytotoxic cell should theoretically lyse only one target. Enumeration of cytotoxic T-cells in this way by counting the number of killed allogenic targets gives an estimate of approximately 1% of the spleen lymphocytes. This high proportion of cells committed to each major histocompatibility specificity is striking and implies a special relationship between T-cells and such antigens. In this context it should be noted that effective killing is only seen when the T-cells are sensitized to the major histocompatibility antigens or a determinant (e.g. viral) recognized in association with these antigens (cf. p. 234).

The anatomical basis of the immune response

The complex cellular interactions which form the basis of the immune response take place within the organized architecture of peripheral, or secondary, lymphoid tissue which includes the lymph glands, spleen and unencapsulated tissue lining the respiratory, alimentary and genito-urinary tracts.

LYMPH NODE

The encapsulated tissue of the lymph node contains a meshwork of reticular cells and their fibres organized into sinuses. These act as a filter for lymph draining the body tissues and possibly bearing foreign antigens which enters the subcapsular sinus by the afferent vessels and diffuses past the lymphocytes in the cortex to reach the medullary sinuses and thence the efferent lymphatics (figures 3.1 and 3.14).

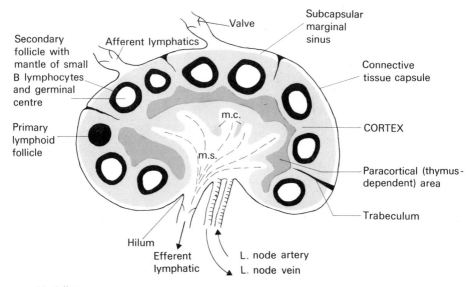

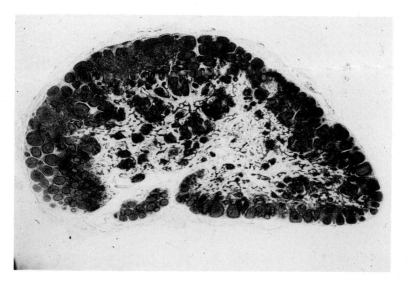

FIGURE 3.14. A human lymph node. (a) (top) Diagrammatic representation (b); (bottom) low power view of histological section, ×10. (Photographed by Dr P.M. Lydyard.)

B-cell areas

The follicular aggregations of B-lymphocytes are a prominent feature of the cortex. In the unstimulated node they are present as spherical collections of cells termed *primary nodules* but after antigenic challenge they form *secondary follicles* (figure 7.15)

72

which consist of a corona or mantle of concentrically packed small B-lymphocytes surrounding a pale-staining *germinal centre* which contains large, often proliferating, lymphoid cells, scattered conventional reticular macrophages and the specialized dendritic macrophages with elongated cytoplasmic processes and few if any lysosomes. Germinal centres are greatly enlarged in secondary antibody responses and it is reasonable to regard them as important sites of B-cell memory. Following antigenic stimulation, differentiating plasmablasts appear and become plasma cells in the medullary cords of lymphoid cells which project between the medullary sinuses.

T-cell areas

Compartmentation of the two major lymphocyte populations occurs in that T-cells are largely confined to a region of the node referred to as the paracortical (or thymus-dependent) area (figure 3.14); if one looks at nodes taken from children with selective T-cell deficiency (figure 7.15) or neonatally thymectomized mice, the paracortical region is seen to be virtually devoid of lymphocytes. Furthermore, when a T-cell-mediated response is elicited in a normal animal, say by a skin graft or by painting chemicals such as picryl chloride on the skin to induce contact hypersensitivity, there is a marked proliferation of cells in the thymus-dependent area and typical lymphoblasts are evident. In contrast, stimulation of antibody formation by the 'thymus-independent' antigen pneumococcus polysaccharide leads to proliferation in the cortical lymphoid follicles with development of germinal centres while the paracortical region remains inactive reflecting the inability to develop cellular hypersensitivity to the polysaccharide. As would be expected, nodes taken from children with congenital hypogammaglobulinaemia associated with failure of B-cell development are conspicuously lacking in primary and secondary follicular structures. This segregation of B- and T-lymphocyte areas tends to favour models of co-operation which involve soluble factors rather than antigen-bridging of T- and B-cells but the separation of cell types is not absolute.

Lymphocyte traffic

Lymphocytes enter the node through the afferent lymphatics and by passage across the specialized cuboidal epithelium of the postcapillary venules (cf. figure 3.1). This traffic of lymphocytes between the tissues, the blood stream and the lymph glands enables antigen-sensitive cells to seek the antigen and to be recruited to sites at which a response is occurring, while the dissemination of memory cells and their progeny enables a more widespread response to be organized throughout the lymphoid system. Thus, antigen-reactive cells are depleted from the circulating pool of lymphocytes within 24 hours of antigen first localizing in the lymph nodes or spleen; several days later, after proliferation at the site of antigen localization, a peak of activated cells appears in the thoracic duct. When antigen reaches a node in a primed animal, there is a dramatic fall in the output of cells in the efferent lymphatics, a phenomenon described variously as 'cell shutdown' or 'lymphocyte trapping' and which probably results from the antigen-induced release of a T-cell soluble factor (cf. the lymphokines, p. 70); this is followed by an output of activated blast cells which peaks at around 80 hours.

SPLEEN

On a fresh section of spleen, the lymphoid tissue forming the white pulp is seen as circular or elongated grey areas within the

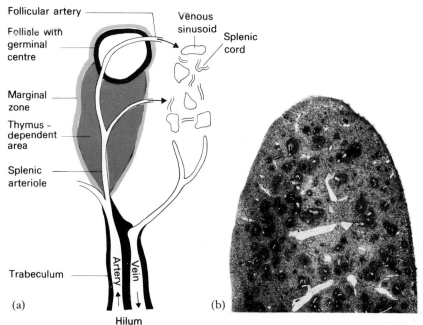

FIGURE 3.15. Human spleen. (a) Diagrammatic representation. The lymphoid cells form a sheath around the arterioles (white pulp). The remainder (red pulp) consists of splenic cords and venous sinusoids filled with erythrocytes. (b) Low power view of histological section, ×35. (Photographed by Dr P.M. Lydyard.)

erythrocyte-filled red pulp consisting of splenic cords lined with macrophages and venous sinusoids. As in the lymph node, T- and B-cell areas are segregated (figure 3.15). The spleen is a very effective blood filter, removing effete red and white cells and responding actively to blood-borne antigens, the more so if particulate. Plasmablasts and mature plasma cells are present in the marginal zone extending into the red pulp.

UNENCAPSULATED LYMPHOID TISSUE

The respiratory, alimentary and genito-urinary tracts are guarded immunologically by subepithelial accumulations of lymphoid tissue which are not constrained by a connective tissue capsule. These may occur as diffuse collections of lymphocytes, plasma cells and phagocytes throughout the lamina propria of the intestinal wall with only isolated solitary follicles (figure 3.16a) or as more clearly organized tissue with well-formed follicles (figure 3.16b). In man, the latter includes the lingual, palatine and pharyngeal tonsils, the small intestinal Peyer's patches and the appendix. It has been suggested that the unencapsulated lymphoid tissue forms a separate inter-connected system, the mucosal-associated lymphoid tissue (MALT), within which cells committed to IgA or IgE synthesis may circulate.

In the gut, cells leave the Peyer's patches, presumably after antigenic stimulation, and ultimately drain into the blood from the thoracic duct and pass into the lamina propria where many

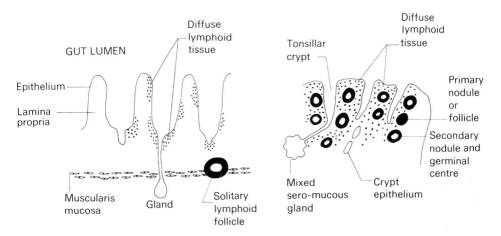

(a) Diffuse lymphoid tissue in lamina propria

(b) Well-formed lymphoid tissue of a tonsil

FIGURE 3.16. Unencapsulated lymphoid tissue.

become IgA-forming cells. This maturation of antibody-forming cells at a site distant from that at which antigen triggering has occurred is seen in the lymph node where plasma cells develop in the medullary cords and the spleen where they are found predominantly in the marginal zone. My guess is that this movement of cells acts to prevent the generation of high local concentrations of antibody in the region of the macrophage-processed antigen, so avoiding neutralization of the antigen and premature shutting off of the immune response.

Another tissue in the human which can support very active antibody synthesis is the bone marrow.

Summary

T-lymphocytes, which mature under the influence of the thymus, mediate cellular immunity and B-lymphocytes, which mature in the bone marrow in mammals (Bursa of Fabricius in birds), become antibody-forming cells responsible for humoral immunity. T- and B-cells are recognized by different surface markers: human T-cells form rosettes with sheep erythrocytes and B-cells have surface Ig which functions as a receptor for antigen.

Macrophages present antigen on their surface for reacting with and triggering antigen-sensitive lymphocytes. In the thymus dependent response to a hapten linked to an immunogenic carrier, T-cells reacting to the carrier help B-cells to be triggered by the hapten to form anti-hapten antibody. In the response to a typical protein, one determinant is like a hapten and the remaining determinants act as carrier. Combination of the antigen with B-cell Ig receptor provides a signal which tolerizes the B-cell unless it is activated by a second signal produced by the T-cell as a result of carrier stimulation. Poorly digested, linear, highly polymeric antigens can stimulate IgM-producing B-cells directly without T-cell help and are termed thymus independent antigens.

Cell-mediated immunity which provides the main defence against intracellular organisms, depends upon the interaction of antigen with specific receptors (not conventional Ig) on the surface of T-lymphocytes. One sub-population of T-cells elaborates soluble factors (lymphokines) whose main function is to recruit and activate cells of the mono-nuclear phagocyte system; another population becomes cytotoxic for target cells bearing the antigen.

The immune response occurs most effectively in structured secondary lymphoid tissue. The lymph nodes filter and screen lymph flowing from the body tissues while spleen filters the blood. B- and T-cell areas are separated. B-cell structures appear in the lymph node cortex as primary follicles or secondary follicles with germinal centres after antigen stimulation; T-cells occupy the paracortical area; plasma cells synthesizing antibody appear in medullary cords which penetrate the macrophage lined medullary sinuses. Lymphoid tissue guarding the gastrointestinal tract is unencapsulated and somewhat structured (tonsils, Peyer's patches, appendix) or present as diffuse cellular collections in the lamina propria. Together with the subepithelial accumulations of cells lining the respiratory and genito-urinary tracts, they form the so-called mucosal associated lymphoid tissue system.

Further reading

See references at the end of chapter 4.

4

The immune response
II—Further aspects

Synthesis of humoral antibody

DETECTION OF ANTIBODY-FORMING CELLS

Immunofluorescence

Cells containing antibody within their cytoplasm can be identified by the 'sandwich' technique (see figure 6.9c). For example, a cell making antibodies to tetanus toxoid if treated first with the antigen will subsequently bind a fluorescein labelled anti-tetanus antibody and can then be visualized in the fluorescence microscope (cf. figure 3.6h).

Plaque techniques

Antibody secreting cells can be counted by diluting them in an environment in which the antibody formed by each individual cell produces a readily observable effect. In one of the most widely used techniques, developed from the original method of Jerne and Nordin, the cells from an animal immunized with sheep erythrocytes are suspended together with an excess of sheep red cells within a shallow chamber formed between two microscope slides. On incubation the antibody-forming cells release their immunoglobulin which coats the surrounding erythrocytes. Addition of complement (cf. p. 134) will then cause lysis of the coated cells and a plaque clear of red cells will be seen around each antibody-forming cell (figure 4.1). Direct plaques obtained in this way largely reveal IgM producers since this antibody has a high haemolytic efficiency. To demonstrate IgG synthesizing cells it is necessary to increase the complement binding of the erythrocyte-IgG antibody complex by first adding a rabbit anti-IgG serum; this develops the 'indirect plaques' and can be used to enumerate cells making antibodies in different immunoglobulin subclasses, provided the appropriate rabbit antisera are available. The method can be extended by coating an antigen such as pneumococcus polysaccharide onto the red cell, or by coupling hapten groups to the erythrocyte surface.

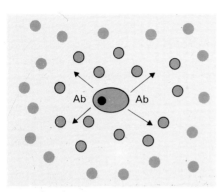

Secreted antibody coats surrounding
red cells

(a)

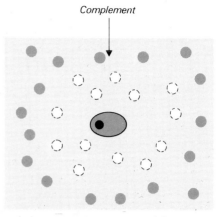

Coated erythrocytes lysed on
adding complement to form plaque
with antibody-forming cell at centre

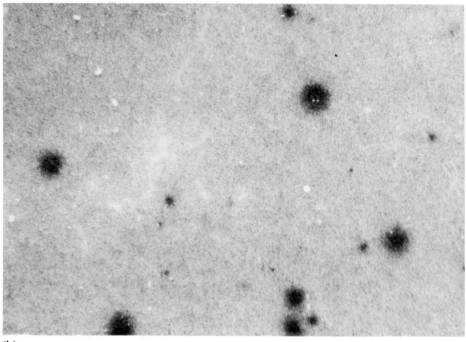

(b)

FIGURE 4.1. Jerne plaque techniques for enumerating antibody-forming cells
(Cunningham modification). (a) The direct technique for cells synthesizing
IgM haemolysin is shown. The indirect technique for visualizing cells
producing IgG haemolysins requires the addition of anti-IgG plus
complement in the final stage. The difference between the plaques obtained
by direct and indirect methods gives the number of 'IgG' plaques.
(b) Photograph of plaques which show as circular dark areas under dark-
ground illumination (courtesy of Mr C. Shapland, Ms P. Hutchings & Dr D.
Male).

In the normal antibody-forming cell there is a rapid turnover of light chains which are present in slight excess. Defective control occurs in many myeloma cells and one may see excessive production of light chains or complete suppression of heavy chain synthesis. Interchain disulphide bridges may form while the heavy chains are still attached to the ribosomes (figure 4.2) but the sequence in which the intermediates arise varies with the nature of the immunoglobulin. Using 'pulse and chase' techniques with radioactive amino acids it was found that the build-up of both light and heavy chains proceeds continuously starting from the N-terminal end. Furthermore, isolation of the mRNA for each type of chain has shown them to be of appropriate size to allow synthesis of the complete peptides. The evidence is, therefore, against the view that either chain can be formed by joining together two preformed lengths of peptide and it is now thought that the messenger regions for variable and constant regions are spliced together before leaving the nucleus.

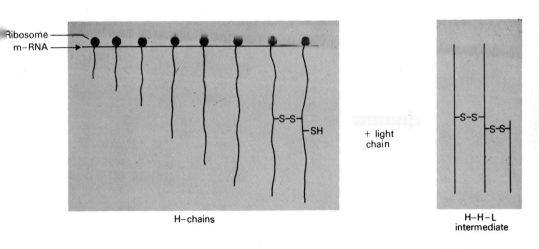

FIGURE 4.2. Synthesis of mouse IgG2a immunoglobulin. As the H-chains near completion, adjacent peptide chains can spontaneously cross-link through their constant regions. It is thought that the light chains may aid release of the terminal chains from the ribosome by forming the L–H–H molecule. Combination with a further light chain would yield the full immunoglobulin L–H–H–L. The order in which the interchain disulphide bridges are formed varies in different immunoglobulins depending on the relative strengths of the bonds as assessed by susceptibility to reduction. (Based on Askonas B.A. & Williamson A.R., (1968) *Biochem. J.* **109**, 637.)

In chapter 2 we discussed the production of unique monoclonal immunoglobulins in multiple myeloma where there is an uncontrolled proliferation of a single clone of Ig-producing plasma cells. IgG, IgA, IgD and IgE myeloma has been reported in frequencies which parallel their serum concentration; Waldenström's macroglobulinaemia represents a closely comparable situation involving monoclonal IgM production. The myeloma or 'M' component in serum is recognized as a tight band on paper electrophoresis (all molecules in the clone are of course identical and have the same mobility) and as an abnormal arc on immunoelectrophoresis with a 'bump' caused by the monoclonal protein (figure 4.3a and b). 'M' bands have been found in the sera of a number of individuals who have no clinical signs of myeloma; the comparative rarity with which invasive multiple myeloma develops in these people and the constant level of the monoclonal protein over a period of years suggests the presence of benign tumours of the lymphocyte-plasma cell series.

Amyloide. Between 10 and 20% of patients with myeloma develop widespread amyloid deposits which contain the variable region of the myeloma light chain. Being identical, the variable region fragments polymerise and form the

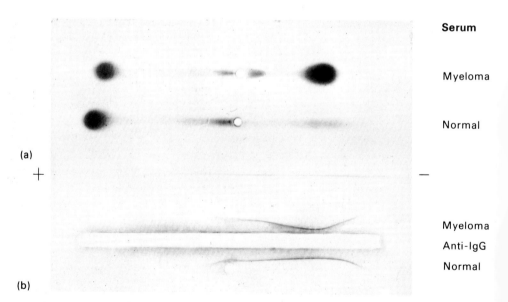

Serum

Myeloma

Normal

(a)

+   —

Myeloma

Anti-IgG

Normal

(b)

FIGURE 4.3. Myeloma serum with an 'M' component. (a) Agar gel electrophoresis showing the strong band in the γ-globulin region. (b) Immunoelectrophoresis against anti-IgG serum revealing the 'bump' or 'bow' in the precipitin arc. (Courtesy of Dr F.C. Hay.)

characteristic amyloid fibrils which are recognizable by their green bire-fringence on staining with Congo Red. Other components in amyloid have not yet been characterized. The fibrils are relatively resistant to digestion and accumulate in the ground substance of connective tissue where they can lead to pathological changes in the kidneys, heart and brain. Amyloid can also be formed secondarily to chronic inflammatory conditions such as rheumatoid arthritis and familial Mediterranean fever but in this case involves the polymerization of a unique substance, Amyloid A (AA) protein derived from the N-terminal part of a serum precursor (SAA) of molecular weight 90,000. SAA behaves as an acute phase protein in that its concentration increases rapidly in response to tissue injury or inflammation. Levels rise with age and the minority of individuals with high values are the most likely to develop amyloid.

MONOCLONAL ANTIBODIES

A fantastic technological revolution has been achieved by Milstein and Köhler who devised a technique for the production of 'immortal' clones of cells making single antibody specificities by fusing normal antibody-forming cells with an appropriate B-cell tumour line. These so-called 'hybridomas' are selected out in a tissue culture medium which fails to support growth of the parental cell types, and by successive dilutions or by plating out, single clones can be established. These clones can be propagated in spinner culture or grown up in the ascitic form in mice when quite prodigious titres of monoclonal antibody can be attained. Remember that even in a good antiserum over 90% of the Ig molecules have little or no avidity for the antigen, and the 'specific antibodies' themselves represent a whole spectrum of molecules with different avidities directed against different determinants on the antigen. What a contrast is provided by the monoclonal antibodies where all the molecules produced by a given hybridoma are identical: they have the same Ig glass and allotype, the same variable regions, structures, idiotypes, affinities and specificities. Furthermore, they have the advantage that theoretically all laboratories throughout the world can use the same reagent since the cell line should be immortal (please God or whoever). Their potential defies the imagination; the separation of individual cell types with specific surface markers (lymphocyte sub-populations, neural cells, etc.), diagnosis of lymphoid and myeloid malignancies, tissue typing, radioimmunossay, sero-typing of micro-organisms, the fine structure of the antibody combining site and the basis for variability, immunological intervention with passive antibody, anti-idiotype inhibition or 'magic bullet' therapy with cytotoxic agents coupled to anti-tumour specific antibody—these and many other areas will all be transformed by hybridoma technology.

Activated T-cells have been fused with T-lymphoma lines to generate hybridomas producing individual suppressor factors for example and the technique is clearly not just confined to cells of immunological importance. Further excitement stems from the description of human cell hybridomas, an advance on the previously available technology in which antigen-enriched lymphocytes are transformed to cell-lines by polyclonal stimulation with EB virus.

IMMUNOGLOBULIN CLASSES

The synthesis of antibodies belonging to the various immunoglobulin classes proceeds at different rates. Usually there is an early IgM response which tends to fall off rapidly. IgG antibody synthesis builds up to its maximum over a longer time period. On secondary challenge with antigen, the time course of the IgM response resembles that seen in the primary though the peak may be higher. By contrast the synthesis of IgG antibodies rapidly accelerates to a much higher titre and there is a relatively slow fall-off in serum antibody levels (figure 4.4). The same probably holds for IgA and in a sense both these immunoglobulin classes provide the main *immediate* defence against future penetration by foreign antigens.

There is evidence that individual cells can switch over from IgM to IgG production. Several days after immunization with salmonella flagella, isolated cells taken into microdrop cultures were shown to produce IgM and IgG immobilizing antibodies. In another study it was shown that antigen challenge of irradiated recipients receiving relatively small numbers of lymphoid cells, produced splenic foci of cells each synthesizing antibodies of different heavy chain class bearing a single idiotype; the common idiotype suggests that each focus is derived from a single precursor cell whose progeny can form antibodies of different class.

Antibody synthesis in certain classes shows considerable dependence upon T-co-operation in that the responses in T-deprived animals are strikingly deficient; such is true of mouse IgG1, IgE and part of the IgM antibody responses and of IgM memory. Immunopotentiation by complete Freund's adjuvant, a water-in-oil emulsion containing antigen in the aqueous phase and a suspension of killed tubercle bacilli in the oily phase (p. 170), seems to occur, at least in part, through the activation of helper T-cells which stimulate antibody production in T-dependent classes. The prediction from this that the response to T-independent antigens (e.g.

84

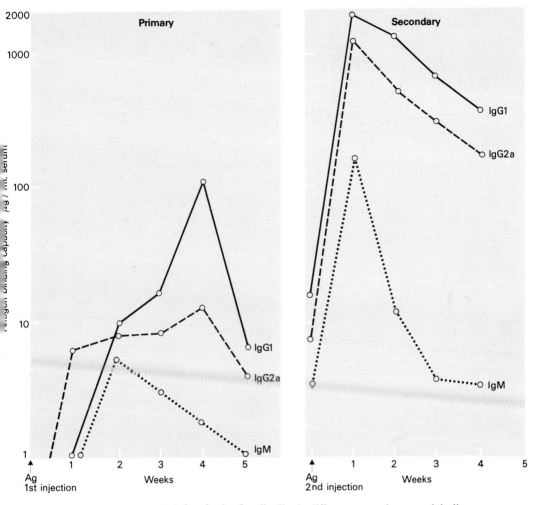

FIGURE 4.4. Synthesis of antibodies in different mouse immunoglobulin classes during the primary and secondary responses to bovine serum albumin. Using more sensitive methods such as agglutination or plaquing, IgM is found to be the first antibody class to be stimulated in the primary response. (Data kindly provided by Dr G. Torrigiani.)

pneumococcus polysaccharide) should not be potentiated by Freund's adjuvant is borne out in practice; furthermore, as would be expected, these antigens evoke primarily IgM antibodies and poorly defined immunological memory as do T-dependent antigens injected into thymectomized hosts. Thus in rodents at least the switch from IgM to IgG appears to be under some degree of thymus or T-cell control. Another class-specific effect which must be mentioned is the tremendous enhancement of IgE responses by helminths and even by soluble extracts derived from them.

Genetic control of the antibody response

GENES AFFECTING GENERAL RESPONSIVENESS

Mice can be selectively bred for high or low antibody responses through several generations to yield two lines, one of which consistently produces high titre antibodies to a variety of antigens and the other, antibodies of relatively low titre (Biozzi & colleagues). Out of the order of ten or so different genetic loci which are involved, one or more affect macrophage behaviour. The two lines are comparable in their ability to clear carbon particles or sheep erythrocytes from the blood by phagocytosis, but macrophages from the high responders retain a far higher proportion of added antigen in an undegraded (and presumably) immunogenic form on their surface (cf. p. 64). On the other hand, the low responders survive infection by *Salmonella typhimurium* better and their macrophages support much slower replication of listeria (cf. p. 158) suggesting a dichotomy in the ability of macrophages to subserve humoral as compared with cell-mediated immunity.

IMMUNE RESPONSE LINKED TO IMMUNOGLOBULIN GENES

In a number of cases where an antigen induces virtually a monoclonal response (e.g. type C streptococcal carbohydrate in rabbits), breeding experiments have shown that the capacity to produce this clone and its idiotype is inherited and is linked to the genetic markers for the immunoglobulin constant region, i.e. there is a gene coding for the variable region of the antibody and it occurs on the chromosome carrying the genes for the constant region. These findings would lead one to suppose that in general we inherit genes which enable us to make particular antibodies and that the capacity to produce an antibody response is limited by the repertoire of specificities encoded by the genes on this chromosome.

IMMUNE RESPONSE LINKED TO THE MAJOR
HISTOCOMPATIBILITY COMPLEX

One genetic region in higher vertebrates termed the major histocompatibility complex (MHC) exerts a predominant influence on the survival of grafts within each species by controlling the synthesis of antigens which provoke intense immunological rejection (see p. 218). The MHC antigens are highly polymorphic (literally 'many shapes') due to the existence of several *alternative* genes (alleles) at each locus, each coding for a different antigen. It has been found that the antibody responses to a number of thymus-dependent antigenically simple substances are determined by genes—the so-called immune response or Ir genes—which are linked chromosomally to the MHC. Thus in mice, where the MHC is referred to as the H-2 region, all strains belonging to the H-2^b group respond well to the the synthetic branched polypeptide antigen (T,G)-A--L (a polylysine backbone with side chains of polyalanine randomly tipped with mixed tyrosine and glutamyl residues), whereas mice of H-2^k specificity which bear a different set of allelic genes in the H-2 region, respond poorly. We say that mice of the H-2^b haplotype (i.e. a particular set of H-2 genes) are high responders to (T,G)-A--L because they possess the appropriate Ir gene. With another synthetic antigen, (H,G)-A--L, having histidine in place of tyrosine, the position is reversed, the 'poor (T,G)-A--L responders' now giving a good antibody response and the 'good (T,G)-A--L responders' a weak one showing that the capacity of a particular strain to give a high or low response varies with the individual antigen (table 4.1). Thus H-2 linked immune responses have been observed not only with relatively simple polypeptides, but also with transplantation antigens from another strain and autoantigens where merely one or two determinants are recognized as foreign by the host.

TABLE 4.1. H-2 linked immune responses to synthetic polypeptide antigens

	Antibody response	
Antigen	H-2^b	H-2^k
(T,G)-A--L	High	Low
(H,G)-A--L	Low	High

See text for definition of terms used.
(After McDevitt H.O. & Sela M.
(1965) *J.Exp.Med.*, **122**, 517.)

H-2I gene control of T–B co-operation

The I region containing the Ir genes has been localized within the H-2 complex close to the H-2K end (figure 4.5). Antisera raised between strains have identified several Ia antigens (i.e. antigens encoded by I region genes) which broadly correspond with five genetic subregions, I-A, I-B, I-J, I-E and I-C; each subregion is multi-allelic and gives rise to a number of different gene products certain of which may endow their host with high responder and others with low responder status to restricted determinants.

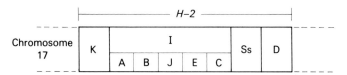

FIGURE 4.5. The major histocompatibility complex in the mouse (H-2). The subregions of I are designated I-A, I-B, etc.

The Ir genes do not appear to affect B-cell triggering by T-independent antigens but rather control the co-operative response to T-dependent antigens. Ia determinants are largely expressed on the surface of B-cells and macrophages, particularly the dendritic variety. Antigens 'processed' by macrophages are presented to T-cells in some form of association with the surface Ia. Helper T-lymphocytes recognize this antigen-Ia complex in much the same way that cytotoxic T-cells have to recognize antigen on the target cell associated with other MHC products, H-2D and H-2K (cf figure 9.12, p 234). The primed helper cells could then be triggered by an Ia-bearing B-cell which had bound the antigen to its surface Ig receptors since it would recognize the same antigen-Ia combination it first saw on the macrophage. The activated T-helper would then presumably deliver the 'second signal' (p. 62) required for B-cell induction (figure 4.6). If the Ia

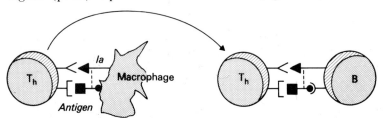

(a) Induction of helper T-cells　　　　(b) Effector phase of T co-operation

FIGURE 4.6. H-2 linked immune response gene product (Ia) and T-B co-operation. Experimentally it can be shown that T-helper cells are most effective when the B-cells bear the same Ia specificity as the macrophages used for priming T-cells. (a) The T-helpers are stimulated by antigen presented by the macrophage in some form of association (-----) with Ia; (b) they can then co-operate with B-cells displaying the same Ia-antigen complex (although in this case the antigen is bound by surface Ig receptors). Other studies indicating the presence of I-A specificities on soluble 'helper' factors suggest the existence of further mechanisms of Ir gene involvement.

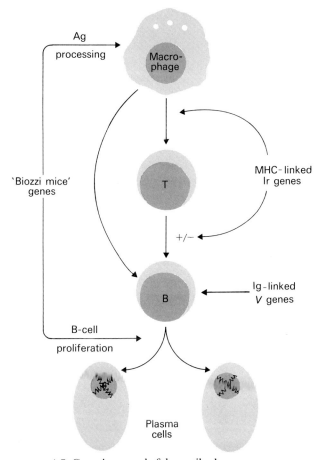

FIGURE 4.7. Genetic control of the antibody response.

product is unable to present antigen effectively or if the T-cells cannot recognize the Ia-antigen complex, the animal will be a poor responder; it is difficult to distinguish these two possibilities.

Other circumstances may also lead to poor antibody responses associated with the MHC. In some instances, low responders carry an I-J gene concerned in the synthesis of dominant amounts of a T-suppressor factor (see below) which acts to limit T-cell co-operation.

Factors influencing the genetic control of the antibody response are summarized diagrammatically in figure 4.7.

Regulation of the immune response

In addition to the genetic factors influencing the immune response discussed above, feedback mechanisms must operate to limit antibody production otherwise after antigenic stimulation we would become overwhelmed by the responding clones of antibody forming cells and their products, a clearly unwelcome state of affairs as may be clearly seen in multiple myeloma where control over lymphocyte proliferation is lost. Since antigen is needed to drive the division and differentiation of lymphocytes, the concentration of antigen must be a major regulating factor. As antigen is catabolized by body enzymes and neutralized or blocked by antibody so will its concentration fall and its ability to sustain the immune response be progressively weakened. The role of antibody in diverting antigen to immunogenically inoffensive sites in the body to prevent primary sensitization is clearly evident from the protection against rhesus immunization afforded by administration of anti-D to mothers at risk (p. 196) and the inhibitory effect of maternal antibody on the peak titres obtained on vaccinating infants. Removal of circulating antibody by plasmapheresis during an ongoing response leads to an increase in synthesis, wheras injection of preformed IgG antibody markedly hastens the fall in the number of antibody-forming cells suggesting that such antibodies must exert an important feedback control on overall synthesis. It is unlikely that this is achieved by simple neutralization of antigen since whole IgG is overwhelmingly more effective than its $F(ab')_2$ fragment in switching off the reaction; perhaps an ability to bind simultaneously to macrophage Fc receptors enables the IgG to combine with immunogenic surface antigen more persistently and so block interaction with lymphocyte receptors.

SUPPRESSOR T-CELLS

T-cells provide a distinct regulatory system. Not only can they amplify the B-cell response through their helper activity, but there is now a body of evidence showing there to be a separate T-cell population with a *suppressor* function. If mice are made unresponsive by injection of a high dose of sheep red cells, their T-cells will suppress specific antibody formation in normal recipients to which they have been transferred (Gershon's 'infectious tolerance'; figure 4.8).

Helper and suppressor T-cells in the mouse have been distinguished in several ways. Suppressors are more vulnerable to adult thymectomy, X-irradiation and cyclophosphamide, and bind to sepharose-linked histamine-albumin conjugates, supposedly through surface histamine receptors. Unlike T-

90

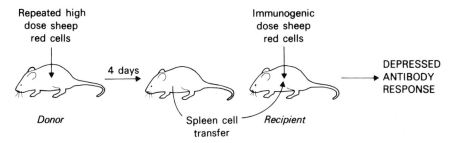

Repeated high
dose sheep
red cells

Immunogenic
dose sheep
red cells

4 days

DEPRESSED
ANTIBODY
RESPONSE

Donor

Spleen cell
transfer

Recipient

FIGURE 4.8. Demonstration of T-suppressor cells. Spleen cells from a donor injected with a high dose of antigen, depress the antibody response of a syngeneic animal to which they have been transferred. The effect is lost if the spleen cells are first treated with anti-Thy1 serum plus complement showing that the suppressors are T-cells. (After Gershon R.K. & Kondo K. (1971) *Immunology*, **21,** 903: in these studies mice were thymectomized, irradiated and reconstituted with bone marrow and thymocytes.)

helpers, they can be depleted by passage down immunosorbent columns containing the specific antigen and whereas helpers have the surface phenotype Ly1, suppressors are Ly2 and bear I-J determinants. In general terms the helper may be looked upon as inducers of the effector cells for humoral and cell-mediated immunity and it now appears that they are also

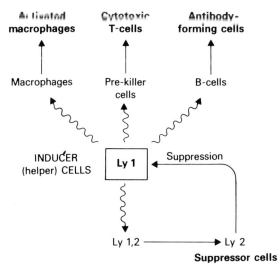

Activated
macrophages

Cytotoxic
T-cells

Antibody-
forming cells

Macrophages

Pre-killer
cells

B-cells

INDUCER
(helper) CELLS

Ly 1

Suppression

Ly 1,2

Ly 2

Suppressor cells

FIGURE 4.9. Immunoregulatory feedback circuit showing the central position of Ly1 cells in the induction (⟶) of T-dependent responses and in the generation of T-suppressors which in turn inhibit the Ly1 cells. A proportion of Ly1 cells express the Qa-1 antigen encoded by genes which map between the H-2D and TL loci (cf. figure 9.4). Both Ly1:Qa-1$^+$ and Ly1:Qa-1$^-$ are involved in optimal collaboration with B-cells but only the former are able to generate suppressors; thus the balance between the Qa-1$^+$ and Qa-1$^-$ subsets may strongly influence the outcome of a given immune response. (After Cantor & Gershon 1979.)

91

responsible for the generation of T-suppressors which exert negative feedback control on the helper cells (figure 4.9). There is evidence that this suppression is mediated by antigen. However, interaction can also occur through recognition of an idiotype on the T-helper receptors by an anti-idiotype on the suppressors ad this will be discussed further in the next section.

Non-antigen specific T-suppression can also occur. Mouse T-lymphocytes when stimulated by the polyclonal activator concanavalin A (cf. p. 207) in culture are able to inhibit a variety of antibody responses. In the human, T-cells with receptors for $Fc\gamma$ (IgG Fc) suppress the help given by T-cells with $Fc\mu$ receptors for the polyclonal stimulation of B-cells by pokeweed nitrogen (cf. p. 207) and these findings may have relevance for the immunosuppressive action of IgG antibody described above and the stimulatory effect of IgM reported by Henry & Jerne.

IDIOTYPIC NETWORKS

The hypervariable loops on the immunoglobulin molecule which go to form the antigen combining site have individual characteristic shapes which can be recognized by the appropriate antibodies as idiotypic determinants (cf. p. 13). There are hundreds of thousands, if not more, different idiotypes in one individual, virtually all of them present in very low concentrations at birth and therefore unlikely to produce self-tolerance.

Jerne reasoned that the great diversity of idiotypes would to a considerable extent mirror the diversity of antigenic shapes in the external world. Thus if lymphocytes can recognize a whole range of foreign antigenic determinants, they should be able to recognize the idiotypes on other lymphocytes. They would therefore form a large network or series of networks depending upon idiotype–anti-idiotype recognition between lymphocytes of the various T- and B-subsets (figure 4.10) and the response to an external antigen perturbing this network would be conditioned by the state of the idiotypic interactions.

There is no doubt that the elements to form an idiotypic network are all there. A whole variety of auto-anti-idiotypes have been generated experimentally and they have been identified during the course of antigen-induced responses. Anti-idiotypic specificities have been associated with both T-helpers and suppressors and Eichman has shown that quite small amounts of anti-idiotypic antibodies can stimulate or inhibit an idiotype response depending on the Ig class of the anti-idiotype.

92

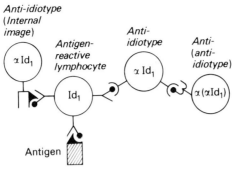

Anti-idiotype
(*Internal image*)

Antigen-reactive lymphocyte

Anti-idiotype

Anti-(anti-idiotype)

αId_1

Id_1

αId_1

$\alpha(\alpha Id_1)$

Antigen

FIGURE 4.10. Elements in an idiotypic network. T-helper, T-suppressor and B-lymphocytes recognize each other through idiotype–anti-idiotype reactions; either stimulation or suppression may result. One of the anti-idiotype sets may bear an idiotype of similar shape to (i.e. provides an *internal image* of) the antigen. The same idiotype (●) may be shared by two receptors of different specificity (since the several hypervariable regions provide a number of potential idiotypic determinants and a given idiotype does not always form part of the epitope binding site), so that the anti-(anti-Id_1) does not necessarily bind the original antigen.

Although outbred rabbits rarely produce the same idiotype (Id_1) in the response to a given antigen, they can be made to do so by preimmunization with anti-idiotype (αId_1) (see figure 4.10), the anti (αId_1) suppresses the αId_1 clone and so allows the Id_1 clone to emerge in response to antigenic stimulation.

It is difficult to assess the extent to which idiotype networks control the immunological system. Is there a complete dynamic network in which messages are constantly passing between all cells including those in a 'resting phase', or are interactions limited largely to the immediate anti-idiotype partners, and then only during clonal expansion of cells bearing the antigen-reactive idiotype? What is the relative importance of antigen and anti-idiotype in regulation of the immune response? Since the body cannot help making anti-idiotypic responses there is bound to be some contribution from the network. However, the dominant effect of one lysozyme determinant in supprressing the response to all other epitopes and the inhibitory effect of a monoclonal antigen-specific suppressor factor on T-help provided by the whole carrier molecule speaks for a major regulatory role of antigen because lymphocytes reacting with *different* determinants on the same molecule can be linked through the antigen itself but not through an idiotype network. It is worth noting that anti-Id may enable immune responses to 'tick over' for extended periods after the complete elimination of antigen. The network provides interesting opportunities for immunological intervention: to give one example, Binz &

93

Wigzell have conditioned rats to accept a skin graft by auto-immunization with the idiotype of the Ig *V* region receptor for the transplantation antigen concerned. It might even be feasible to immunize people against certain infections with a monoclonal anti-idiotype should this prove easier to obtain in bulk than the microbial antigen itself and if successful, the strategy could be extended to tumour-associated antigens.

At this stage, if the reader is feeling a little groggy, try a glance at figure 4.11 which attempts a summary of the main factors currently thought to modulate the immune response.

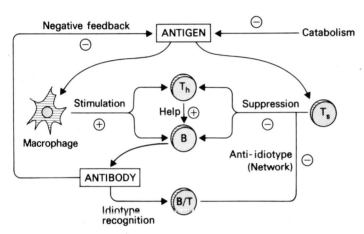

FIGURE 4.11. Regulation of the immune response. T_h, T-helper cell; T_s, T-suppressor cell. T-help for cell-mediated immunity will be subject to similar regulation. Some of these mechanisms may be interdependent; for example one could envisage anti-idiotypic antibody acting in concert with a suppressor T-cell by binding to its Fc receptor, or suppressor T-cells with specificity for the idiotype on T_h or B-cells.

Immunological tolerance

AT BIRTH

Over 20 years ago Owen made the intriguing observation that non-identical (dizygotic) twin cattle, which shared the same placental circulation and whose circulations were thereby linked, grew up with appreciable numbers of red cells from the other twin in their blood; if they had not shared the same circulation at birth, red cells from the twin injected in adult life would be rapidly eliminated by an immunological response. From this finding Burnet & Fenner conceived the notion that potential antigens which reach the lymphoid cells during their developing immunologically immature phase in the perinatal

94

period can in some way specifically suppress any future response to that antigen when the animal reaches immunological maturity. This, they considered, would provide a means whereby unresponsiveness to the body's own constituents ('self') could be established and thereby enable the lymphoid cells to make the important distinction between 'self' and 'non-self'. On this basis, any foreign cells introduced into the body around the perinatal period should trick the animal into treating them as 'self' components in later life and the studies of Medawar and his colleagues have shown that *immunological tolerance* or unresponsiveness can be artificially induced in this way. Thus neonatal injection of CBA mouse cells into newborn A strain animals suppresses their ability to immunologically reject a CBA graft in adult life (figures 4.12 and 4.13). Tolerance can also be induced with soluble antigens; for example, rabbits injected with bovine serum albumin at birth fail to make antibodies on later challenge with this protein.

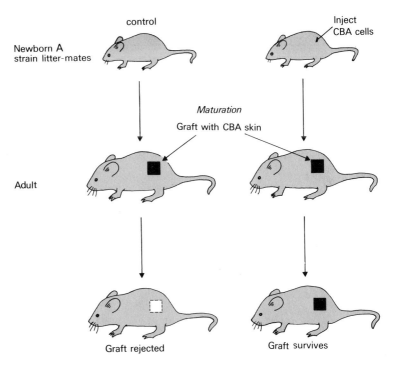

FIGURE 4.12. Induction of tolerance to foreign CBA skin graft in A strain mice by neonatal injection of antigen. (After Billingham R., Brent L. & Medawar P.B.)

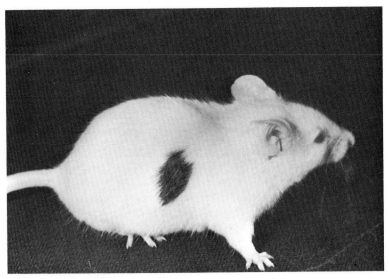

FIGURE 4.13. CBA skin graft on a fully tolerant A strain mouse showing healthy hair growth 8 weeks after grafting (courtesy of Professor L. Brent).

IN THE ADULT

It is now recognized that tolerance can be induced in the adult as well as the neonate, although in general much higher doses of antigen are required. Surprisingly, repeated injection of *low* doses of certain antigens such as bovine serum albumin (BSA) which are weakly immunogenic, established a state of tolerance as revealed by a poor antibody response on challenge with BSA in a strongly antigenic form (in complete Freund's adjuvant— see p. 170). It was shown subsequently that this 'low zone tolerance' could also be achieved with more powerful antigens provided an immunosuppressive drug such as cyclophos· phamide were given to inhibit antibody synthesis during the low dose treatment.

Thus, there is a 'low zone' and a 'high zone' in terms of antigen predosage for tolerance induction. Elegant studies by Weigle and co-workers have pinpointed the T-cell as the target for tolerance at low antigen levels while both B- and T-lymphocytes are made unresponsive at high antigen dose (table 4.2). Thus, for 'thymus-dependent' antigens at dose levels where the T-cells play a major co-operative role in antibody formation, the overall immunological performance of the animal will reflect the degree of reactivity of the T-cell population. In other words, the T-cells guide the reaction and when they are tolerant the B-cells will not respond.

Protein antigens are more tolerogenic (able to induce

TABLE 4.2. Effect of antigen dose on tolerance induction in T- and B-cells

Tolerogen administered (mg)	% tolerance induced		
	T-cells	B-cells	Donor spleen
0.1	96	9	62
0.5	99	56	97
2.5	99	70	99

After induction of tolerance to aggregate-free human IgG in mice, the reactivity of thymocytes and bone marrow cells (containing B-cells) was assessed by transfer to irradiated recipients with either bone marrow or thymus respectively from normal donors. The degree of tolerance induced in the donor is shown in the final column. Low antigen doses tolerize the T-cells. B-cells become unresponsive at higher doses. The T-cell activity largely dictates the response of the spleen as a whole. (From Chiller J.M., Habicht G.S. & Weigle W.O. (1971) *Science*, **171**, 813.)

tolerance) when in a soluble rather than an aggregated or particular form which can be readily taken up by macrophages and it seems that molecules are more likely to be tolerogenic if they escape processing by macrophages before presentation to the lymphocyte. Persistence of antigen is required to maintain tolerance. In Medawar's experiments the tolerant state was long-lived because the injected CBA cells survived and the animals continued to be chimaeric (i.e. they possessed both A and CBA cells). With non-living antigens such as BSA, tolerance is gradually lost, the most likely explanation being that in the absence of antigen, newly recruited immunocompetent cells which are being generated throughout life, are not being rendered tolerant. Since recruitment of newly competent T-lymphocytes is drastically curtailed by removal of the thymus, it is of interest to note that the tolerant state persists for much longer in thymectomized animals.

MECHANISMS

Genetic unresponsiveness. If an animal lacks the genetic programmes which enable it to recognize certain self-determinants it will be 'immunologically silent'. This would be the case if there are no genes coding for the appropriate lymphocyte receptors; analysis of the experimentally induced autoantibody response to cytochrome c suggests that only those parts of the molecule which show species variation are autoantigenic whereas the highly conserved regions do appear to be silent. It is conceivable that unresponsiveness might arise from an inability to present certain self-components on the surface of a macrophage in an immunogenic form in association with Ia.

Clonal deletion. The exceptional vulnerability of the neonate to tolerance induction has led to the suggestion that during lymphocyte development, the cell goes through a phase in which contact with antigen leads to death or permanent inactivation.

T-suppression. Low zone tolerance to protein antigens has been shown in at least one case to be mediated by T-suppressors directed against T-helpers and a suppressor mechanism will probably prove to be the most common basis for this phenomenon. The inferior immunogenicity of soluble as distinct from aggregated or particulate antigen, may be ascribed to weak stimulation of T-helpers through poor macrophage processing in contrast to effective activation of suppressor cells which do not require macrophage presentation. T-suppression has been recognized to be a major factor in transplantation tolerance in *adults* induced by a cocktail of donor antigen, pertussis vaccine and antilymphocyte serum.

Helplessness. T-cells are more readily tolerized than B-cells and, as a result, a number of self-reacting B-cells are present in the body which cannot be triggered by T-dependent self-components since the T-cells required to provide the necessary T-B help are already tolerant—you might describe the B-cells as helpless. If we think of the determinant on a self-component which combines with the receptors on a self-reacting B-cell as a hapten and another determinant which has to be recognized by a T-cell as a carrier (cf. figure 3.11), then tolerance in the T-cell to the carrier will prevent the provision of T-cell help and the B-cell will be unresponsive.

It is likely that self-tolerance involves all these mechanisms to

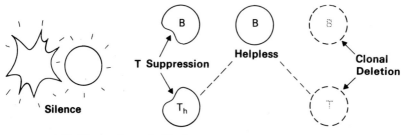

FIGURE 4.14. Mechanisms of self-tolerance.

varying degrees and that while clonal deletion is of prime importance early in life, T-suppression becomes a dominant factor later (figure 4.14). It should be stressed that these terms early and late apply to the life of the lymphocyte not of the host. If an adult is irradiated and reconstituted with immature lymphocytes in the form of bone marrow cells, the animal behaves as a neonate with respect to the ease of tolerance induction with low doses of antigen.

Ontogeny of the immune response

Haemopoiesis originates in the early yolk sac but as embryogenesis proceeds, this function is taken over by the fetal liver and finally by the bone marrow where it continues throughout life. The haemopoietic stem cell which gives rise to the formed elements of the blood and the cells of the lymphoreticular system (figure 4.15) can be shown to be multipotent, to seed other organs and to renew itself through the creation of further stem cells.

Stem cells attracted to the thymus by a chemotactic factor, differentiate within the microenvironment of the epithelioid cells where they proliferate extensively and acquire characteristic early T-cell markers (figure 4.16). Under the influence of the epithelioid cells, and in some cases also the dendritic reticular cells of the medulla, the thymocytes differentiate further to form distinct functional subpopulations with the competence to respond in the mixed lymphocyte reaction (p. 220), mediate allograft cytotoxicity (p. 67), generate carrier-specific help for B-cells and produce lymphokines for cell-mediated immunity ('delayed-type hypersensitivity' cells); cortisone-sensitive cells with potential suppressor function appear in the cortex. The ability to recognize self-MHC specificities which provide the basis for haplotype restricted T-cell responses to antigen (p. 235) is also acquired at this stage. Some cells move directly from the cortex into the periphery and others (future helper and delayed-type hypersensitivity cells which must learn to react with macrophages?) migrate to the medulla, a proportion staying there for a curiously long time.

Earlier experiments on the partial restitution of immunocompetence in thymectomized females through pregnancy were taken to imply that a soluble thymic product (derived from the fetal thymuses) was responsible, at least in part, for the influence of the gland on T-cell maturation. Several different soluble thymic extracts have been prepared and active

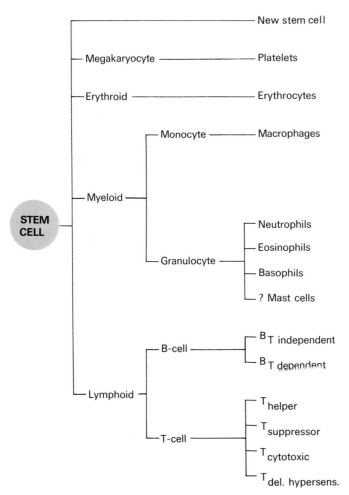

FIGURE 4.15. The multipotent haemopoietic stem cell. The classification of B- and T-cell subsets is still tentative as is the relationship between basophils and mast cells.

preparations isolated usually on the basis of their ability to promote the appearance of T-cell differentiation markers (Thy1 in the mouse, sheep cell receptors in the human) on culture with bone marrow cells *in vitro*. Of the four major candidates for the role of thymic hormone, 'thymosin', 'thymopoietin', 'thymic humoral factor' and 'facteur thymique serique' (FTS), only FTS (J.F.Bach) is a single molecular species. It is a nona-peptide of molecular weight 847 which can be detected in the cytoplasm of thymic epithelial cells by immuno-fluorescence and which binds to specific receptors on T-cells to cause an increase in cAMP formation. High doses are said to stimulate mature T-suppressor cells. Blood levels of FTS fall steadily with age as the thymus involutes (? and the cells wearily

100

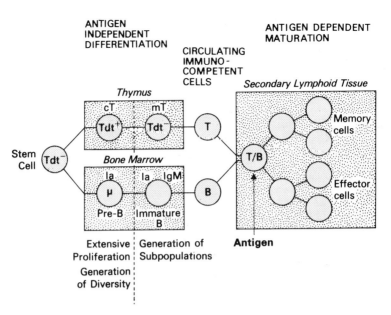

ANTIGEN
INDEPENDENT
DIFFERENTIATION

CIRCULATING
IMMUNO-
COMPETENT
CELLS

ANTIGEN DEPENDENT
MATURATION

Secondary Lymphoid Tissue

Thymus

Stem Cell

Bone Marrow

Extensive Proliferation | Generation of Subpopulations

Generation of Diversity

Antigen

FIGURE 4.16. Differentiation and maturation of human B- and T-cells. Tdt, terminal deoxynucleotidyl transferase; cT, cortical T-cell surface antigen; mT, mature T-cell surface antigen. The early replicating cells in the thymus and bone marrow are in the majority. Thymocytes are educated to recognize self-MHC haplotype (cf. p. 234). Tolerance to self-antigens is induced in the immature B- and T-cells within the primary lymphoid organs. Ia$^+$, μ^- pre-B cells precursors are Tdt$^+$; the Tdt enzyme may be involved as one of the mechanisms controlling the generation of diversity. In the mouse, the earliest thymocytes acquire surface Thy1; this then increases in surface density and is accompanied by the TL antigen (p. 219); cells ready to leave the thymus have lost TL and have a reduced Thy1.

approach their Hayflick number), and precipitously in certain autoimmune disorders (SLE and NZB mice—chapter 10) at a time corresponding roughly with the onset of disease.

The microenvironment for the differentiation of B-cells is provided by the Bursa of Fabricius in the chicken and the bone marrow itself in mammalian species (a nameless immunologist regularly slays his students by recalling that 'the bursa is strictly for the birds'). The early, rapidly dividing pre-B cells display cytoplasmic μ chains but no light chains (figure 4.16). It is likely that the genetic mechanisms responsible for the generation of receptor diversity (in T-cells as well) operate at this stage. In the immature B-cell, the receptor for which the cell is finally programmed is inserted into the plasma membrane as a specific IgM molecule. As immune competence emerges, the ability to mount an antibody response to each of a defined series of antigens appears sequentially and in the same order in different members of the same species, suggesting that

101

the individual genes in the antibody V gene repertoire are recruited for receptor synthesis in a predetermined fashion.

At the next stage of differentiation, the cell develops a commitment to producing a particular antibody class and either bears surface IgM alone or in combination with IgA or IgG. The further addition of surface IgD now marks the readiness of the virgin B-cell for priming by antigen. Some cells, therefore, bear surface Ig of three different classes, M, G and D or M, A and D, but all Ig molecules on a single cell have the same idiotype and therefore are derived from the same V_H and V_L genes. IgD is lost on antigenic stimulation so that memory cells lack this Ig. At the terminal stages in the life of a fully mature plasma cell, virtually all surface Ig is shed. Injection of anti-μ (anti-IgM heavy chain) into chick embryos prevents the subsequent maturation of IgM and IgG antibody producing cells, whereas anti-γ inhibits only IgG development. Whether the switch from IgM production to other classes is partly antigen-driven (cf. p. 84) or occurs entirely as a result of microenvironmental factors is still unresolved. In the embryonic chicken bursa, a regular switch from IgM to IgG is observed and it seems possible that local influences in the gut will prove to be responsible for the predominant development of

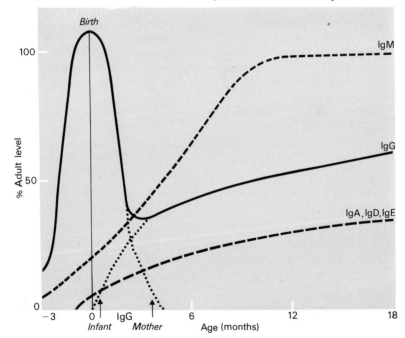

FIGURE 4.17. Development of serum immunoglobulin levels in the human. (After Hobbs J.R. (1969) In *Immunology and Development*, p. 118. Adinolfi M. (ed.). Heinemann, London).

IgA bearing cells. These cells are generated in Peyer's patches, pass into the blood via the thoracic duct and return to populate the diffuse lymphoid tissue in the lamina propria of the gut.

Lymph node and spleen remain relatively underdeveloped in the human even at birth except where there has been intra-uterine exposure to antigens as in congenital infections with rubella or other organisms. The ability to reject grafts and to mount an antibody response is reasonably well developed by birth but the immunoglobulin levels with one exception are low particularly in the absence of intra-uterine infection. The exception is IgG which is acquired by placental transfer from the mother, a process dependent upon Fc structures specific to this Ig class. This material is catabolized with a half-life of approximately 30 days and there is a fall in IgG concentration over the first three months accentuated by the increase in blood volume of the growing infant. Thereafter the rate of synthesis overtakes the rate of breakdown of maternal IgG and the overall concentration increases steadily. The other immunoglobulins do not cross the placenta and the low but significant levels of IgM in cord blood are synthesized by the baby (figure 4.17). IgM reaches adult levels by 9 months of age. Only trace levels of IgA, IgD and IgE are present in the circulation of the newborn.

Lymphoid malignancies

Lymphoid cells at almost any stage in their differentiation or maturation may become malignant and proliferate to form a clone of cells which are virtually 'frozen' in the developmental stage of the parent cell and bear the markers of the normal cell type from which they are derived. Thus, chronic lymphocytic leukaemia cells which originate from mature B-lymphocytes all stain for surface Ig and Ia and bear identical idiotypes in a given patient.

Summary

Antibody-forming cells can be recognized by immunofluorescence or plaque techniques. Ig peptide chains are synthesized as a single unit starting at the N-terminal end. In myeloma, the monoclonal protein shows as a sharp 'M' band on paper electrophoresis or a 'bump' on the precipitin arc in immunoelectrophoresis; in some cases heavy chains with a central deletion are excreted in the urine. Myeloma light chain dimers appear as Bence-Jones protein in the urine and the variable regions can polymerize to form amyloid deposits. Immortal cell lines making monoclonal antibodies provide powerful new immunological reagents. IgM antibody responses reach an early peak and decline; IgG levels are quantitatively much higher and more persistent. Some Ig classes are particularly thymus dependent. Freund's adjuvant which stimulates T-cell activity only improves the response to thymus-dependent antigens.

Approximately ten genes control the overall antibody response to complex antigens: some affect macrophage antigen handling and some the rate of proliferation of differentiating B-cells. Genes coding for antibodies of given specificities may be inherited together with (i.e. linked to) genetic markers for the heavy chain. Immune response genes linked to the major histocompatibility locus define products (with Ia specificities) on the T- and B-cells and macrophages which control the interactions required for T-B collaboration.

Regulation of the antibody response is strongly influenced by antigen concentration; since the response is antigen-driven, as effective antigen levels fall through catabolism and antibody feedback, the synthesis of antibody wanes. T-cells regulate B-lymphocyte responses not only through co-operative help but also by T-cell suppressor activity. Clonal proliferation is blocked by the development of an immune response to the antibody idiotype; an interlocking network based on recognition of idiotypes within the lymphocyte system provides a regulatory mechanism (Jerne).

Immunological tolerance can be induced by exposure to antigens in neonatal and (less readily) in adult life. T-cells are more readily tolerized than B-cells leaving T-dependent B-cells 'helpless'. Elimination of specific cells or generation of T-suppressors may occur.

Multipotent haemopoietic stem cells from the bone marrow differentiate within the thymus to become immuno-competent T-cells. In mammals the bone marrow itself provides the microenvironment for differentiation of B-cells. In man, maternal IgG is the only class to cross the placenta.

Lymphoid cells may become malignant and proliferate clonally, maintaining the developmental stage and specific markers of the parent cell.

Further reading

Beer A.E. & Billingham R.E. (1976) *The Immunobiology of Mammalian Reproduction*. Prentice-Hall, Hemel Hempstead.
Bevan M.J., Parkhouse R.M.R., Williamson A.R. & Askonas B.A. (1972) Biosynthesis of immunoglobulins. *Prog. Biophys. Mol.Biol.*, **25**, 131.

Cantor H. & Gershon R.K. (1979) Immunological circuits: cellular composition. *Fed. proc.*, **38**, 2058.

Cooper M. *et al.* (eds) (1979) *B Lymphocytes in the Immune Response.* Developments in Immunology, vol. 3. Elsevier/North-Holland, New York.

Dresser D.W. (ed.) (1976) Immunological tolerance. *Brit.med.Bull.*, **32**, No. 2.

Fougereau M. & Dausset J. (eds) (1980) *Progress in Immunology IV.* Academic Press, London.

Greaves M.J. & Janossy G. (1978) Patterns of gene expression and the cellular origins of human leukaemias. *Biochem. biophys. Acta*, **516**, 193.

Hildemann W.H. & Reddy A.L. (1973) Phylogeny of immune responsiveness: marine invertebrates. *Fed.Proc.*, **32**, 2188.

Jerne N.K. (1973) The immune system (Network theory). *Scient. Am.* 52.

Marchalonis J.J. (ed.) (1976) *Comparative Immunology.* Blackwell Scientific Publications, Oxford.

Melchers F. *et al.* (1978) *Lymphocyte hybridomas.* (Milstein's technique of fusion to establish monoclonal cell lines). *Current Topics in Microbiol. and Immunol.* **81**. Springer-Verlag, Berlin.

Milstein C. *et al.* (1979) Monoclonal antibodies and cell surface antigens. In *Human Genetics, Possibilities and Realities.* p. 251. Ciba Foundation Series 66. Excerpta Medica, New York.

Moller G. (ed.) (1978) Acquisition of the T cell repertoire. *Immunol.Rev.* **42**.

Moller G. (ed.) (1978) Role of macrophages in the immune response. *Immunol.Rev.* **40**.

Porter R. & Knight J. (eds) (1972) *Ontogeny of Acquired Immunity.* Ciba Foundation Symposium. Elsevier, Amsterdam.

Quesenberry P. & Levitt L. (1979) Haemopoietic stem cells. *N. Engl. J Med* **301**. 755, 819 & 868.

Taniguchi M., Takei I. & Tada T. (1980) Functional and molecular organization of an antigen-specific suppressor factor from a T-cell hybridoma. *Nature*, **283**, 227.

Uhr J.W. *et al.* (1979) Organization of the immune response genes. *Science*, **206**, 292.

Watson J., Trenkner E. & Cohn M. (1973) The use of bacterial lipopoly-saccharides to show that two signals are required for the induction of antibody synthesis. *J.exp.Med.*, **138**, 699. (Note that these authors do not consider cross-linking of receptors to be a necessary condition for induction.)

Zucker–Franklin D., Greaves M.F., Grossi C.E. & Marmont A.M. (1980) *Atlas of Blood Cells. Function and Pathology.* E.E., Milan.

5

The immune response
III—Theoretical aspects

Instructive theory

The ability of animals to synthesize antibodies directed against determinants such as dinitrobenzene and sulphanilic acid, which were so unlikely to occur in nature, made it difficult to accept the idea based on Ehrlich's earlier views that the body has preformed antibodies whose production is further stimulated by the entry of antigen. Instead attention turned to theories in which the antigen acted instructively as a template around which a standard unfolded γ-globulin chain could be moulded to provide the appropriate complementary shape. The molecule would be stabilized in this configuration by disulphide linkages, hydrogen bonds and so forth; on separation from the template the molecule would now have a specific combining site for antigen (figure 5.1).

Selective theory

An alternative view holds that the information required for the synthesis of the different antibodies is already present in the genetic apparatus. The gene which codes for a specific antibody is selected and 'switched on' by contact of antigen with the cell, and through transcription and translation of the appropriate messenger RNA, immunoglobulin peptide chains with corresponding individual primary amino acid sequences are synthesized; based on the sequence, these chains then fold spontaneously to a preferred globular configuration which possesses the specific antigen-combining sites (figure 5.1).

An analogy may help in the comparison of these two theories. If we consider the purchase of a suit, two courses of action are open. We may *instruct* the tailor to make the suit to measure, in which case we act as a template for the suit to be made on. Alternatively the tailor may be an enterprising fellow who has already made up to 10^4 different suits, one of which is almost certain to fit any intending purchaser; all we have to do is *select* the best fit for ourselves. Although in both cases the know-how of making suits (cf. protein synthesis) is there, in the first instance we provide essential information for the final shape (as

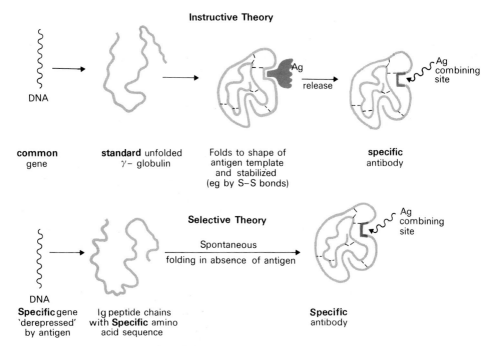

common gene   **standard** unfolded γ- globulin   Folds to shape of antigen template and stabilized (eg by S–S bonds)   **specific** antibody

DNA

Ag combining site

Selective Theory

Spontaneous folding in absence of antigen

Ag combining site

Specific gene 'derepressed' by antigen   Ig peptide chains with **Specific** amino acid sequence   **Specific** antibody

FIGURE 5.1. Comparison of instructive and selective theories for generating a specific antigen-combining site.

the antigen does), whereas in the second situation the tailor himself had the foresight to make a whole variety of differently shaped suits (information already in the DNA) before seeing the customer (antigen).

Evidence for a selective theory

ABSENCE OF ANTIGEN FROM PLASMA CELLS

Using autoradiography to visualize highly radioactive antigens combined with immunofluorescence to identify cells making specific antibody, Nossall has shown that nearly all cells which contain intracellular antibody do not have demonstrable antigen molecules. This is clearly at variance with the idea of antigen acting as a template.

AMINO ACID SEQUENCE OF ANTIBODIES

Purified antibodies show differences in amino acid sequence. As mentioned previously, myeloma proteins which represent individual immunoglobulin molecules show considerable variability in the sequences of the N-terminal part of both light

108

and heavy chains. Indeed of the many human myeloma light chains so far sequenced, none have proved to have identical structures. These differences in amino acid sequence reflect differences in DNA nucleotide sequences strongly implicating genetic control of specificity.

GENETIC STUDIES

Immune responsiveness to certain defined antigens has indeed been associated with genetic constitution, not only with respect to MHC-linked genes controlling the synthesis of antigen specific Ia molecules concerned in T-cell regulation of the antibody response but in particular with the Ig-allotype linked genes encoding certain antibody clones and idiotypes which provides strong evidence for the view that the capacity to form particular antibodies is inherited through the possession of Ig V-region genes (p. 86).

Clonal selection model

The evidence clearly favours a genetic theory and we should now examine how this can be expressed in cellular terms. Clonal selection, based largely on the ideas elaborated by Burnet, is generally regarded as an acceptable working model for antibody synthesis.

It is envisaged that each lymphocyte is genetically programmed to make one particular antibody and molecules of that antibody are built into the cell-surface membrane as receptors. Different lymphocytes make different antibodies so that all the body lymphocytes between them present antibodies with a wide spectrum of specificities. Antigen will combine with those lymphocytes carrying antibody on their surface which is a good fit, and these cells will be stimulated by the reaction on the plasma membrane to differentiate and divide to form a clone of cells synthesizing antibody with the same specificity as that on the surface of the parent lymphocyte (figure 5.2). Some of the progeny revert to small lymphocytes and become memory cells.

Evidence for clonal selection model

ONE CELL/ONE IMMUNOGLOBULIN

With immunofluorescent techniques, cells producing immunoglobulin can be stained for either κ- or λ-chains but not both, and in the heterozygous rabbit, for the maternal allotypic

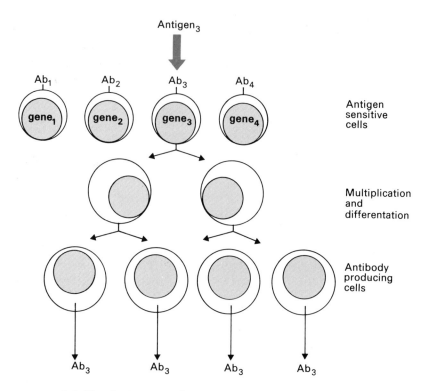

FIGURE 5.2. Clonal selection model. Each lymphocyte expresses the genes coding for one specific antibody, several molecules of which are built into the surface membrane to act as receptors. In the diagram, antigen₃ combines with the cell capable of making the complementary antibody₃ and this reaction at the cell surface leads to the formation of a clone of daughter cells making and exporting that specific antibody.

marker or the paternal but never both together (*allelic exclusion*). Furthermore plasma cell tumours only produce one, and not more than one, myeloma protein. Similar restrictions apply to the staining of surface Ig on B-lymphocytes described in an earlier chapter (p. 63).

That these surface immunoglobulins can behave as antibodies is suggested by the ability of a small percentage of lymphocytes to bind specific antigens such as sheep cells (forming 'rosettes') or radioactive salmonella flagellin. This binding can be blocked by anti-immunoglobulin sera. Humphrey has further shown that the percentage of cells binding antigen is increased in primed and decreased in tolerant animals.

When a soluble antigen like polymerized flagellin binds to a specific cell it causes patching and capping of the surface Ig in just the same way as an anti-Ig serum (cf. p. 63). If the antigen-capped cells are now stained with fluorescent anti-Ig, all the Ig is found in the cap, there being none on the remainder of the lymphocyte surface, i.e. when antigen reacts with a cell, all the Ig molecules on the cell surface combine with the antigen showing that they have similar specificity. In summary, the surface Ig of each B-lymphocyte represents the product of only one of the two chromosomes which code for each Ig chain and behaves as antibody of a single specificity.

RELATION OF SURFACE ANTIBODY TO
FUTURE PERFORMANCE

When cells are taken from an animal which has given a primary response to both ovalbumin and bovine serum albumin (BSA) and are passed down a column of glass beads coated with BSA, they retain the ability to give a secondary antibody response to ovalbumin but are unresponsive to BSA. Thus the BSA-responsive cells have anti-BSA receptors on their surface which cause them to stick to the BSA-coated beads (figure 5.3).

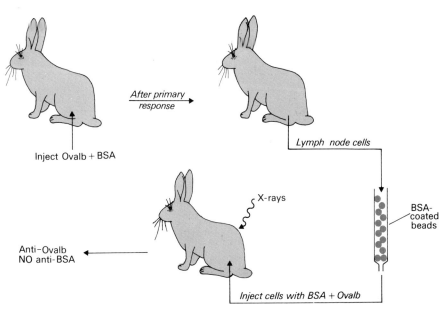

FIGURE 5.3. Absorption of antibody-forming cell precursors on antigen coated column. Lymph node cells primed to ovalbumin (ovalb) and bovine serum albumin (BSA) are run down a column of BSA-coated glass beads and injected into an irradiated recipient. On secondary challenge anti-ovalb but no anti-BSA is produced showing that the cells destined to make anti-BSA were bound to the column presumably through their specific anti-BSA receptors on the surface. (Based upon the work of Wigzell H. & Anderson B., (1969) *J.exp.Med.*, **129,** 23.)

Validity of the clonal selection model

Antibody affinity and antigen dosage

The combination of antigen and antibody is reversible and the complex may readily dissociate, depending upon the strength of binding. This can be defined broadly through the equilibrium constant of the reaction:

$$Ag + Ab \rightleftharpoons AgAb$$

and the reactants will behave according to the laws of mass action (cf. chapter 1, p. 11). If the antigen and antibody fit together very closely, the equilibrium will lie well over to the right; we refer to such antibodies which bind strongly to the antigen as *high-affinity antibodies* (strictly *high avidity* in the case of multivalent antigens, cf. p. 14). Experimentally it is found that injection of *small* amounts of antigen leads to the production of *high*-affinity antibodies whereas *larger* amounts of antigen give more antibody of *lower* affinity. How can we account for this on the clonal selection model?

It may be supposed that when an appropriate number of antigen molecules are bound to the antibody receptors on the cell surface, the lymphocyte will be stimulated to develop into an antibody-producing clone. When only small amounts of antigen are present, only those lymphocytes with high-affinity antibody receptors will be able to bind sufficient antigen for stimulation to occur and their daughter cells will, of course, also produce high-affinity antibody. Consideration of the antigen–antibody equilibrium equation will show that as the concentration of antigen is increased, even antibodies with relatively low affinity will bind more antigen; therefore at high doses of antigen the lymphocytes with lower affinity antibody receptors will also be stimulated and these are more abundant than those with receptors of high affinity.

Feedback inhibition of antibody synthesis

It was mentioned earlier (p. 90) that the injection of pre-formed antibody could inhibit an immune response to antigen and that this suggests a possible negative feedback model for control of antibody synthesis *in vivo*. The higher the affinity of the injected IgG antibody used to inhibit the immune response, the more effective it is. On the basis of the clonal selection model it may be argued that there will be a competition between injected antibody and the lymphocyte receptors for antigen and only cells with receptors of higher affinity than the administered antibody will be triggered. The higher the affinity of the antibody, the smaller will be the percentage of the total cells available.

Increase of affinity during immunization

As immunization proceeds, only lymphocytes with higher and higher affinity receptors can be triggered because the concentration of available antigen steadily falls and feedback inhibition by synthesized antibody will 'turn off' cells with equal or lower affinity receptors.

Immunological tolerance

The clonal selection model readily provides a basis for the mechanism of tolerance induction. It has only to be postulated that under the conditions known to cause unresponsiveness, contact with antigen causes death or long-term inactivation of the antigen-sensitive cell rather than its stimulation. Although we are uncertain of the mechanism, the idea that deletion or inactivation' of specific clones is responsible for tolerance induction is attractive. For example, it can account for the development of self-tolerance since all lymphocytes having receptors capable of reacting with circulating or accessible

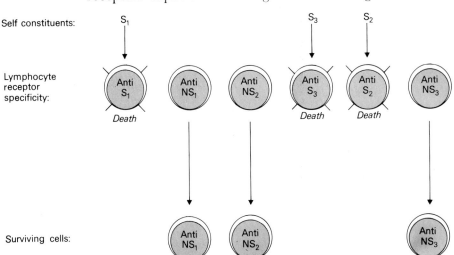

FIGURE 5.4. Induction of tolerance to self-constituents (S_1–S_3) by selective elimination of lymphocytes with self-reacting surface receptors. These cells are either killed or inactivated or inhibited by specific T suppressors. Surviving cells are able to react only with non-self (NS) foreign antigens of specificity NS_1, NS_2, NS_3, etc.

self-components would be eliminated or suppressed leaving only those cells with receptors for non-self determinants in the immunological armamentarium (figure 5.4).

Genetic theories of antibody variability

The variation in primary amino acid sequence of different antibodies, the differences between animal strains in their immunological responsiveness to selected synthetic and viral antigens and the plausibility of the clonal selection model all speak for a genetic basis underlying antibody variability. Similarities in amino acid sequence (homology) between the loops formed by intrachain disulphide bonds in the constant parts of heavy and light chains (figure 2.12) and to some extent between variable and constant parts, suggest that the existing genes controlling immunoglobulin structure are derived from a primitive smaller gene—perhaps coding for a peptide half the length of a light chain—by a process of duplication and translocation with early divergence of V genes.

Rough estimates place the total repertoire of different antibody molecules which can be synthesized by a given individual, at around 10^8 or perhaps even more. To help us understand the genetic basis for this quite remarkable diversity, we should first review the current status of our knowledge concerning the form and number of inherited (i.e. germ line) genes encoding antibody molecules.

GENES CODING FOR ANTIBODY

These fall into three clusters on three different chromosomes coding for κ, λ and heavy chains respectively. There appears to be only one variable region (V) gene for mouse λ chain and the genetic basis for the synthesis of this peptide is illustrated in figure 5.5. In common with other eukaryotic proteins, the chain is encoded in multiple distinct gene segments separated by intervening nucleotide sequences, *introns,* which are removed either by DNA translocation or by excision of the corresponding mRNA sequence. There is a leader sequence required for passage of the peptide through the endoplasmic reticulum, a V_λ segment coding for amino acid residues 1 to 98, a joining segment (J—not to be confused with the J peptide in IgM and IgA) encoding the remaining 11 amino acids of the variable region, and a C_λ gene segment giving rise to the constant region. As a lymphocyte undergoes differentiation to become an immunocompetent cell capable of synthesizing λ chains, there

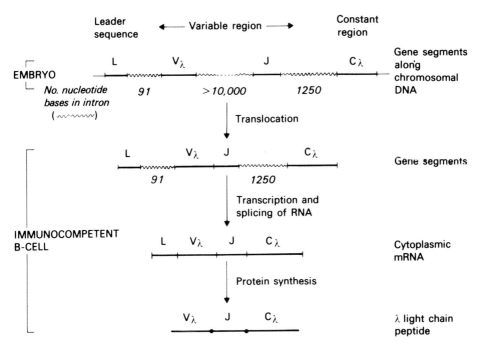

FIGURE 5.5. Genetic basis for synthesis of mouse λ chain. The variable region gene segment formed by the combination of V_λ with the joining segment J, is separate from the gene encoding the constant region as originally predicted by Dreyer and Bennett. In the human, the V_λ genes are more complex (cf. V_κ genes below).

is a rearrangement or translocation of the DNA bringing the V_λ and J segments together but still separated from the C_λ by an intron of 1250 nucleotides. Splicing of the transcribed RNA in the nucleus produces an mRNA which can now be used for the synthesis of a continuous λ chain peptide.

The same general principles apply to the arrangement of κ and heavy chain genes although they exist in far greater variety. The V_κ genes occur as a series of 50–100 clusters or sets each containing 6–8 closely related individual genes. There are five different J segments but just a single constant region gene. The heavy chain constellation shows additional features: the sub-class constant region genes form a single cluster and there is evidence for a highly variable sequence (D segment) inserted between the V and J regions. The D and J segments together encode almost the entire third hypervariable region which forms one side of the combining site groove (figure 2.10).

The arrangement of heavy chain genes would clearly permit a given V–J variable region to associate sequentially with different constant region genes and account for class switch during the antibody response. Whether this occurs at the DNA or mRNA level is still unresolved.

115

The problem of generating 10^8 or more different antibody molecules is now seen as a problem of generating 10^8 or more different combining sites since the V genes in any cluster can all link with the same constant region segment and it is therefore only necessary to have single C region genes. There are essentially two possibilities. Either: (a) we inherit *all* variable region genes—*the germ line theory*, or (b) we inherit just a few V genes from which diversity is generated by *somatic mutation* (figure 5.6).

Germ line concepts were initially criticized on the basis that 10^8 or so different V genes could not possibly be accommodated within the available genetic material. However, the finding through analysis of monoclonal proteins and DNA sequencing that light and heavy chain gene clusters each may have 5×10^2 or more V segments and around five separate J segments, leads to an explanation of diversity based upon random combinations of these genetic elements which may occur in the following ways:

(1) *Intra-chain amplification* of V and J segments by random DNA combination would lead to approximately 2.5×10^3 V–J

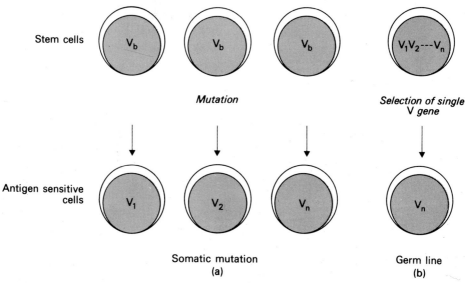

Stem cells

V_b V_b V_b $V_1 V_2 \text{---} V_n$

Mutation

Selection of single V gene

Antigen sensitive cells

V_1 V_2 V_n V_n

Somatic mutation
(a)

Germ line
(b)

FIGURE 5.6. Somatic mutation and germ line theories of antibody diversity: (a) a basic gene V_b undergoes somatic mutation during evolution from a stem cell to give different genes, one in each lymphocyte, coding for different antibodies with specificities from 1 to n; (b) each lymphocyte has the full range of genes coding for specificities 1 to n but only expresses one of these genes as it differentiates to immunocompetence.

regions ($5 \times 10^2 V \times 5J$), and because the J chain may have an influence on the combining site, this would represent 2.5×10^3 different combining specificities. Variation in the N-terminal codon of the J segment caused by variation in the way a given V and J region are combined (at least in the κ chain) would increase this figure to around 10^4.

(2) *Inter-chain amplification* occurs by random association of heavy and light chains so that 10^4 heavy and 10^4 light chain V–J regions would code for 10^8 ($10^4 \times 10^4$) antibody specificities.

In other words, random interactions between 10^3 or so basic gene segments could allow the expression of around 10^8 different antibodies and it seems likely that diversity can be accounted for largely on the basis of germ line genes. Nonetheless, there is evidence that somatic mutation may play some role. To summarize, a body of germ line V and J genes may provide virtually the full diversity of antibody response needed but somatic mutation could increase this variation further.

Summary

Antigen does not act as a template for antibody production; the complete information for antibody synthesis is already in the genome. Folding of the antibody molecule and hence specificity, depends upon the primary amino acid structure and differences in amino acid sequence between different antibodies reflect differences in DNA nucleotide sequence. Immune responsiveness is genetically controlled.

The clonal selection model assumes that each immunocompetent lymphocyte is programmed to synthesize one immunoglobulin which is inserted into the plasma membrane as a surface receptor. An antigen which reacts strongly with this surface antibody will be bound selectively, trigger the cell and cause clonal amplification and differentiation to provide a large population of cells all making antibody of the required specificity plus an expanded population of memory cells. The model accounts for the inverse relation between antigen dose and antibody affinity, the greater effectiveness of high affinity antibody in feedback inhibition of the immune response and the increase in affinity with immunization; it envisages immunological tolerance in terms of deletion or inactivation of specific clones.

There are three distinct clusters of genes coding for κ, λ and heavy Ig peptide chains. In each cluster there are multiple V and J (joining) gene segments but only single genes encoding the constant region. Random joining of V and J segments occurs as the lymphocyte differentiates to a committed cell; since the V–J combined gene segment encodes the variable region, this mechanism provides for the generation of $V \times J$ specificities. Additional amplification occurs through random association of heavy and light chains; p heavy plus q light chain genes would produce $p \times q$ different antibodies. The 1000 or so different gene segments in the germ line could give rise to around 10^8 different antibodies by such mechanisms. Somatic mutation could increase this variation further. In the secreting cell, coupling between the V–J and the constant region is effected by splicing the nuclear mRNA; a switch to coupling with another C gene leads to production of antibody with the same specificity but different class or subclass.

Further reading

Cunningham A.J. (ed.) (1976) *The Generation of Antibody Diversity. A New Look.* Academic Press, London.

Edelman G. (ed.) (1974) *Cellular Selection and Regulation in the Immune Response.* Soc.Gen.Physiol.Series, **29**. Raven Press, New York.

Fudenberg H.H., Pink J.R.L., Stites D.P. & Wang A-C. (1977) *Basic Immuno genetics,* 2nd edn. Oxford University Press, New York.

Hofmann G.W. (1975) A theory of regulation and self–non-self discrimination in an immune network. *Eur.J.Immunol.,* **5**, 638.

Marx J.L. (1978) Antibodies: new information about gene structure. *Science,* **202**, 298 & 412.

Schilling J., Clevinger B., Davie J.M. & Hood L. (1980) Amino acid sequence of homogeneous antibodies to dextran and DNA rearrangements in heavy chain V-region gene segments. *Nature,* **283**, 35.

Siskind G.W. & Benacerraf B. (1969) Cell selection by antigen in the immune response. *Adv. Immunol.,* **10**, 1.

Williamson A.R. (1979) Control of antibody formation: certain uncertainties. *J.clin.Path.,* **32**, Suppl. (Roy. Coll. Path.) **13**, 76.

6

Interaction of antigen and antibody

The primary interaction between an antigenic determinant and the combining site of an antibody, governed by the affinity, gives rise to a number of secondary phenomena such as precipitation, agglutination, phagocytosis, cytolysis, neutralization and so on. In this chapter we consider the practical implications of this interaction and begin to explore its consequences.

Precipitation

Multivalent antigens mixed with bivalent antibodies in solution can combine to form complexes which aggregate and precipitate. As described in chapter 1 (p. 7) the amount of precipitate varies with the proportions of the reagents and, generally speaking, insoluble complexes are formed in *antibody excess* while the complexes generated in *antigen excess* tend to be soluble. A variety of techniques depend upon visualization of the precipitation reaction in gels.

PRECIPITATION IN GELS

In the double diffusion method of Ouchterlony, antigen and antibody placed in wells cut in agar gel, diffuse towards each other and precipitate to form an opaque line in the region where they meet in optimal proportions. A preparation containing several antigens will give rise to multiple lines. The immunological relationship between two antigens can be assessed by setting up the precipitation reactions in adjacent wells; the lines formed by each antigen may be completely confluent indicating immunological identity, they may show a 'spur' as in the case of partially related antigens, or they may cross, indicative of unrelated antigens (figure 6.1). The origins of these patterns are explained in figure 6.2. It should be emphasized that even in the case of confluent lines this can only indicate immunological identity in terms of the antiserum used, not necessarily molecular identity. For example, purified antibodies to the dinitrobenzene hapten would give a line of confluence when set up against dinitrobenzene–ovalbumin and dinitrobenzene–serum albumin conjugates placed in adjacent wells.

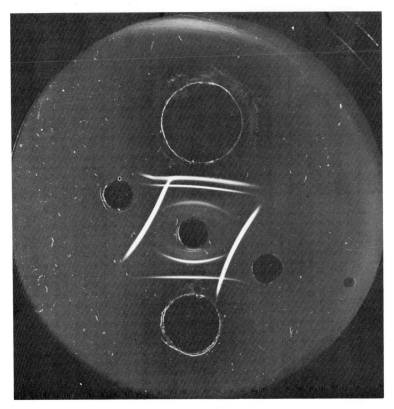

Antiserum in centre well

FIGURE 6.1. Multiple lines formed in the Ouchterlony test (double-diffusion precipitation) when rabbit antiserum (centre well) reacts in agar gel with four different antigen preparations (peripheral wells). Non-identity and partial identity of antigens are shown respectively by crossing over and spur formation between precipitin lines.

Where reagents are present in balanced proportions, the line formed will generally be concave to the well containing the reactant of higher molecular weight, be it antigen or antibody. This is a consequence of the usually slower diffusion rate of larger sized molecules.

The gel precipitation method can be made more sensitive by incorporating the antiserum in the agar and allowing the antigen to diffuse into it; up to 90% serum in agar may be employed (Feinberg). This method of single radial immunodiffusion is used for the quantitative estimation of antigens.

SINGLE RADIAL IMMUNODIFFUSION (SRID)

When antigen diffuses from a well into agar containing suitably diluted antiserum, initially it is present in a relatively high

120

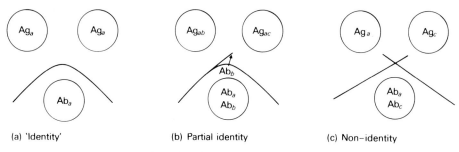

| (a) 'Identity' | (b) Partial identity | (c) Non-identity |

FIGURE 6.2. (a) Line of confluence obtained with two antigens which cannot be distinguished by the antiserum used.

(b) Spur formation by partially related antigens having a common determinant a but individual determinants b and c reacting with a mixture of antibodies directed against a and b. The antigen with determinants a and c can only precipitate antibodies directed to a. The remaining anti-bodies (Ab_b) cross the precipitin line to react with the antigen from the adjacent well which has determinant b giving rise to a 'spur' over the precipitin line.

(c) Crossing over of lines formed with unrelated antigens.

concentration and forms soluble complexes; as the antigen diffuses further the concentration continuously falls until the point is reached at which the reactants are nearer optimal proportions and a ring of precipitate is formed. The higher the concentration of antigen, the greater the diameter of this ring (figure 6.3). By incorporating, say, three standards of known antigen concentration in the plate, a calibration curve can be obtained and used to determine the amount of antigen in the unknown samples tested (figure 6.4). The method is used routinely in clinical immunology, particularly for immuno-globulin determinations, and also for substances such as the third component of complement, transferrin, C-reactive protein and the embryonic protein, α-foetoprotein, which is associated with certain liver tumours.

IMMUNOELECTROPHORESIS

The principle of this has been described earlier (p. 27). The method is of value for the identification of antigens by their electrophoretic mobility, particularly when other antigens are also present. In clinical immunology, semiquantitative infor-mation regarding immunoglobulin concentrations and identifi-cation of myeloma proteins is provided by this technique.

There have been some felicitous developments of the prin-ciple combining electrophoresis with immunoprecipitation in which movement in an electric field drives the antigen directly into contact with antibody. *Countercurrent immunoelectrophoresis* may be applied to antigens which migrate towards the positive

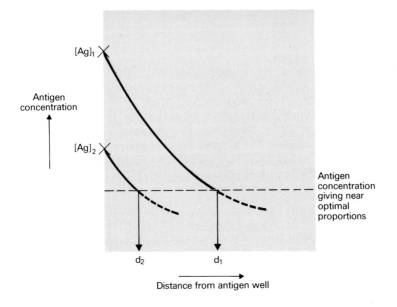

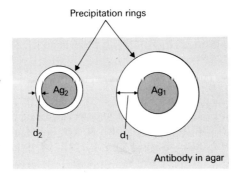

FIGURE 6.3. Single radial immunodiffusion: the relation of antigen concentration to the size of precipitation ring formed. Antigen at higher concentrations diffuses further from the well before it falls to the level giving precipitation with antibody near optimal proportions.

pole in agar (see figure 6.5). This qualitative technique is much faster and considerably more sensitive than double diffusion (Ouchterlony) and is used for the detection of hepatitis B antigen or antibody, DNA antibodies in SLE (p. 250), auto-antibodies to soluble nuclear antigens in mixed connective tissue disease, and *Aspergillus* precipitins in cases with allergic bronchopulmonary aspergillosis. *Rocket electrophoresis* is a quantitative method which involves electrophoresis of antigen into a gel containing antibody. The precipitation arc has the appearance of a rocket, the length of which is related to antigen concentration (figure 6.6). Like countercurrent electrophoresis this is a rapid method but again the antigen must move to the

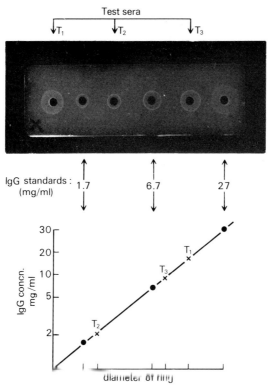

FIGURE 6.4. Measurement of IgG concentration in serum by single radial immuno-diffusion. The diameter of the standards (●) enables a calibration curve to be drawn and the concentration of IgG in the sera under test can be read off: T_1—serum from patient with IgG myeloma; 15 mg/ml; T_2—serum from a patient with hypogammaglobulinaemia; 2.6 mg/ml; T_3—normal serum; 9.6 mg/ml. (Courtesy of Dr F.C. Hay.)

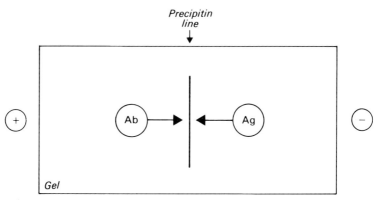

FIGURE 6.5. Countercurrent immunoelectrophoresis. Antibody moves 'backwards' in the gel on electrophoresis due to endosmosis; an antigen which is negatively charged at the pH employed will move towards the positive pole and precipitate on contact with antibody.

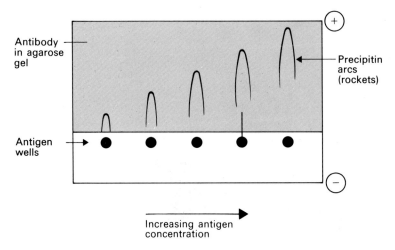

Antibody in agarose gel

Precipitin arcs (rockets)

Antigen wells

Increasing antigen concentration

FIGURE 6.6. Rocket electrophoresis. Antigen is electrophoresed into gel containing antibody. The distance from the starting well to the front of the rocket shaped arc is related to antigen concentration.

positive pole on electrophoresis; it is therefore suitable for proteins such as albumin, transferrin and caeruloplasmin but immunoglobulins are more conveniently quantitated by single radial immunodiffusion.

Radioactive binding techniques

MEASUREMENT OF ANTIBODY

These methods assess antibody level either by determining the capacity of an antiserum to complex with radioactive antigen or by measuring the amount of immunoglobulin binding to an insoluble antigen preparation. Perhaps the point should be made that it is not possible to define the *absolute* concentration of antibody in a given serum because each serum contains immunoglobulins with a range of binding affinities and the estimation of the amount of antigen bound to antibody depends upon the concentration and affinities of the antibodies as well as the nature and sensitivity of the test. With this proviso, the quantitative tests described do give a measure of the antibody content of a serum which is of practical value.

Using radioactive antigen

The two methods to be considered involve the addition of excess radio-labelled antigen to the antiserum followed by assessment of the amount of antigen which has been complexed with antibody (this being the antigen binding capacity). This is achieved either by: (a) *the Farr technique* in which complexed antigen is separated from that in the free form by precipitation with 50% ammonium sulphate (only applicable to those antigens soluble at this salt concentration), or (b) *the antiglobulin co-precipitation technique* in which the antigen bound to antibody is precipitated together with the rest of the immunoglobulin by an antiglobulin serum, leaving free antigen in the supernatant (figure 6.7). By using antibodies to different immunoglobulin classes and subclasses as the antiglobulin reagent, it is possible to determine the distribution of antibody activity among the classes. For example, addition of a radioactive antigen to human serum followed by a precipitating rabbit antihuman IgA, would indicate how much antigen had been bound to the serum IgA. The data documented in figure 4.4 on p. 85 were obtained by similar methods.

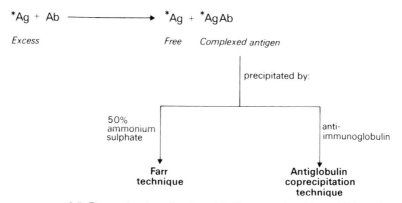

FIGURE 6.7. Determination of antigen-binding capacity. After addition of excess radioactive antigen (*Ag), that part bound to antibody as a complex is precipitated either by ammonium sulphate (Farr) or by an antiglobulin (antiglobulin co-precipitation).

Using insoluble antigen

The antibody content of a serum can be assessed by the ability to bind to antigen which has been insolubilized either by coupling to an immunoadsorbent or by physical adsorption to a plastic tube; the bound immunoglobulin may then be estimated by addition of a radiolabelled anti-Ig raised in another species (figure 6.8). Consider, for example, the determination of DNA autoantibodies in systemic lupus erythematosus (cf. p. 250). When a patient's serum is added to a plastic tube coated with antigen (in this case DNA), the autoantibodies will bind to the

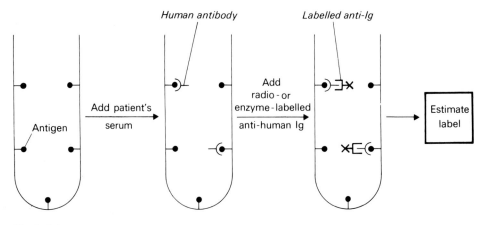

Human antibody   Labelled anti-Ig

Antigen   Add patient's   Add radio- or enzyme-labelled   Estimate label
serum   anti-human Ig

Plastic tube

FIGURE 6.8. The 'tube test' for quantitative determination of antibody.

tube and remaining serum proteins can be readily washed away. Bound antibody can now be estimated by addition of ^{125}I-labelled purified rabbit anti-human IgG; after rinsing out excess unbound reagent, the radioactivity of the tube will clearly be a measure of the autoantibody content of the patient's serum. The distribution of antibody in different classes can obviously be determined by using specific antisera. Take the radio-allergosorbent test (RAST) for IgE antibodies in allergic patients. The allergen (e.g. pollen extract) is covalently coupled to a paper disc which is then treated with patient's serum. The amount of specific IgE bound to the paper is then estimated by addition of labelled anti-IgE.

MEASUREMENT OF ANTIGEN

Radioimmunoassay

The binding of radioactively labelled antigen to a limited fixed amount of antibody can be partially inhibited by addition of unlabelled antigen and the extent of this inhibition can be used as a measure of the unlabelled material added. With the development of methods for labelling antigens to a high specific activity, very low concentrations down to the 10^{-12} g/ml level can be detected and most of the protein hormones can now be assayed with this technique. One disadvantage is that these methods cannot distinguish active protein molecules from biologically inactive fragments which still retain antigenic determinants.

126

Because of health hazards, the expense of counting equipment and the deterioration of labelled reagents through radiation damage, other types of label have been sought. Enzymes such as peroxidase and phosphatase which give a coloured reaction product have been successfully employed particularly in the ELISA (enzyme-linked immunosorbent assay), an immuno-metric assay for antibody (figure 6.8) or antigen. Chemi-luminescent and new fluorescent tags are under active scrutiny but almost the ultimate in sensitivity (around 10^3 molecules of antigen) is claimed for a method combining enzyme label with radioactive substrate.

Immunohistochemistry

IMMUNOFLUORESCENCE

Fluorescent dyes such as fluorescein and rhodamine can be coupled to antibodies without destroying their specificity. Coons showed that such conjugates would combine with anti-gen present in a tissue section and that the bound antibody could be visualized in the fluorescence microscope. In this way the distribution of antigen throughout a tissue and within cells can be demonstrated. Looked at another way, the method can also be used for the detection of antibodies directed against antigens already known to be present in a given tissue section or cell preparation. There are three general ways in which the test is carried out.

(1)   Direct test

The antibody to the tissue substrate is itself conjugated with the fluorochrome and applied directly (figure 6.9a). For example, suppose we wished to show the tissue distribution of a gastric autoantigen reacting with the autoantibodies present in the serum of a patient with pernicious anaemia. We would isolate IgG from the patient's serum, conjugate it with fluorescein, and apply it to a section of human gastric mucosa on a slide. When viewed in the fluorescence microscope we would see that the cytoplasm of the parietal cells was brightly stained. By using antisera conjugated to dyes which emit fluorescence at different wavelengths, two different antigens can be identified simul-taneously in the same preparation. In figure 3.6h (p. 57), direct staining of fixed plasma cells with a mixture of rhodamine-labelled anti-IgG and fluorescein-conjugated anti-IgM craftily demonstrates that these two classes of antibody are produced by different cells.

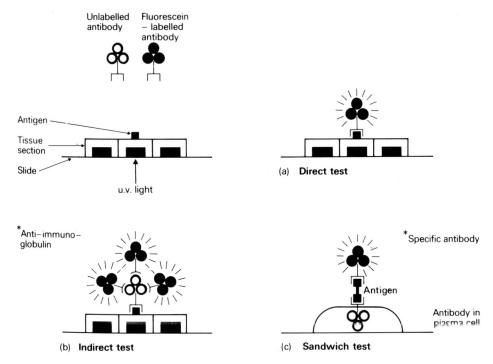

FIGURE 6.9. Fluorescent antibody tests. *Fluorescein labelled.

(2) *Indirect test*

In this double layer technique, the unlabelled antibody is applied directly to the tissue substrate and visualized by treatment with a fluorochrome-conjugated anti-immunoglobulin serum (figure 6.9b). In this case, in order to find out whether the serum of a patient has antibodies to gastric parietal cells, we would first treat a gastric section with the serum, wash well and then apply a fluorescein-labelled, rabbit, anti-human immunoglobulin; if antibodies were present, there would be staining of the parietal cells (figure 6.10a).

This technique has several advantages. In the first place the fluorescence is brighter than with the direct test since several fluorescent anti-immunoglobulins bind onto each of the antibody molecules present in the first layer (figure 6.9b). Secondly, since the conjugation process is lengthy, much time can be saved when many sera have to be screened for antibody because it is only necessary to prepare a single labelled reagent, viz. the anti-immunoglobulin. Furthermore, the method has great flexibility. For example, by using conjugates of antisera to individual immunoglobulin heavy chains, the distribution of antibodies among the various classes and subclasses can be assessed at least semi-quantitatively.

Applications of the indirect test may be seen in figure 6.10a and in chapter 10 (e.g. figure 10.2, pp. 252–3).

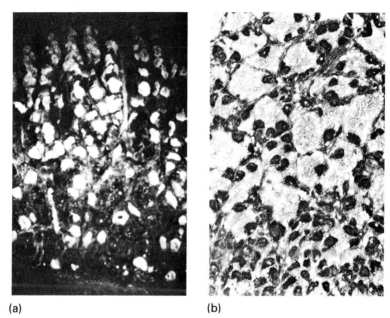

(a)   (b)

FIGURE 6.10. Staining of gastric parietal cells by (a) fluorescein and (b) peroxidase linked antibody. The sections were sequentially treated with human parietal cell autoantibodies and then with the conjugated rabbit anti-human IgG. The enzyme was visualized by the peroxidase reaction. (Courtesy of Miss V. Petts.)

(3) Sandwich test

This is a double layer procedure designed to visualize specific antibody. If, for example, we wished to see how many cells in a preparation of lymphoid tissue were synthesizing antibody to pneumococcus polysaccharide, we would first fix the cells with ethanol to prevent the antibody being washed away during the test, and then treat with a solution of the polysaccharide antigen. After washing, a fluorescein labelled antibody to the polysaccharide would then be added to locate those cells which had specifically bound the antigen (figure 6.9c). The name of the test derives from the fact that antigen is sandwiched between the antibody present in the cell substrate and that added as the second layer.

In place of fluorescent markers, other workers have evolved methods in which enzymes such as peroxidase or phosphatase are coupled to antibodies and these can be visualized by conventional histochemical methods at both light microscope (figure 6.10b) and electron microscope (figure 6.11) level.

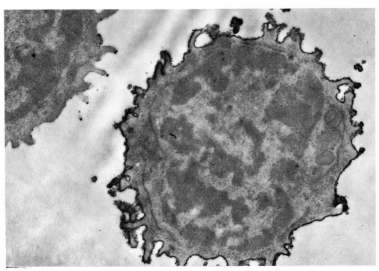

FIGURE 6.11. Electron microscopic visualization of human IgG on the surface of a B-lymphocyte by treatment of viable cell suspensions with peroxidase coupled anti-IgG. Note the adjacent unstained lymphocyte. (Courtesy of Miss V. Petts.)

Reactions with cell surface antigens

BINDING OF ANTIBODY

Surface antigens can be detected and localized by the use of labelled antibodies. Because antibodies cannot readily penetrate living cells except by endocytosis, treatment of cells with labelled antibody in the cold (to minimize endocytosis) should lead to staining only of antigens on the surface. Such studies have been carried out using antibodies labelled with peroxidase (figure 6.11) and with fluorescein (figures 3.9 and 6.12). The amount of fluorescent antibody bound to the cell can be quantified by flow cytofluorography.

After combination with antibody, many antigens are removed from the cell surface either through capping and endocytosis, or shedding into the extracellular medium as

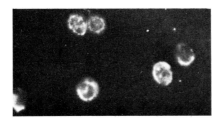

FIGURE 6.12. Antigens on the surface of viable human thyroid cells as demonstrated with thyroid autoantibodies in the indirect test. Note the patchy distribution. (Courtesy of Mrs H. Lindqvist; after Fagreus A. & Jonsson J.)

complexes. This 'stripping' process may have deleterious consequences for the host if it makes virally infected cells or tumours refractory to immunological attack.

AGGLUTINATION

Whereas the cross-linking of multivalent protein antigens by antibody leads to precipitation, cross-linking of cells or large particles by antibody directed against surface antigens leads to agglutination. Since most cells are electrically charged, a reasonable number of antibody links between two cells is required before the mutual repulsion is overcome. Thus agglutination of cells bearing only a small number of determinants may be difficult to achieve unless special methods such as further treatment with an antiglobulin reagent are used. Similarly, the higher avidity of multivalent IgM antibody relative to IgG (cf. p. 39) makes the former more effective as an agglutinating agent, molecule for molecule.

Agglutination reactions are used to identify bacteria and to type red cells; they have been observed with leucocytes and platelets and even with spermatozoa in certain cases of male infertility due to sperm agglutinins. Because of its sensitivity and convenience, the test has been extended to the identification of antibodies to soluble antigens which have been artificially coated onto various types of particle. Red cells have been popular and they can be coated with proteins after first modifying their surface with tannic acid or chromium chloride. The tests are usually carried out in the wells of plastic agglutination trays where the settling pattern of the cells on the bottom of the cup may be observed (figure 6.13); this provides a more sensitive indicator than macroscopic clumping. Inert particles such as bentonite and polystyrene latex have also been coated with antigens for agglutination reactions, particularly those used to detect the rheumatoid factors (figure 6.14).

131

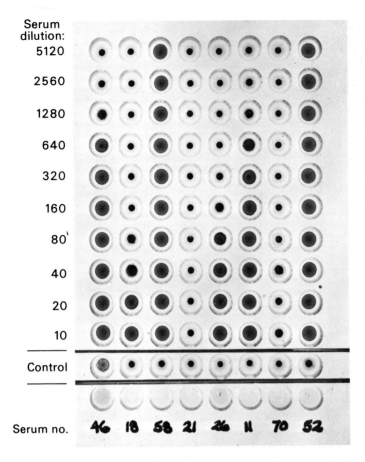

Serum dilution:
5120
2560
1280
640
320
160
80'
40
20
10
Control

Serum no.   46   18   58   21   26   11   70   52

FIGURE 6.13. Tanned red cell haemagglutination test for thyroglobulin autoantibodies. Thyroglobulin-coated cells were added to dilutions of patients' sera. Uncoated cells were added to a 1:10 dilution of serum as a control. In a positive reaction, the cells settle as a carpet over the bottom of the cup. Because of the 'V'-shaped cross-section of these cups, in negative reactions the cells fall into the base of the 'V', forming a small easily recognizable button. The reciprocal of the highest serum dilution giving an unequivocally positive reaction is termed the *titre*. The titres reading from left to right are: 640, 20, > 5120, neg, 40, 320, neg, > 5120. The control for serum No. 46 was slightly positive and this serum should be tested again after absorption with uncoated cells.

OPSONIC (Fc) ADHERENCE

On combination with IgG antibodies, antigens develop an increased adherence to polymorphonuclear leucocytes and macrophages through the specific IgG Fc binding sites on the surface of these cells. To take one example, bacteria coated with antibody become *'opsonized'* — i.e. 'ready for the table' or 'tasty for the phagocytes'—and will adhere to phagocytic cells; this in turn facilitates the engulfment and subsequent digestion of the

132

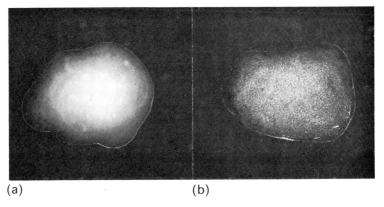

(a)   (b)

FIGURE 6.14. Macroscopic agglutination of latex coated with human IgG by serum from a patient with rheumatoid arthritis. This contains rheumatoid factor, an autoantibody directed against determinants on IgG. (a) Normal serum, (b) patient's serum.

micro-organisms. Opsonic adherence and the related *immune adherence* reactions which involve binding through complement components (see below) are of major importance in the defence against infection. They may also be concerned in the removal of lymphocytes from the circulation by anti-lymphocyte serum and of red cells by the autoantibodies in autoimmune haemolytic anaemia. The *extracellular killing* of antibody-coated target cells (cf. p. 193) depends upon adherence to Fc receptors on the effector cell surface. IgE-mediated degranulation of mast cells by antigen which triggers acute inflammatory responses and sometimes anaphylaxis, provides an interesting contrast, since in this case the Ig molecules are already firmly bound to their Fc receptors before the reaction with antigen.

STIMULATION

A quite unexpected phenomenon has been observed in that antibodies to cell-surface components may sometimes lead not to cytotoxic reactions as discussed below, but to actual stimulation of the cell. This problem occurs if the antibodies are directed against receptors on the surface which can generate a stimulatory signal when triggered by combination with the antibody. Examples are:

(1) The transformation and mitosis induced in small lymphocytes by anti-lymphocyte serum and anti-immunoglobulin sera *in vitro*. The latter combine with the immunoglobulin antigen receptors on the cell surface and mimic the configurational changes produced by antigen which activate the cell.

133

(2) Degranulation of human mast cells by anti-IgE serum. The anti-IgE brings about the same sequence of changes as would specific antigen combining with the surface bound IgE molecules.

(3) Stimulation of thyroid cells by autoantibodies present in the serum of patients with thyrotoxicosis.

CYTOTOXIC REACTIONS

If antibodies directed against the surface of cells are able to fix certain components present in the extracellular fluids, collectively termed *complement*, a cytotoxic reaction may occur. Historically, complement activity was recognized by Bordet who showed that the lytic activity against red cells of freshly drawn rabbit anti-sheep erythrocyte serum was lost on ageing or heating to 56°C for half-an-hour but could be restored by addition of fresh serum from an unimmunized rabbit. Thus, for haemolysis one requires a relatively heat stable factor, the antibody, plus a heat labile factor, complement, present in all fresh sera.

Complement

NATURE OF COMPLEMENT

The classical activity ascribed to complement (C') depends upon the operation of nine protein components $(C1-C9)$ acting in sequence of which the first consists of three major sub-fractions termed $C1q$, $C1r$ and $C1s$. Some of the characteristics of the three most abundant components are given in table 6.1.

TABLE 6.1.

	C1q	C4	C3
Serum concn., $\mu g/ml$	100–200	400	1200
Molecular weight	400,000	230,000	185,000
Thermolability	+	−	−
Immunoelectrophoresis	γ	β_{1E}	β_{1C}

When the first component is activated by an immune complex (e.g. antibody bound to a red cell), it acquires the ability to activate several molecules of the next component in the sequence; each of these is then able to act upon the next

134

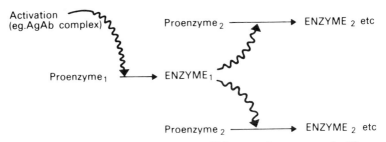

FIGURE 6.15. Enzymic basis of the amplifying complement cascade. The activated *enzyme₁* splits a peptide fragment from several molecules of *proenzyme₂* which all become active *enzyme₂* molecules capable of splitting *proenzyme₃* and so on.

component and so on, producing a cascade effect with amplification. In this way, the triggering of one molecule of C1 can lead to the activation of thousands of the later components. At each stage, activation is accompanied by the appearance of a new enzymic activity and since one enzyme molecule can process several substrate molecules, so each complement factor can cause the processing or activation of many molecules of the next component in the sequence (figure 6.15). The terminal components of the complement cascade have the ability to punch a 'functional hole' through the cell membrane on which they are fixed, presumably by some perturbation of phospholipid structure, and this leads to cell death. Thus, through this sequential amplification process, the activation of one C1 molecule can lead to a macroscopic event, namely the lysis of a cell. As will be seen later, the intermediate stages in the complement sequence also give rise to other biological activities which are of importance in health and disease. Like the blood clotting, kallikrein and fibrinolytic systems which also involve enzyme cascades, the complement components have a complex system of inhibitors to regulate activation.

Complement is measured as an activity as are other enzyme systems and is expressed in terms of the degree of lysis of a standard suspension of antibody coated sheep red cells produced within a fixed time (figure 6.16).

ACTIVATION OF COMPLEMENT

The activation of C1 is initiated by binding through C1q to C_H2 sites on the immunoglobulins forming a complex with antigen. Aggregation of immunoglobulin as by heating to 60°C for 20 minutes also leads to the changes in structure which allow complement activation. Different immunoglobulin classes have

135

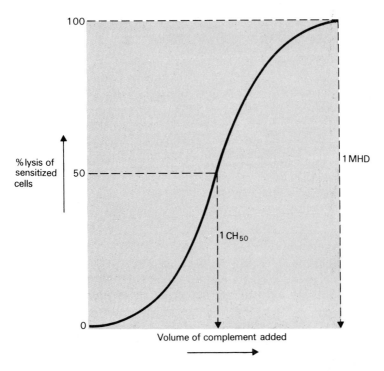

FIGURE 6.16. Relationship of added complement to percentage lysis of standard suspension of sensitized red cells. At the 50% lysis point, the curve is steep and the amount of C' giving 50% lysis ($1\ CH_{50}$) can be accurately determined. The curve only gradually reaches 100% lysis and the amount of C' giving 100% lysis (1 Minimum Haemolytic Dose: 1 MHD) is less precisely assessed. The MHD is nonetheless adequate for routine serological purposes but for more accurate work the CH_{50} unit is preferred.

different Fc structures and only IgG and IgM can bind C1. There are differences even within the IgG subclasses: IgG1 and IgG3 fix complement well, IgG2 modestly and IgG4 poorly, if at all. C1q is polyvalent with respect to Ig binding and consists of a central collagen-like stem branching into six peptide chains each tipped by an Ig binding subunit (resembling the blooms on a bunch of flowers). At least two of these subunits must bind to immunoglobulin C_H2 sites for activation of C1q. With IgM this is less of a problem since several Fc regions are available within a single molecule, although these only become readily accessible when the $F(ab')_2$ arms bend out of the plane of the inner Fc region on combination with antigen (cf. figure 2.16). On the other hand, IgG antibodies will only fix complement when two or more molecules are bound to closely adjacent sites on the antigen. It is for this reason that IgM antibodies to red cells have a high haemolytic efficiency since a 'single hit' will

136

produce full complement activation and cell death. With IgG antibodies, a far larger number of 'hits' will be required before, by chance, two IgG antibodies are bound at adjacent sites and are then able to initiate the complement sequence.

Complement can be activated by another route, the so-called *alternative pathway* (see below). This can be stimulated by certain cell wall polysaccharides such as bacterial endotoxin and yeast zymosan, by some aggregated immunoglobulins such as human IgA and guinea pig IgG1 known to be ineffective for C1q binding, and, as we shall see later, by a feedback mechanism from the classical pathway.

THE COMPLEMENT SEQUENCE

Classical pathway (figure 6.17)

Let us analyse the sequence of events which take place when IgM or IgG antibodies combine with the surface membrane of a cell in the presence of complement. C1q is linked in a tri-molecular complex through calcium to C1r and C1s. After the binding of C1q to the Fc regions of the immune complex, C1s acquires esterase activity and brings about the inactivation and transfer to sites on the membrane (or immune complex) of first C4 and then C2 (unfortunately components were numbered before the sequence was established). This complex has 'C3-

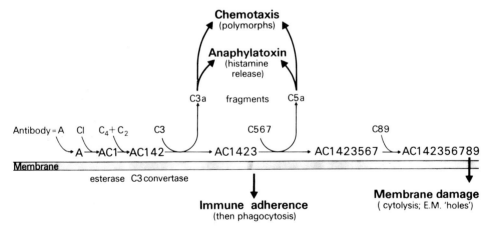

FIGURE 6.17. Sequence of classical complement activation by membrane-bound antibody showing formation of C3a and C5a fragments chemotactic for polymorphs and with anaphylatoxin activity causing histamine release. Immune adherence through C3 to macrophages, platelets or red cells facilitates phagocytosis. Fixation of C8 and 9 generates cytolytic activity. Fragments released during the activation of C4 and C2 are thought to have chemotactic and kinin-like activity respectively.

convertase' activity and splits C3 in solution to produce a small peptide fragment (C3a) and a residual molecule (C3b) which have quite distinct functions:

(1) C3a is chemotactic for polymorphonuclear leucocytes and has *anaphylatoxin* activity in that it causes histamine release from mast cells.

(2) C3b, like C2 and C4, exposes an internal thioester bond immediately after proteolytic cleavage of the parent C3 which enables it to react with adjacent regions on the membrane. By this means a large number of C3b molecules may be transferred to the surface membrane through the action of the convertase. There are specific receptors for this membrane-bound C3b on polymorphs and macrophages (all mammalian species studies), platelets (rabbits) and red cells (primates) which allow *immune adherence* of the antigen–antibody-C3b complex to these cells so facilitating subsequent phagocytosis (figure 6.17). The bound C3 presents a new structural configuration not present on the native molecule which can provoke the formation of the autoantibody *immunoconglutinin*. Control of C3b levels is maintained through the action of a C3b inactivator (Factor I). C3b readily combines with Factor H to form a complex which is broken down by Factor I and loses its haemolytic and immune adherence properties; it then becomes highly susceptible to attack by trypsin-like enzymes present in the body fluids and splits to form the fragments C3c and C3d (figure 6.18).

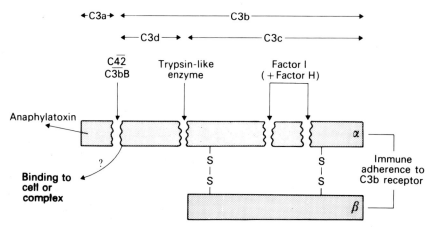

FIGURE 6.18. The structural basis for the cleavage of C3 by C3 convertases and the inactivation of C3b by successive action of C3b inactivator and a protease. Factor I was previously termed C3bina and before that KAF; Factor H was originally called β_{1H}.

Alternative pathway

In the classical pathway we have just discussed, the active C3b fragment is formed by the action of C142 convertase. Another C3 convertase, C$\overline{\text{3bB}}$, can be generated by a distinct series of reactions collectively termed the alternative pathway (figure 6.19) which can be triggered by extrinsic agents, in particular microbial polysaccharides such as endotoxin, acting independently of antibody. The convertase is formed by the action of Factor D on C3b and Factor B. This creates an interesting positive feedback loop in which the product of C3 breakdown helps to form more of the cleavage enzyme.

The present view is that the low concentrations of C3b in plasma can give rise to C$\overline{\text{3bB}}$ convertase under normal conditions; however, the lability of C$\overline{\text{3bB}}$ and the action of C3b inactivator prevent the system from getting out of hand and

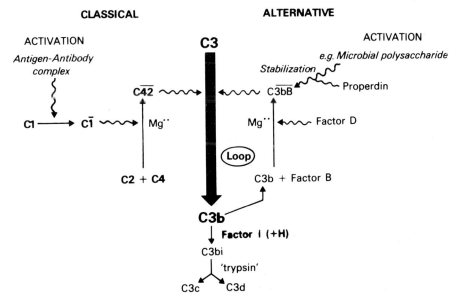

FIGURE 6.19. The alternative complement pathway showing points of similarity with the classical sequence. Both pathways generate a C3 convertase, C$\overline{42}$ in one case and C$\overline{\text{3bB}}$ in the other, which activates C3 to provide the central event in the complement system. The C3b inactivator may split C4b in the same manner as it does C3b. C3 and C4 resemble each other structurally as do C2 and Factor B. The alternative pathway is probably the older of the two in phylogenetic terms. ⤳ represents an activation process. The convention of using a horizontal bar above a complement component to designate its activation is used. The activated components are usually fragments of the original molecules, e.g. the alternative pathway convertase is actually C$\overline{\text{3bBb}}$, but in the interests of simplicity in a complicated system, such details have been omitted.

allow the feedback loop to 'tick over' quietly. Microbial polysaccharides and other initiators of the alternative pathway boost the levels of $\overline{C3bB}$ convertase by providing a surface upon which the enzyme is stabilized (probably with the help of properdin).

The alternative pathway can be studied independently of the classical sequence under circumstances where the latter is inoperative as, for example, in C4-deficient serum or in a serum treated with Mg-EGTA to complex Ca^{2+} and inactivate C1.

The solubilization of immune complexes by coating with C3b appears to be due to activation of the alternative pathway, perhaps through stabilization of convertase on the surface of the complex. An unexpected finding was the observation that factor B can be detected on the surface of B-lymphocytes. Is this connected with a role for C3b as a second signal for lymphocyte induction?

Post C3 pathway

The sequence reaches its full amplitude at the C3 stage which represents the essential heart of the complement system. Thereafter C5 is split by C3b to give C5a and C5b fragments. C5a degranulates mast cells and is the dominant polymorph chemotactic agent in the complement system; it also brings about the extracellular secretion of leucocyte lysosomal enzymes. Both C3a and C5a are inactivated by a carboxypeptidase which removes the terminal arginine. Meanwhile, the C5b binds as a complex with C6 and 7 to form a thermostable site on the membrane which recruits the final components C8 and C9 and these administer the coup de grâce by generating *membrane damage*. The cytolytic component is C8 but C9 enhances its activity (figure 6.17); incredibly just one molecule of C8 is sufficient to lyse a red cell.

Yet more complexity is introduced by the phenomenon of *reactive lysis* (Lachmann & Thomson); a proportion of the activated C5b67 complexes formed remain free and not only are they chemotactic for neutrophils but they are also able to bind to 'innocent' cells in the vicinity. Once fixed to the cell surface they can complete the complement sequence by binding C8, 9 with resultant cell lysis.

Cytolysis

The full complement system leading to membrane damage can cause bacteriolysis in Gram-negative organisms by allowing lysozyme to reach the plasma membrane where it destroys the mucopeptide layer (p. 155). Negatively stained preparations in the electron microscope shows the 'pits' on the surface (figure 6.20) which correspond with individual sites of complement activation and which resemble those seen on the red cell.

Immune (C3b) adherence

This plays a major role in facilitating the phagocytosis of micro-organisms after coating with antibody and C' or after activation of the alternative complement pathway. Since many C3 molecules are bound onto the surface at each site of C' activation, adherence to macrophages and polymorphs may operate largely through C3 binding although it should be noted that subsequent phagocytosis is provoked to a greater extent by IgG rather than C3b. Purified C3b has been shown to trigger extracellular release of lysosomal enzymes from macrophages and it is possible, but not yet established, that this could damage adhering micro-organisms.

Immunoconglutinin

This may play a role by agglutinating relatively small complexes containing bound C3 thereby making them more susceptible to phagocytosis.

Acute inflammation

The fragments produced during complement consumption stimulate two helpful features of the acute inflammatory response. First, the chemotactic factors attract phagocytic neutrophil polymorphs to the site of C' activation, and secondly anaphylatoxin, through histamine release, increases vascular permeability and hence the flow of serum antibody and more C' to the infected area.

ROLE IN DISEASE

Complement is implicated in disease processes involving

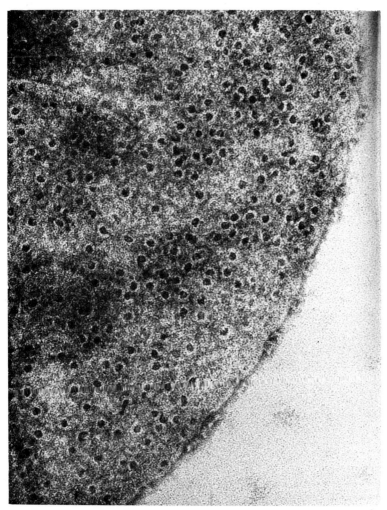

FIGURE 6.20. Multiple lesions in the cell wall of *Escherichia coli* bacterium caused by interaction with IgM antibody and complement. Each lesion is caused by a single IgM molecule and shows as a 'dark pit' due to penetration by the 'negative stain'. This is somewhat of an illusion since in reality these 'pits' are like volcano craters standing proud of the surface, and are each single complexes containing one each of the terminal C5-8 components plus six molecules of C9. C8 opens and shuts a transmembrane channel which eventually causes lysis, and C9 acts to jam this channel open. Comparable results may be obtained in the absence of antibody since the cell wall endotoxin can activate the alternative pathway. Magnification ×400,000. (Courtesy of Drs R. Dourmashkin and J.H. Humphrey.)

cytotoxic and immune-complex mediated hypersensitivities which will be discussed in more detail in chapter 8. Cytotoxic reactions are seen in nephrotoxic nephritis and autoimmune haemolytic anaemia. Complexes formed in antibody excess giving rise to immune vasculitis of the Arthus type are seen, for example, in Farmer's lung and cryoglobulinaemia with cutaneous vasculitis; soluble complexes formed in antigen excess give 'serum sickness' type reactions with considerable deposition in the kidney glomcruli as found in many forms of chronic glomerulonephritis.

COMPLEMENT DEFICIENCIES

The importance of C′ in defence against infections is emphasized by the occurrence of repeated infections in a patient lacking C3b inactivator. Because of his inability to destroy C3b there is continual activation of the alternative pathway through the feedback loop leading to very low C3 and Factor B levels with normal C1, 4 and 2. On the other hand, permanent deficiencies in C5, C6 and C7 have all been described in man yet in virtually every case the individuals are healthy and not particularly prone to infection. Thus full operation of the C′ system up to C8,9 does not appear to be essential for survival and adequate protection must be afforded by opsonizing antibodies and the immune adherence mechanism.

An inhibitor of active C1 is grossly lacking in hereditary angioneurotic oedema and this can lead to recurring episodes of acute circumscribed non-inflammatory oedema. The patients are heterozygotes and synthesize small amounts of the inhibitor which can be raised to useful levels by administration of testosterone or, in critical cases, of the purified inhibitor itself.

Summary

The formation of single bands of precipitate when antigen and antibody react in gels can be used qualitatively to study the number of reacting components and the immunological relationship between different antigens (Ouchterlony double diffusion system) and the electrophoretic mobility of the antigens (immunoelectrophoresis). Quantitative measurement of antigen concentration is made by single radial immuno-diffusion, 'rocket' electrophoresis and two-dimensional electro-phoresis.

Radioisotopic techniques for assessing the antibody content

of serum include: (a) addition of radiolabelled antigen and determination of the amount bound to antibody by ammonium sulphate or a second antibody precipitation (antigen-binding capacity) and (b) determination of the amount of antibody binding to insoluble antigen by addition of a labelled anti-Ig (e.g. 'tube test'). Radioimmunoassay of antigen is a form of saturation analysis in which the test material competes with labelled antigen for a limited amount of antibody, the amount of label displaced being a measure of the antigen in the test sample.

The localization of antigens in tissues, within cells or on the cell surface can be achieved microscopically using antibodies tagged with fluorescent dyes or enzymes such as peroxidase whose reaction product can be readily visualized. In the direct test, the labelled antibody is applied directly to the tissue; in the indirect test the label is conjugated to an anti-Ig used as a second amplifying antibody. Fluorescent antibody bound to the surface of single cells, e.g. lymphocytes, can be quantified by flow cytofluorography. For ultrastructural studies, antibodies are usually tagged with peroxidase.

Reaction of antibody with a cell surface antigen can lead to agglutination, enhancement of phagocytosis or extracellular killing, metabolic stimulation and mitosis, and complement-mediated cytotoxicity.

Complement, like the blood coagulation, fibrinolytic and kallikrein systems, involves a multicomponent enzymic cascade in which the first component, on activation, splits a small peptide from several molecules of the second component each of which is now an active enzyme able to act on the third component, etc.; a small number of initiating events leads to a large effect through this amplification method. The most abundant component, C3, is split by a convertase enzyme generated either by the *classical pathway* (C1,4,2) which is initiated by antibody, or by the alternative pathway (properdin, Factors B and D) which is initiated in the absence of antibody by material such as bacterial polysaccharides. One split product, C3a, is chemotactic for polymorphonuclear leucocytes and increases vascular permeability through histamine release from mast cells and basophils. The other product, C3b, binds non-specifically to the antigen surface and increases the efficiency of binding to the polymorphs (attracted by C3a) because of C3b receptors on the surface of these phagocytic cells. C3b also activates C5 to release C5a (with similar properties to C3a) and generates C5b which fires the remainder of the sequence to C8 and 9 thereby leading to cell death through membrane damage.

144

Through these effects complement plays an important role in the defence against infection. It is also concerned in certain hypersensitivity reactions involving combination of antibody with surfaces (e.g. nephrotoxic nephritis) and immune complexes (e.g. Farmer's lung, chronic glomerulonephritis). Massive activation of complement by microbial products can lead to disseminated intravascular coagulation. Deficiency in complement components predisposes to the development of SLE. Like the blood clotting system, inhibitors play a crucial role and if they are defective, disease may result, e.g. hereditary angioneurotic oedema (C1 inhibitor) or repeated infection (C3b inactivator).

Further reading

Clausen J. (1969) *Immunochemical Techniques for the Identification and Estimation of Macromolecules*. North-Holland, Amsterdam.

Hudson L. & Hay F.C. (1980) *Practical Immunology*, 2nd edn. Blackwell Scientific Publications, Oxford.

Lachmann P.J. (1982) Complement. In *Clinical Aspects of Immunology*, 4th edn. Lachmann P.J. & Peters K. (eds). Blackwell Scientific Publications, Oxford.

Nairn R.C. (1976) *Fluorescent Protein Tracing*, 4th edn. Churchill Livingstone, Edinburgh.

Rose N.R. & Friedman H. (eds) (1976) *Manual of Clinical Immunology*. American Society of Microbiology, Washington, D.C.

Thompson R.A. (1974) *The Practice of Clinical Immunology*, Edward Arnold, London.

Weir D.M. (ed.) (1973) *Handbook of Experimental Immunology*, 2nd edn. Blackwell Scientific Publications, Oxford.

Williams C.A. & Chase M.W. (1967–71) *Methods in Immunology and Immunochemistry*, vols I–IV. Academic Press, London.

7 Immunity to infection

Aside from ill-understood constitutional factors which make one species innately susceptible and another resistant to certain infections, a number of non-specific anti-microbial systems (e.g. phagocytosis) have been recognized which are *'innate'* in the sense that they are not intrinsically affected by prior contact with the infectious agent. We shall discuss these systems and examine how, in the state of *specific acquired immunity*, their effectiveness can be greatly increased by both B- and T-cell activity.

Innate immunity

PREVENTING ENTRY

The simplest way to avoid infection is to prevent the micro-organisms from gaining access to the body (figure 7.1). The major line of defence of course is the skin which, when intact, is impermeable to most infectious agents. Furthermore most bacteria fail to survive for long on the skin because of the direct inhibitory effects of lactic acid and fatty acids in sweat and sebaceous secretions and the low pH which they generate. An exception is *Staphylococcus aureus* which often infects the relatively vulnerable hair follicles and glands.

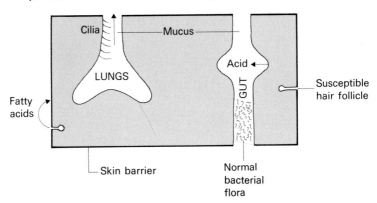

FIGURE 7.1. The first lines of defence against infection: protection at the external body surfaces.

147

Mucus, secreted by the membranes lining the inner surfaces of the body, acts as a protective barrier and can inhibit the penetration of cells by viruses through competition with cell surface receptors for the viral neuraminidase. Microbial and other foreign particles trapped within the adhesive mucus are removed by mechanical stratagems such as ciliary movement, coughing and sneezing. Among other mechanical factors which help protect the epithelial surfaces, one should also include the washing action of tears, saliva and urine. Many of the secreted body fluids contain bactericidal components, e.g. acid in gastric juice, spermine in semen and lysozyme in tears, nasal secretions and saliva.

A totally different mechanism is that of microbial antagonism associated with the normal bacterial flora of the body. These suppress the growth of many potentially pathogenic bacteria and fungi at superficial sites by competition for essential nutrients or by production of inhibitory substances such as colicins or acid.

COUNTER-ATTACK AGAINST THE INVADERS

When micro-organisms do penetrate the body, two main defensive operations come into play, the destructive effect of soluble chemical factors such as bactericidal enzymes and the mechanism of phagocytosis — literally 'eating' by the cell.

Humoral factors

Of the soluble bactericidal substances elaborated by the body, perhaps the most abundant and widespread is the enzyme lysozyme, a muramidase which splits the mucopeptide wall of susceptible bacteria. A number of plasma components, C-reactive protein (CRP), α_1 anti-trypsin, α_2-macro-globulin, fibrinogen, caeruloplasmin, C9 and factor B, collectively termed *acute phase proteins*, show a dramatic increase in concentration in response to infection or tissue injury. For example, CRP is released from the liver in response to endogenous pyrogen derived from endotoxin stimulated macrophages, and its concentration can rise 1000-fold. CRP shows a Ca-dependent binding to a number of micro-organisms which contain phosphoryl choline in their membranes, the complex having the useful property of activating complement by the classical pathway. We remember of course that many microbes activate the alternative pathway directly and we will explore the consequences in more detail below; suffice it to say under this head

148

that such activation can result in damage to the outer membrane of the infective agent mediated by the terminal components C8 and C9.

Lastly we should include the non-specific antiviral agent *α-interferon* which inhibits intracellular viral replication and is itself synthesized by cells in response to viral infection. Viral interference, the resistance of an animal or cell infected with one virus to superinfection with a second unrelated virus, may be attributed to interferon. In children given live measles vaccine, smallpox vaccine will not take if inoculated at the height of interferon production. It must be presumed that interferon plays a significant role in the recovery from, as distinct from the prevention of, viral infections. The finding that interferon heightens the activity of non-specific killer cells (NK; p. 239) could have considerable significance if these are shown to be generally cytotoxic for virally infected cells since this would constitute a nicely integrated system.

Phagocytosis

The engulfment and digestion of micro-organisms is assigned to two major cell types recognized by Metchnikoff at the turn of the century as *micro-* and *macrophages*. The smaller polymorphonuclear neutrophil (cf. figure 3.6f) is a non-dividing short-lived cell with granules containing a wide range of bactericidal factors and glycogen stores which can be utilized by glycolysis under anaerobic conditions. It is the dominant white cell in the blood stream. Macrophages derive from bone marrow promonocytes which, after differentiation to blood monocytes, finally settle in the tissues as mature macrophages where they constitute the so-called *reticuloendothelial system*. They are present throughout the connective tissue and around the basement membrane of small blood vessels and are particularly concentrated in the lung (alveolar macrophages), liver (Kupffer cells), and lining of spleen sinusoids and lymph node medullary sinuses where they are strategically placed to filter off foreign material. Other examples are mesangial cells in the kidney glomerulus, brain microglia and osteoclasts in bone. Unlike the polymorphs, they are long-lived cells with significant rough-surfaced endoplasmic reticulum and mitochondria and whereas the polymorphs provide the major defence against pyogenic (pus-forming) bacteria, as a rough generalization it may be said that macrophages are at their best in combating those bacteria, viruses and protozoa which are capable of living within the cells of the host.

149

Before phagocytosis can occur, the microbe must first adhere to the surface of the polymorph or macrophage, an event mediated by some rather primitive recognition mechanism on the part of the phagocytic cells. Depending upon its nature, a particle attached to the membrane may initiate the ingestion phase in which it becomes engulfed by cytoplasmic processes and comes to lie within a vacuole termed a phagosome (figures 7.2 & 3.7g–j). A lysosomal granule then fuses with the vacuole to form a phagolysosome in which the ingested microbe is slaughtered by a battery of mechanisms (table 7.1). Dominant among these are the oxygen-dependent systems. Phagocytosis is associated with a dramatic increase in activity of the hexose monophosphate shunt providing NADPH and a burst of oxygen consumption as this is metabolized by a plasma membrane NADPH oxidase which is activated on contact with the microbe during ingestion and continues to function on the inner surface of the phagolysosome. The oxygen is converted to superoxide anion, hydrogen peroxide, singlet oxygen and hydroxyl radicals, all powerful microbicidal agents. The combination of peroxide, myeloperoxidase and halide ions constitutes a potent halogenating system capable of killing both bacteria and viruses. Low pH, lysozyme, lactoferrin and the cationic proteins constitute a series of bacteriostatic and bactericidal factors which are oxygen-independent and can therefore function under anaerobic circumstances. The rich

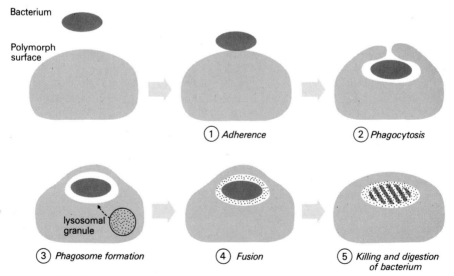

FIGURE 7.2. Phagocytosis of bacterium by neutrophil leucocyte (see also figure 3.7g–j).

TABLE 7.1. Antimicrobial systems in phagocytic vacuoles

Oxygen dependent mechanisms:

$$\text{Glucose} + \text{NADP}^+ \xrightarrow[\text{shunt}]{\text{hexose monophosphate}} \text{Pentose phosphate} + \text{NADPH}$$

$$\text{NADPH} + \text{O}_2 \xrightarrow{\text{oxidase}} \text{NADP}^+ + \mathbf{O_2^-}$$

} O_2 burst + generation of superoxide anion

$$2\text{O}_2^- + 2\text{H}^+ \xrightarrow[\text{dismutation}]{\text{spontaneous}} \mathbf{H_2O_2} + {}^1\mathbf{O_2}$$

$$\text{O}_2^- + \text{H}_2\text{O}_2 \longrightarrow \cdot\mathbf{OH} + \text{OH}^- + {}^1\mathbf{O_2}$$

} Spontaneous formation of further microbicidal agents

$$\text{H}_2\text{O}_2 + \text{Cl}^- \xrightleftharpoons{\text{myeloperoxidase}} \mathbf{OCl}^- + \text{H}_2\text{O}$$

$$\text{OCl}^- + \text{H}_2\text{O} \qquad\qquad {}^1\mathbf{O} + \text{Cl}^- + \text{H}_2\text{O}$$

} Myeloperoxidase generation of micro-bicidal molecules

$$2\text{O}_2^- + 2\text{H}^+ \xrightarrow[\text{dismutase}]{\text{superoxide}} \text{O}_2 + \text{H}_2\text{O}_2$$

$$2\text{H}_2\text{O}_2 \xrightarrow{\text{catalase}} 2\text{H}_2\text{O} + \text{O}_2$$

} Protective mechanisms used by host + many microbes

Oxygen independent mechanisms:

Low pH (lactic acid formation)	Not a microbial paradise
Lysozyme	Splits mucopeptide in bacterial cell wall
Lactoferrin	Deprives bacteria of iron
Cationic proteins (leukin, phagocytin)	Damage to microbial membranes
Proteolytic enzymes (including elastase)	} Digestion of killed organisms
Variety of other hydrolytic enzymes	

* Microbicidal species in bold type.
O_2^-, superoxide anion; ${}^1\text{O}_2$, singlet (activated) oxygen; $\cdot\text{OH}$, hydroxyl free radical.

variety of proteolytic and other hydrolytic enzymes present are concerned in the digestion of the killed organisms.

To some extent there is an extracellular release of lysosomal constituents during phagocytosis which may play an amplifying role. The basic polypeptides, for example, stimulate an acute inflammatory reaction with increased vascular permeability, transudation of serum proteins and egress of leucocytes from blood vessels by diapedesis. The release of an endogenous pyrogen from the polymorphs may explain, in part

151

at least, the fever which often accompanies an infection and the output of acute phase proteins from liver.

It is clear then, that the phagocytic cells possess an impressive anti-microbial potential, but when an infectious agent gains access to the body, this formidable array of weaponry is useless until some way is found to enable the phagocyte to 'home onto' the micro-organism. The body has solved this problem with the effortless ease that comes with a few million years of evolution by developing the complement system.

THE ROLE OF COMPLEMENT

As we argued in chapter 6, the surface carbohydrates of many microbial species are able to activate the alternative pathway thereby generating C3 convertase activity The convertase now splits C3 to give C3b which binds tò the surface of the microbe, and the small peptide C3a which provides the answer we need through its ability to attract polymorphs (a later product of the sequence of C5a, has similar powers, cf. p. 140). The polymorphs move up the chemotactic C3a gradient until suddenly they come face to face with the C3b-coated micro-organisms to which they become attached by virtue of their surface C3b receptors so thoughtfully placed there by the subtle processes of evolution.

The formation of C3a and C5a (the anaphylatoxins) has

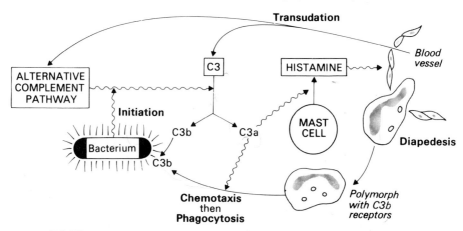

FIGURE 7.3. The role of complement in the defence against infection showing the consequences of activation of the alternative pathway by a bacterium, with generation of an *acute inflammatory reaction* involving increased vascular permeability through separation of capillary endothelial cells and an influx of polymorphs. C5a is also chemotactic and the terminal components C8 and C9 may be lytic.

further ramifications through their action on the mast cell which releases histamine and causes transudation of complement components and movement of polymorphs from the local blood vessels into the surrounding tissue providing the ingredients of an acute inflammatory reaction (figure 7.3).

Adherence to the surface of the phagocyte having been achieved, it remains only for the cell to be stimulated by its contact with the micro-organism for the ingestion phase to be initiated. How splendid—but what happens if the micro-organism should be of such physical and chemical constitution that it lacks the decency either: (a) to activate the alternative complement pathway, or (b) to be able to stimulate phagocytic ingestion? Once again the body has produced an ingenious solution: it has devised a variable adaptor molecule.

Acquired immunity

Looking at the problem teleologically (which usually gives the right answer for the wrong reasons), the body had to develop a molecule with the intrinsic ability to activate complement and phagocytosis but which could be adapted to stick onto any one of a host of different micro-organisms so that each would then become susceptible to the combined complement – phagocyte defence system. And lo and behold, it came to pass, and we marvelled and called it—ANTIBODY! An immunoglobulin of the appropriate class, e.g. human IgG1, activates complement by a separate pathway (classical) through binding C1q to its C_H2 domain thereby generating a C3 convertase; the C_H3 domain binds to specific Fc receptors on the phagocyte and presumably initiates ingestion (cf. figure 2.12, p. 33). The whole molecule is attached to the foreign invader through the antigen binding region of the variable domains, the body making sure of its defences by manufacturing antibody molecules with a wide range of combining specificities.

The B-lymphocyte system developed in order to produce antibodies, and by allowing each lymphocyte to synthesize only one type of antibody great flexibility could be introduced. Although there are sufficient lymphocytes to produce a wide range of different antibodies, it would be wasteful to maintain large numbers of lymphocytes capable of reacting with antigens which the body did not encounter. The system of clonal triggering and formation of memory cells ensures that the body only concentrates its main energies on antigens which it actually meets while retaining the potential to react against some obscure microbe which might infect the body at any time in the future. The ability to generate memory cells in response to a particular infection is, of course, the basis of *acquired* as distinct from *innate* immunity but it should be perfectly plain that antibody, as one agent of acquired immunity, acts to enhance the mechanisms of innate immunity.

Immunity to bacterial infection

ROLE OF HUMORAL ANTIBODY

Enhancing phagocytosis

Many virulent forms of bacteria resist engulfment by phagocytic cells: for example, encapsulated forms of pneumococci do not stick readily to these cells and virulent strains of staphylococci and streptococci elaborate antiphagocytic substances including certain toxins. In accord with our previous discussion, antibody has a dramatic effect on phagocytosis and the

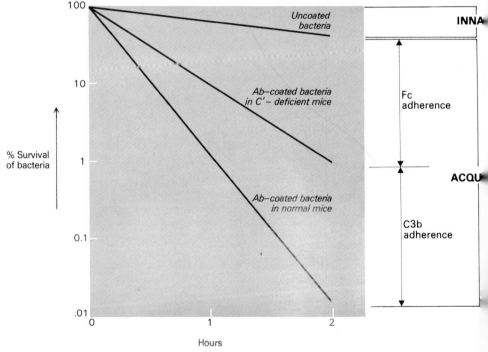

FIGURE 7.4. Effect of opsonizing antibody and complement on the rate of clearance of virulent bacteria from the blood. The uncoated bacteria are phagocytosed rather slowly (innate immunity) but on coating with antibody, adherence to phagocytes is increased many-fold (acquired immunity). The adherence is somewhat less effective in animals temporarily depleted of complement.

154

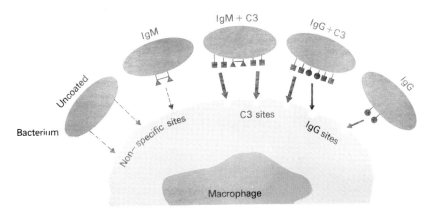

FIGURE 7.5. Immunoglobulin and complement coats greatly increase the adherence of bacteria (and other antigens) to macrophages and polymorphs. Uncoated or IgM (⊢⊣) coated bacteria adhere relatively weakly to non-specific sites but there are specific receptors for IgG (Fc) (◆) and C3 (◀) on the macrophage surface which considerably enhance the strength of binding. The augmenting effect of complement is due to the fact that two adjacent IgG molecules can fix many C3 molecules thereby increasing the number of links to the macrophage (cf. 'bonus' effect of multivalency; p. 14). Although IgM does not bind specifically to the macrophage, it promotes adherence through complement fixation.

rate of clearance of such organisms from the blood stream is strikingly enhanced when they are coated with specific Ig (figure 7.4). The less effective removal of coated bacteria in complement-depleted animals emphasizes the synergism between antibody and complement for 'opsonization' (cf. pp. 36 & 142) which is mediated through specific high affinity receptors for IgG and C3b on the phagocyte surface (figure 7.5). It is clearly advantageous that the subclasses which bind strongly to these Fc receptors (e.g. IgG1 and 3 in the human) also fix complement well.

Bacteria may also be captured by antibody already fixed to the Fc receptor site (cytophilic antibody) but it is probable that adherence is mediated more through opsonization than through the prior binding of cytophilic antibody to the phagocyte. Complexes containing C3 may show immune adherence to primate red cells and rabbit platelets to provide phagocytosable aggregates.

Some strains of Gram-negative bacteria which have a lipo-protein outer wall resembling mammalian surface membranes in structure are susceptible to the bactericidal action of fresh serum containing antibody. The antibody initiates the development of a complement-mediated lesion producing similar 'holes' to those caused by complement in mammalian

155

cells (figure 6.20); this allows access of serum lysozyme to the inner wall of the bacterium with resulting cell death. Activation of complement through union of antibody and bacterium will also generate the C3a and C5a anaphylatoxins leading to extensive transudation of serum components including more antibody, and to the chemotactic attraction of polymorphs to aid in phagocytosis. In other words the series of events described in figure 7.3 can be entirely recreated by substituting the antibody-initiated classical complement sequence in place of the alternative pathway.

Protecting external surfaces

IgA antibodies afford protection in the external body fluids, tears, saliva, nasal secretions and those bathing the surfaces of the intestine (so-called 'coproantibodies') and lung, by coating bacteria and viruses and preventing their adherence to mucosal surfaces. It might be anticipated that in order to fulfil this function, secretory IgA molecules would themselves have very little innate adhesiveness for cells and certainly no high affinity Fc receptors for this Ig class have yet been described. If an infectious agent succeeds in penetrating the IgA barrier, it comes up against the next line of defence of the MALT system (p. 75) which is manned by IgE. Although present in low concentration, IgE is bound very firmly to the Fc receptors of the mast cell (p. 190) and contact with antigen leads to the release of mediators which effectively recruit agents of the immune response. Thus histamine, by increasing vascular permeability, causes the transudation of IgG and complement into the area while chemotactic factors for neutrophils and eosinophils attract the effector cells needed to dispose of the infectious organism coated with specific IgG and C3b (figure 7.6). Where the opsonized organism is too large for phagocytosis, these cells can kill by an extracellular mechanism after attachment by their Fcγ receptors. This phenomenon, termed antibody-dependent cell-mediated cytotoxicity (ADCC) is discussed further in the following chapter but there is evidence for its involvement in parasitic infections. There are obvious parallels between the ways in which complement-derived anaphylatoxins and IgE utilize the mast cell to cause local amplification of the immune defences.

Toxin neutralization

In addition to their role in removal of microbes, circulating

156

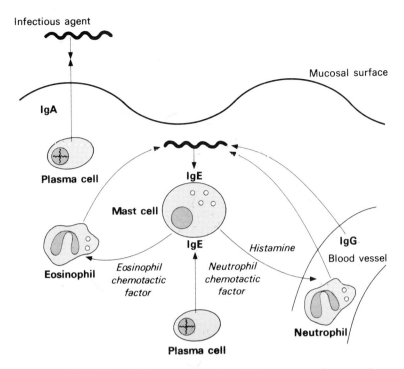

FIGURE 7.6. Defence of the mucosal surfaces. IgA prevents adherence of organisms to the mucosa. IgE recruits agents of the immune response by firing the release of mediators from mast cells.

antibodies act to neutralize the soluble exotoxins (e.g. phospholipase C of *Clostridium welchii*) released by bacteria. Combination near the biologically active site of the toxin would stereochemically block reaction with the substrate, particularly if it were macromolecular; combination distant from the active site may also cause inhibition through allosteric conformational changes. In its complex with antibody, the toxin may be unable to diffuse away rapidly and will be susceptible to phagocytosis, especially if the complex can be increased in size by the action of naturally occurring antibodies to altered IgG (antiglobulin factors) and altered C3 (immunoconglutinin).

Specific organisms

Let us see how these considerations apply to the defence against infection by common organisms such as streptococci and staphylococci. β-Haemolytic streptococci were classified by Lancefield according to their carbohydrate antigen and the most important from the standpoint of human disease are those belonging to group A. However the most immunogenic surface

157

component is the M-protein (variants of which form the basis of the Griffith typing). This protein inhibits phagocytosis and the protection afforded by antibodies to the M-component is attributable to the striking increase in phagocytosis which they induce. High titred antibodies to the streptolysin O exotoxin (ASO) are indicative of recent streptococcal infection. The erythrogenic toxin elaborated by strains which give rise to scarlet fever is neutralized by antibody and the erythematous intradermal reaction to the injected toxin is only seen in individuals lacking antibody (Dick reaction).

Virulent forms of staphylococci, of which *S. aureus* is perhaps the most common, resist phagocytosis. This may be due partly to capsule formation *in vivo* and partly to the elaboration of factors such as protein A which combines with the Fc portion of IgG (except for subclass IgG3) and inhibits binding to the polymorph Fc receptor. *S. aureus* is readily phagocytosed in the presence of adequate amounts of antibody but a small proportion of the ingested bacteria survive and they are difficult organisms to eliminate completely. Where the infection is inadequately controlled, severe lesions may occur in the immunized host as a consequence of type IV delayed hypersensitivity reactions. Thus, staphylococci were found to be avirulent when injected into mice passively immunized with antibody but caused extensive tissue damage in animals previously given sensitized T-cells (Glynn).

IgA produced in genital secretions in response to gonococcal infection appears to be capable of inhibiting the attachment of the organisms, through their pili, to mucosal cells. Nonetheless, such antibody does not protect against reinfection, perhaps due to the ability of gonococcal protease to split IgA dimers, or to the existence of multiple non-cross-reacting serotypes.

ROLE OF CELL-MEDIATED IMMUNITY
(CMI)

Some strains of bacteria such as the tubercle and leprosy bacilli, and listeria and brucella organisms, are able to live and continue their growth within the cytoplasm of macrophages after their uptake by phagocytosis. In an elegant series of experiments, Mackaness has demonstrated the importance of CMI reactions for the killing of these intracellular facultative parasites and the establishment of an immune state. Animals infected with moderate doses of *M. tuberculosis* overcome the infection and are immune to subsequent challenge with the bacillus. Surprisingly, if they are given an unrelated organism such as *Listeria monocytogenes* at *the same time* as the second infection with tubercle bacillus, they are resistant and can kill the listeria which have been engulfed by macrophages. Without the prior immunity to *M. tuberculosis* or the second challenge with this organism, the animal would have succumbed to listeria infection. In the same way, an animal immune to listeria can rapidly kill tubercle bacilli given at the same time as a second infection with listeria (table 7.2). Thus the triggering of a specific secondary immune response to one organism may endow the animal with a simultaneous but transient non-specific resistance to unrelated microbes of similar growth habits.

TABLE 7.2. Induction of non-specific immunity by a CMI reaction

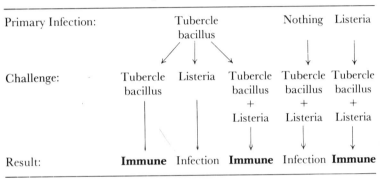

Primary Infection:	Tubercle bacillus			Nothing	Listeria
Challenge:	Tubercle bacillus	Listeria	Tubercle bacillus + Listeria	Tubercle bacillus + Listeria	Tubercle bacillus + Listeria
Result:	**Immune**	Infection	**Immune**	Infection	**Immune**

Immunity—both specific and non-specific—can be transferred to a normal recipient with lymphocytes but not macrophages or serum from an immune animal (figure 7.7). This strongly suggests that the specific immunity is mediated by T-cells. In support of this view is the greater susceptibility to infection with tubercle and leprosy bacilli of mice in which the T-lymphocytes have been depressed by thymectomy plus anti-lymphocyte serum.

The intracellular organisms survive because they are able to thwart the killing mechanisms of the host macrophage. During a CMI reaction when sensitized T-lymphocytes are stimulated by contact with specific antigen, one of the many soluble factors released (e.g. MAF—p. 70) confers on these macrophages the power to kill the ingested organisms and it may be relevant to note that the oxygen-dependent microbicidal systems of such cells are enhanced. Thus the specificity lies at the level of the initial reaction of T-cell with its antigen; the non-specific initial reaction of the T-cell with its antigen; the non-specific

159

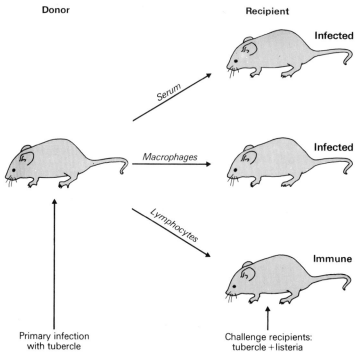

Donor   Recipient

Infected

Serum

Infected

Macrophages

Lymphocytes

Immune

Primary infection
with tubercle

Challenge recipients:
tubercle + listeria

FIGURE 7.7. Transfer of specific and non-specific immunity by lymphocytes from an immune animal. The syngeneic recipient of the lymphocytes resisted simultaneous challenge with tubercle and listeria organisms. The recipients were not immune to listeria given without the tubercle. The lymphocytes lost their power to confer passive immunity on the recipients if treated with a cytotoxic anti-T cell serum plus complement prior to injection. Serum or macrophages were ineffective in transferring immunity. (After Mackaness.)

macrophage to kill almost *any* organism it has phagocytosed (figure 7.8).

Where the host has difficulty in effectively eliminating such organisms, the chronic CMI response to locally released antigen leads to the accumulation of densely packed macrophages which release fibrogenic factors and stimulate the formation of granulation tissue and ultimately fibrosis. The resulting structure, termed a granuloma, represents an attempt by the body to isolate a site of persistent infection.

Immunity to viral infection

Genetically controlled constitutional factors which render a host or certain of his cells non-permissive (i.e. resistant to takeover of their replicative machinery by virus) play a dominant role in influencing the vulnerability of a given individual to infection. Macrophages may readily take up

160

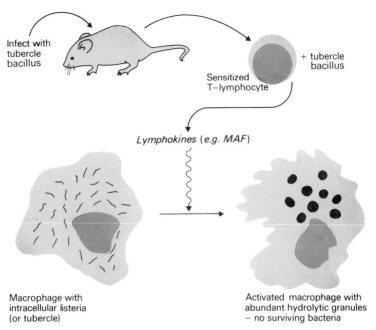

Infect with
tubercle
bacillus

Sensitized
T–lymphocyte

+ tubercle
bacillus

Lymphokines (e.g. MAF)

Macrophage with
intracellular listeria
(or tubercle)

Activated macrophage with
abundant hydrolytic granules
– no surviving bacteria

FIGURE 7.8. Macrophage killing of intracellular bacteria triggered by specific cell-mediated immunity reaction.

viruses non-specifically and kill them. However, in some instances the macrophages allow replication and if the virus is capable of producing cytopathic effects in various organs, the infection may be lethal; with non-cytopathic agents such as lymphocytic choriomeningitis, Aleutian mink disease and equine infectious anaemia viruses, a persistent infection will result.

PROTECTION BY SERUM ANTIBODY

The antibody molecule can neutralize viruses by a variety of means. It may stereochemically inhibit combination with the receptor site on cells thereby preventing penetration and subsequent intracellular multiplication, the protective effect of antibodies to influenza viral neuraminidase providing a good example. It may lyse a virus particle directly through activation of the classical complement pathway or lead to aggregation, enhanced phagocytosis and intracellular death by mechanisms already discussed.

Relatively low concentrations of circulating antibody can be effective and one is familiar with the protection afforded by poliomyelitis antibodies, and by human γ-globulin given prophylactically to individuals exposed to measles. The most clear-cut protection is seen in diseases with long incubation times where the virus has to travel through the blood stream before it reaches the tissue which it finally infects. For example, in poliomyelitis the virus gains access to the body via the gastrointestinal tract and eventually passes through the circulation to reach the brain cells which become infected. Within the blood, the virus is neutralized by quite low levels of specific antibody while the prolonged period before the virus infects the brain allows time for a secondary immune response in a primed host.

LOCAL FACTORS

With other viral diseases, such as influenza and the common cold, there is a short incubation time related to the fact that the final target organ for the virus is the same as the portal of entry and no intermediate stage involving passage through the body occurs. There is little time for a primary antibody response to be mounted and in all likelihood the rapid production of interferon is the most significant mechanism used to counter the viral infection. Experimental studies certainly indicate that after an early peak of interferon production, there is a rapid fall in the titre of live virus in the lungs of mice infected with influenza

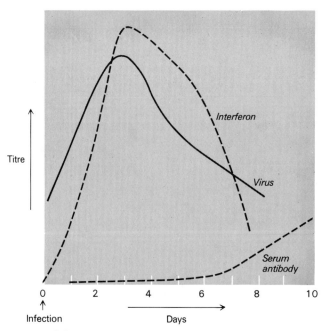

FIGURE 7.9. Appearance of interferon and serum antibody in relation to recovery from influenza virus infection of the lungs of mice. (From Isaacs A. (1961) *New Sci.*, **11**, 81.)

(figure 7.9). Antibody, as assessed by the *serum* titre, seems to arrive on the scene much too late to be of value in aiding recovery. However, recent investigations have shown that antibody levels may be elevated in the *local* fluids bathing the infected surfaces, e.g. nasal mucosa and lung, despite low serum titres and it is the production of antiviral antibody (most prominently IgA) by locally deployed immunologically primed cells which may prove to be of great importance for the *prevention* of subsequent infection. Unfortunately, in so far as the common cold is concerned, a subsequent infection is likely to involve an antigenically unrelated virus so that general immunity to colds is difficult to achieve.

CELL-MEDIATED IMMUNITY

Local or systemic antibodies can block the spread of cytolytic viruses but alone they are usually inadequate to control those viruses which modify the antigens of the cell membrane and bud off from the surface as infectious particles. Included in this group are: oncorna (=oncogenic RNA virus, e.g. murine leukaemogenic), orthomyxo (influenza), paramyxo (mumps, measles) toga (dengue), rhabdo (rabies), arena (lymphocytic choriomeningitis), adeno, herpes (simplex, varicella, zoster, cytomegalo, Epstein-Barr, Marek's disease), pox (vaccinia), papova (SV40, polyoma) and rubella viruses. The importance of cell-mediated immunity for recovery from infection with these agents is underlined by the inability of children with primary T-cell immunodeficiency to cope with such viruses whereas patients with Ig deficiency but intact cell-mediated immunity are not troubled in this way.

T-lymphocytes from a sensitized host are directly cytotoxic to cells infected with viruses from this group, the new surface antigens on the target cells being recognized by specific receptors on the aggressor lymphocytes. Strikingly, these lymphocytes are not cytotoxic for cells infected with the same virus but carrying different major histocompatibility antigens (cf. figure 9.12, p. 234). The sensitized T-cells must therefore recognize: (a) virally modified histocompatibility antigen, (b) a complex of histocompatibility antigen with virally associated antigen, or (c) *both* virally associated *and* self-histocompatibility antigens.

This direct attack on the cell will effectively limit the infection if the surface antigen changes appear before full replication of the virus, otherwise the organism will spread by two major routes. The first, involving free infectious viral particles released by budding from the surface, can normally be checked by humoral antibody. The second, which depends upon the passage of virus from one cell to another across intercellular junctions, cannot be influenced by antibody but is countered by cell-mediated immunity. Macrophages, attracted to the site by chemotactic factors released by the interaction of T-cells with virally associated antigen, appear to discourage the formation of these intercellular bridges, a capability which may be enhanced by other T-cell lymphokines such as macrophage-activating factor. Furthermore, γ-interferon, produced either by the reacting T-cell itself or by the lymphokine-stimulated macrophage will render the contiguous cells non-permissive for

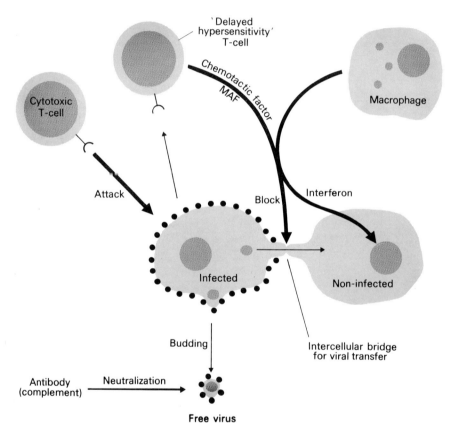

FIGURE 7.10. Control of infection by 'budding' viruses. Cytotoxic T-cells kill virally infected targets directly after recognition of new surface antigen (—•—•—•—). Interaction with a separate sub-population of T-cells releases lymphokines which attract macrophages to inhibit intercellular virus transfer and prime contiguous uninfected cells with interferon. Free virus released by budding from the cell surface is neutralized by antibody (which if thymus-dependent points to yet another contribution by the T-cell to viral immunity).

164

the replication of any virus acquired by intercellular transfer (figure 7.10). It may also increase the non-specific cytotoxicity of NK cells (p. 239) for infected cells. The generation of 'immune interferon' in response to non-nucleic acid viral components provides a valuable back-up mechanism when dealing with viruses which are intrinsically poor stimulators of interferon synthesis.

The neutralization of free virus particles by antibody is relatively straightforward but the interaction with infected cells is rather more complex. Access to the surface antigens by T-cells would be denied were they blocked by coating with antibody. Nonetheless, these antibodies should be able to initiate type II hypersensitivity reactions. Antibody-dependent cell mediated cytotoxicity (ADCC; p. 193) has been reported with herpes and mumps-infected target cells while Oldstone has described the complement-mediated killing of measles infected cells by $F(ab')_2$ antibody fragments via the alternative pathway (? suggesting a role for the C_H1 domain as an initiator of this sequence). Antibody may play a different tune, however, since in the case of measles-infected cells, although 10^6 antibody molecules per cell permit complement-mediated cytotoxicity, 10^5 molecules do not kill but cause capping and shedding of surface antigen (cf. p. 62) leaving the cell resistant to attack by any immunological mechanism.

Prophylaxis

The control of infection is approached from several directions. One method of breaking the chain of infection has been achieved in the U.K. with rabies and psittacosis by controlling the importation of dogs and parrots respectively. Improvements in public health—water supply, sewerage systems, education in personal hygiene—prevent the spread of cholera and many other diseases. And of course when other measures fail we can fall back on the induction of immunity.

PASSIVELY ACQUIRED IMMUNITY

Temporary protection against infection can be established by giving preformed antibody from another individual of the same or a different species. As the acquired antibodies are utilized by combination with antigen or catabolized in the normal way, this protection is gradually lost.

165

Homologous antibodies

Maternal. In the first few months of life while the baby's own lymphoid system is slowly getting under way, protection is afforded by maternally derived antibodies acquired by placental transfer and by intestinal absorption of colostral immunoglobulins.

γ-Globulin. Preparations of pooled human adult γ-globulin are of value to modify the effects of chicken pox or measles, particularly in individuals with defective immune responses such as premature infants, children with primary immunodeficiency or protein malnutrition or patients on steroid treatment. Contacts with cases of infectious hepatitis and smallpox may also be afforded protection by γ-globulin, especially when in the latter case the material is derived from the serum of individuals vaccinated some weeks previously. Human anti-tetanus immunoglobulin is preferable to horse antitoxin which can cause serum reactions.

Heterologous antibodies

Horse globulins containing anti-tetanus and anti-diphtheria toxins have been extensively employed prophylactically, but at the present time the practice is more restricted because of the complication of serum sickness developing in response to the foreign protein. This is more likely to occur in subjects already sensitized by previous contact with horse globulin; thus individuals who have been given horse anti-tetanus (e.g. for immediate protection after receiving a wound out in the open) are later advised to undergo a course of active immunization to obviate the need for further injections of horse protein in any subsequent emergency.

ACTIVE IMMUNIZATION

In the case of tetanus, immunization is of benefit to the individual but not to the community since it will not eliminate the organism which is formed in the faeces of domestic animals and persists in the soil as highly resistant spores. Where a disease depends on human transmission, immunity in just a proportion of the population can help the whole community if it leads to a fall in the reproduction rate (i.e. the number of further cases produced by each infected individual) to less than one; under these circumstances the disease will die out, witness for example the disappearance of diphtheria from communities in which around 75% of the children have been immunized.

166

The objective of vaccination is to provide effective immunity by establishing adequate levels of antibody and a primed population of cells which can rapidly expand on renewed contact with antigen. The first contact with antigen during vaccination obviously should not be injurious and the manoeuvre is to modify the pathogenic effect without losing important antigens:

(1) *Toxoids.* Bacterial exotoxins such as those produced by diphtheria and tetanus bacilli can be successfully detoxified by formaldehyde treatment without destroying the major immunogenic determinants (figure 7.11). Immunization with the *toxoid* will therefore provoke the formation of protective anti-

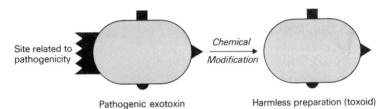

FIGURE 7.11. Modification of toxin to harmless toxoid without losing many of the antigenic determinants (■●▲). Thus antibodies to the toxoid will react well with the original toxin. Utilizing a similar principle, microorganisms can be rendered harmless by killing or attenuating to non-virulent but still living forms.

bodies which neutralize the toxin by stereochemically blocking the active site and encourage removal by phagocytic cells. The toxoid is generally given after adsorption to aluminium hydroxide which acts as an adjuvant and produces higher antibody titres.

(2) *Killed organisms.* Dead bacteria and viruses which have been inactivated provide a safe antigen for immunization. Examples are typhoid (in combination with the relatively ineffective paratyphoid A and B), cholera and killed poliomyelitis (Salk) vaccines. The success of the Salk vaccine was slightly marred by a small rise in the incidence and deaths from poliomyelitis in 1960–1 (figure 7.12) but this has now been attributed to poor antigenicity of one of the three different strains of virus used and present-day vaccines are far more potent. In other instances, the immunity conferred by killed vaccines, even when given with adjuvant (see below), is often inferior to that resulting from infection with live organisms. This must be partly because the replication of the living

167

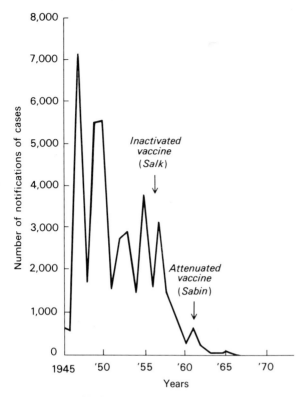

FIGURE 7.12. Notifications of paralytic poliomyelitis in England and Wales showing the beneficial effects of community immunization with killed and live vaccines. (Reproduced from Dick (1978), with kind permission of author and publishers.)

microbes confronts the host with a larger and more sustained dose of antigen and that with budding viruses, infected cells are required for the establishment of good cytotoxic T-cell memory. Another significant advantage is that the immune response takes place largely at the site of the natural infection. As an example cholera infection will be most efficiently dealt with by antibodies produced locally by the gut wall ('copro-antibodies') yet injected *killed* vaccine may stimulate antibody synthesis in the spleen and perhaps many lymph nodes without initiating an adequate response in the intestinal lymphoid system. Ideally immunity would be best established by infection with a modified but live (attenuated) form of cholera bacillus which would multiply at the site of the natural infection without producing disease. This is well illustrated by the nasopharyngeal IgA response to immunization with polio vaccine. In contrast with the ineffectiveness of parenteral injection of killed vaccine, intranasal administration evoked a good local antibody response; but whereas this declined over a period of

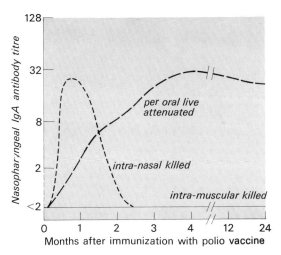

FIGURE 7.13. Local IgA response to polio vaccine. Local secretory antibody synthesis is confined to the specific anatomical sites which have been directly stimulated by contact with antigen. (Data from Ogra *et al*. In *Viral Immunology and Immunopathology*, p. 67. Notkins A.L. (ed.). Academic Press, London.)

two months or so, per oral immunization with *live attenuated* virus established a persistently high IgA antibody level (figure 7.13).

(3) *Attenuated organisms*. Pasteur first achieved the production of live but non-virulent forms of chicken cholera bacillus and anthrax by such artifices as culture at higher temperatures and under anaerobic conditions, and was able to confer immunity by infection with the attenuated organisms. A virulent strain of *Mycobacterium tuberculosis* became attenuated by chance in 1908 when Calmette and Guérin at the Institut Pasteur, Lille, added bile to the culture medium in an attempt to achieve dispersed growth. After 13 years of culture in bile-containing medium, the strain remained attenuated and was used successfully to vaccinate children against tuberculosis. The same organism, BCG (Bacille, Calmette, Guérin), is widely used today for immunization of tuberculin negative individuals; it may also bestow a reasonable degree of protection against *Mycobacterium leprae*.

Attenuated vaccines for poliomyelitis (Sabin), measles and rubella have gained general acceptance.

Adjuvants

For practical and economic reasons prophylactic immunization should involve the minimum number of injections and the least amount of antigen. We have referred to the undoubted advantages of replicating attenuated organisms in this respect but non-living organisms frequently require an adjuvant which by definition is a substance incorporated into or injected simultaneously with antigen which potentiates the immune response (L *adjuvare*—to help). The mode of action of adjuvants may be considered under several headings:

(1) *Depot effects.* Free antigen usually disperses rapidly from the local tissues draining the injection site and an important function of the so-called repository adjuvants is to counteract this by providing a long-lived reservoir of antigen, either at an extracellular location or within macrophages. The most common adjuvants of this type used in man are aluminium compounds (phosphate and hydroxide) and Freund's incomplete adjuvant (in which the antigen is incorporated in the aqueous phase of a stabilized water in paraffin oil emulsion). Both types increase the antibody response but the emulsions tend to produce higher and far more sustained antibody levels with a broadening of the response to include more of the epitopes in the antigen preparation.

(2) *Macrophage activation.* Under the influence of the repository adjuvants, macrophages form granulomata which provide sites for interaction with antibody-forming cells. The maintenance by the depot of consistent antigen concentrations, particularly on the macrophage surface, ensures that as antigen-sensitive cells divide within the granuloma, their progeny are highly likely to be further stimulated by antigen. Virtually all adjuvants stimulate macrophages, the majority probably through direct action, but complete Freund's adjuvant appears to act on the macrophage through the T-cell (cf. p. 84; it will be recalled that complete Freund's is made from the incomplete adjuvant by addition of killed mycobacterium, or more recently the water soluble muramyl dipeptide, MDP, isolated from its active components). The activated macrophages are thought to act by improving immunogenicity through an increase in the amount of antigen on their surface and the efficiency of its presentation to lymphocytes, by the provision of accessory signals to direct lymphocytes towards an immune response rather than tolerance, and by the secretion of soluble stimulatory factors (e.g. interleukin I) which influence the proliferation of lymphocytes.

(3) *Specific effects on lymphocytes.* The immunopotentiating and

other effects of the mycobacterial component in complete Freund are so striking that their use in man is not normally countenanced; enhancement of T-cell function is seen in helper activity, delayed type hypersensitivity and the production of autoimmune disease. In man, BCG is a potent stimulator of T,B and reticuloendothelial cell activity. Levamisole boosts delayed hypersensitivity while polyanions such as poly A:U, and the fungal polysaccharide lentinan, promote T-helper cells. By contrast, bacterial lipopolysaccharide and polyanions such as dextran sulphate are B-cell mitogens with a preferential effect on $B\mu$ cells.

(4) *Anti-tumour action.* This will be discussed in chapter 9 but one may summarize by saying that the major effect is mediated through a cytostatic action of activated macrophages on tumours with the stimulation of specific T-cell immunity to the tumour antigens as a further possibility.

Recent interest has centred on the use of small lipid membrane vesicles (liposomes) as agents for the presentation of antigen to the immune system. It may be that the liposome acts as a storage vacuole within the macrophage or perhaps fuses with the macrophage membrane to provide a suitably immunogenic complex. One envisages the possibility of selecting the type of lymphocyte activated by incorporating accessory signalling agents into the liposome membrane, e.g. MDP derivatives, polyanions or levamisole to stimulate T-cells, components of ascaris or *Bordetella pertussis* to exaggerate IgE production, T-cell soluble factors for the triggering of Bγ cells, C3b for homing to lymph node follicles and so on.

Some general problems

Vigorous public health immunization programmes have virtually eliminated diseases like diphtheria and poliomyelitis from many communities (figures 7.12 & 7.14), while a global effort by the World Health Organisation combining widespread vaccination and selective epidemiological control methods, has eradicated smallpox. With certain vaccines there is a very small, but still real, risk of developing complications such as the encephalitis which can occur following rabies or measles immunization. With live viral vaccines there is a possibility that the nucleic acid might be incorporated into the host's genome or that the strain may revert to a virulent form, although to some extent this latter eventuality can be countered by injection of appropriate antiserum. Another disadvantage of

171

attenuated strains is the difficulty and expense of maintaining appropriate cold storage facilities. In diseases such as viral hepatitis and cancer, the dangers associated with live vaccines would make their use unthinkable. Generally speaking, the risk of complication must be balanced against the expected chance of contracting the disease. Where this is minimal some may prefer to avoid general vaccination and to rely upon a crash course backed up if necessary by passive immunization in the localities around isolated outbreaks of infectious disease.

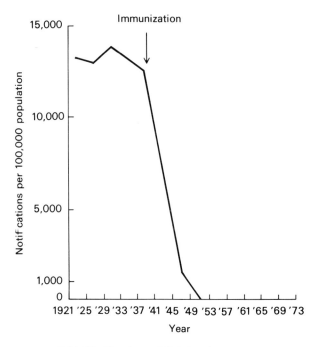

FIGURE 7.14. Notifications of diphtheria in England and Wales per 100,000 population showing a dramatic fall after immunization. (Reproduced from Dick (1978), with kind permission of author and publishers.)

It is important to recognize those children with immuno-deficiency before injection of live organisms; a child with impaired T-cell reactivity can become overwhelmed by BCG and die. Perhaps this is only a sick story, but it is said that in one particular country there are no adults with T-cell deficiency. The reason? All children had been immunized with live BCG as part of a community health programme(!) The extent to which children with partial deficiencies are at risk has yet to be assessed. It is also inadvisable to give live vaccines to patients being treated with steroids, immuno-suppressive drugs or radiotherapy or who have malignant conditions such as

172

TABLE 7.3. Classification of immunodeficiency states with examples

Deficiency	Example	Immune response		Infection	Treatment
		Humoral	Cellular		
Comple-ment	C$_3$ deficiency	Normal	Normal	Pyogenic bacteria	Antibiotics
Myeloid cell	Chronic granulo-matous disease	Normal	Normal	Catalase-positive bacteria	Antibiotics
B-cell	Infantile sex-linked a-γ-globulinaemia (Bruton)	↓↓	Normal	Pyogenic bacteria Pneumocystis carinii	γ-Globulin
T-cell	Thymic hypoplasia (DiGeorge)	↓	↓↓	Certain viruses Candida	Thymus graft
Stem cell	Severe combined deficiency (Swiss-type)	↓↓	↓↓	All the above	Bone marrow graft

lymphoma and leukaemia; pregnant mothers must also be included here because of the vulnerability of the fetus.

Primary immunodeficiency

In accord with the dictum that 'most things that can go wrong, do', a multiplicity of immunodeficiency states in man have been recognized. These are classified in table 7.3 together with some of the most clear-cut (and correspondingly rare) examples. We have earlier stressed the manner in which the interplay of complement, antibody and phagocytic cells constitutes the basis of a tripartite defence mechanism against pyogenic (pus-forming) infections with bacteria which require prior opsoniza-tion before phagocytosis. It is not surprising then, that deficiency in any one of these factors may predispose the individual to repeated infections of this type. Patients with T-cell deficiency of course present a markedly different pattern of infection, being susceptible to those viruses and moulds which are normally eradicated by cell-mediated immunity.

A relatively high incidence of malignancies and of auto-antibodies with or without autoimmune disease, have been documented in patients with immunodeficiency but the reason for this association is not yet clear, although failure of T-cell regulation or inability to control key viral infections are among the suggestions canvassed.

In chronic granulomatous disease the monocytes and polymorphs fail to produce hydrogen peroxide due to a defect in the
NADPH oxidase normally activated by phagocytosis. Many
bacteria oblige by generating H_2O_2 through their own
metabolic processes but if they are catalase positive, the
peroxide is destroyed and the bacteria will survive. Thus,
polymorphs from these patients readily take up catalase
positive staphylococci in the presence of antibody and
complement but fail to kill them intracellularly. In Chediak–
Higashi disease (what a lovely name!), the lysosomes are
structurally and functionally abnormal and the patients suffer
from pyogenic infections which can be fatal. Among other rare
conditions, myeloperoxidase deficiency is associated with
susceptibility to systemic candidiasis, while a defective
polymorph response to chemotactic stimuli characterizes the
lazy leucocyte syndrome.

Defects in complement, the other major components of the
innate system, were dealt with in chapter 6.

B-cell deficiency

In Bruton's congenital agamma globulinaemia the production
of immunoglobulin in affected males is grossly depressed and
there are few lymphoid follicles or plasma cells in lymph node
biopsies. The children are subject to repeated infection by
pyogenic bacteria—*Staphylococcus aureus, Streptococcus pyogenes*
and *pneumoniae, Neisseria meningitidis, Haemophilus influenzae*—
and by a rare protozoon, *Pneumocystis carinii*, which produces a
strange form of pneumonia. Cell-mediated immune responses
are normal and viral infections such as measles and smallpox
are readily brought under control. Therapy involves repeated
administration of human γ-globulin to maintain adequate
concentrations of circulating immunoglobulin.

IgA deficiency is encountered with relative frequency and
these patients often have detectable antibodies to IgA. It is
uncertain whether these antibodies prevented development of
the IgA system or whether lack of tolerance resulting from an
absent IgA system allowed the body to make antibodies to
exogenous determinants immunologically related to IgA.

The most common form of immunodeficiency, late onset
hypogammaglobulaemia (also known as common, variable
immunodeficiency), probably includes many entities. The
marrow contains normal numbers of immature B-cells, but a

third of the patients lack circulating B-cells with surface Ig and of the remainder, half have subnormal numbers. Where present they are unable to differentiate to plasma cells in some cases or to secrete antibody in others. T-cells are also affected however; each lymphocyte has a low surface 5-nucleotidase, the T_M cells lack the characteristic non-specific esterase spot, around 30% have poor responses to PHA and a small proportion have marked suppressor activity for B-cells. Thus there are maturation defects in the lymphocyte populations which affect B-cell performance predominantly.

Immunoglobulin deficiency occurs naturally in human infants as the maternal IgG level wanes and may become a serious problem in very premature babies.

T-cell deficiency

The DiGeorge and Nezelof syndromes are characterized by a failure of the thymus to develop properly from the third and fourth pharyngeal pouches during embryogenesis (DiGeorge children also lack parathyroids and have severe cardiovascular abnormalities). Consequently, stem cells cannot differentiate to become T-lymphocytes and the 'thymus dependent' areas in lymphoid tissue are sparsely populated; in contrast lymphoid follicles are seen but even these are poorly developed (figure 7.15). Cell-mediated immune responses are undetectable and although the infants can deal with common bacterial infections they may be overwhelmed by vaccinia or measles, or by BCG if given by mistake. Humoral antibodies can be elicited but the response is subnormal presumably reflecting the need for the co-operative involvement of T-cells. (The similarity of this condition to neonatal thymectomy and of B-cell deficiency to neonatal bursectomy in the chicken should not go unmentioned.) Treatment by grafting neonatal thymus leads to restoration of immunocompetence but unless graft and donor are well matched, the thymus is ultimately rejected by the ungrateful host cells it has helped to maturity; in any event, some matching between the major histocompatibility antigens on the non-lymphocytic thymus cells and peripheral cells is essential for the proper functioning of the T-lymphocytes (p. 235).

Complete absence of the thymus is pretty rare and more often one is dealing with a 'partial DiGeorge' in which the T-cells may rise from 6% at birth to around 30% of the total circulating lymphocytes by the end of the first year; antibody responses are adequate. Selective T-cell depression can arise from deficiency

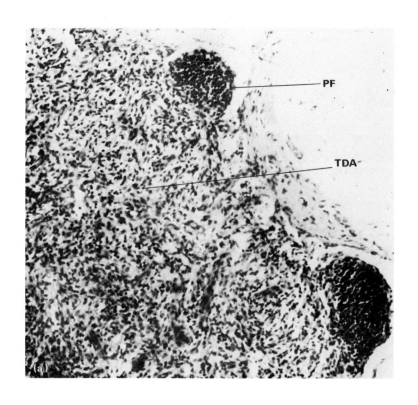

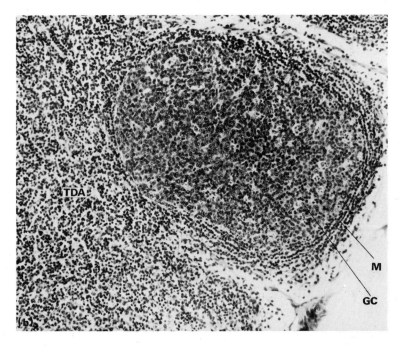

in the enzyme, purine nucleoside phosphorylase. Their poor T-cell responses make them especially susceptible to infection with varicella and vaccinia viruses but despite having less than 10% circulating T-cells, they have normal B-cell immunity suggesting that T-B collaboration can operate at much lower T-cell levels in the human than in the mouse.

Cell-mediated immunity is depressed in immunodeficient patients with ataxia telangiectasia or with thrombocytopenia and eczema (Wiskott-Aldrich syndrome) and it is of great interest that in both conditions about 10% of the patients so far studied have died of malignancies of the lymphoid system or of epithelial tumours. Wiskott-Aldrich is associated with a low IgM and poor antibody responses to many polysaccharides; evidence that a vital defect in macrophage presentation of antigen underlies the disorder has been presented. The concomitant lack of IgE with IgA may be partly responsible for the greater susceptibility to upper respiratory infections in ataxia telangiectasia as compared with individuals deficient in IgA alone. Treatment by injection of transfer factor has been attempted and some success reported.

Isolated cases of T-cell deficiency have been described where the serum contains a lymphocytotoxic antibody which presumably must be selective for T- rather than B-lymphocytes.

Stem-cell deficiency

Without proper differentiation of the common lymphoid stem cell, both T- and B-lymphocytes will fail to develop and there will be a severe combined immunodeficiency of cellular and humoral responses. Normal immune function can be established in the children by grafting with histocompatible bone marrow from a sibling. Cells from other donors too readily initiate a potentially lethal graft-vs-host reaction (cf. p. 220) even when reasonably well-matched, unless steps are first taken to rid the graft of any immunocompetent T-lymphocytes. Some patients lack the enzyme adenosine deaminase which affects both B- and T-cells but predominantly the latter. Half the patients do well on transfusions of normal red cells containing the enzyme whereas others with a longer-standing more severe

---

FIGURE 7.15. Lymph node cortex. (a) From patient with DiGeorge syndrome showing depleted thymus-dependent area (TDA) and small primary follicles (PF); (b) from a normal subject: the populated T-cell area and the well-developed secondary follicle with its mantle of small lymphocytes (M) and pale staining germinal centre (GC) provide a marked contrast. (DiGeorge material kindly supplied by Dr D. Webster; photograph by Mr C.J. Sym.)

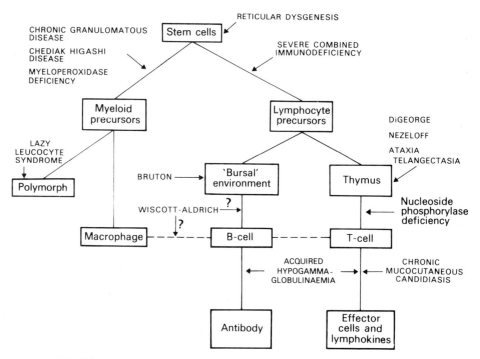

FIGURE 7.16. The cellular basis of immunodeficiency. The arrow indicates the cell type or differentiation process which is defective.

deficiency which might have affected the thymus epithelium, also require treatment with thymic extracts (thymosin).

The rapidly fatal variant of severe combined immuno-deficiency associated with lack of myeloid cell precursors is termed reticular dysgenesis. An attempt has been made to summarize the cellular basis of the various deficiency states in figure 7.16.

Recognition of immunodeficiencies

Defects in immunoglobulins can be assessed by quantitative estimations; levels of 200 mg/100 ml arbitrarily define the practical lower limit of normal. The humoral immune response can be examined by first screening the serum for natural antibodies (A and B isohaemagglutinins, heteroantibody to sheep red cells, bactericidins against *E. coli*) and then attempting to induce active immunization with diphtheria, tetanus, pertussis and killed poliomyelitis — but no live vaccines.

Patients with T-cell deficiency will be hypo- or unreactive in skin tests to such antigens as tuberculin, candida, tricophytin, streptokinase/streptodornase and mumps. Active skin sensitization with dinitrochlorobenzene may be undertaken. The reactivity of peripheral blood mononuclear cells to phyto-haemagglutinin is a good indicator of T-lymphocyte reactivity as is also the one-way mixed lymphocyte reaction (see chapter 9). Enumeration of T-cells is most readily achieved by counting the number of cells forming spontaneous rosettes with sheep erythrocytes (cf. p. 55).

In vitro tests for complement and for the bactericidal and other functions of polymorphs are available while the reduction of nitroblue tetrazolium (NBT) provides a measure of the oxidative enzymes associated with active phagocytosis.

SECONDARY IMMUNODEFICIENCY

Immune responsiveness can be depressed non-specifically by many factors. Cell-mediated immunity in particular may be impaired in a state of malnutrition even of the degree which may be encountered in urban areas of the more affluent regions of the world. Iron deficiency is particularly important in this respect.

Viral infections are not infrequently immunosuppressive and in the case of measles in man this has been attributed to a direct cytotoxic effect of virus on lymphoid cells.

Many agents such as X-rays, cytotoxic drugs and cortico-steroids, although often used in a non-immunological context, can nonetheless have dire effects on the immune system (p. 228). B-lymphoproliferative disorders like chronic lymphatic leukaemia, myeloma and Waldenström's macroglobulinaemia are associated with varying degrees of hypo-γ-globulinaemia and impaired antibody responses. Their common infections with pyogenic bacteria contrast with the situation in Hodgkin's disease where the patients display all the hallmarks of defective cell-mediated immunity—susceptibility to tubercle bacillus, brucella, cryptococcus and herpes zoster virus.

Summary

Micro-organisms are kept out of the body by the skin, the secretion of mucous, ciliary action, the lavaging action of bactericidal fluids (e.g. tears), gastric acid and microbial antagonism. If penetration occurs, bacteria are destroyed by soluble factors such as lysozyme and by phagocytosis with intracellular digestion. By activating the alternative comp-lement pathway, phagocytic cells are attracted to the bacteria which adhere to the C3b receptors and are engulfed if they activate the surface of the polymorph. Complement activation

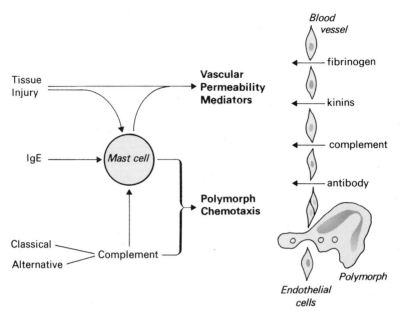

FIGURE 7.17. Production of a protective acute inflammatory reaction by microbes either: (a) through tissue injury (e.g. bacterial toxin) or direct activation of the alternative complement pathway; or (b) by antibody-dependent triggering of the classical complement pathway or mast cell degranulation.

also causes mast cell release of a further polymorph chemotactic factor and mediators of vascular permeability which increase the flow of more complement and antibody to the site. The influx of polymorphs and the increase in vascular permeability constitute the potent antimicrobial *acute inflammatory response* (figure 7.17). The antibody molecule is designed as a flexible adaptor to attach to foreign substances which fail to activate the alternative pathway or the surface of the phagocytic cell; the Ig domains fix complement by the classical pathway and stimulate the phagocyte through its Fc receptor.

Humoral immunity to bacteria depends largely upon this opsonizing mechanism of antibody to enhance phagocytosis, the lysis of cells through the terminal complement components plus lysozyme, and the neutralization of bacterial toxins. Intracellular facultative parasites such as the tubercle bacillus can grow happily within the macrophage which only becomes able to kill the organisms it harbours if activated by a lymphokine released by the reaction of sensitized T-cells with the antigen: this is one mechanism of cell-mediated immunity.

Antibodies can neutralize viruses by blocking their combination with cellular receptor sites and by encouraging their destruction by mechanisms similar to those described for

180

bacteria. Antibodies are very effective in *preventing* reinfection with many viruses, serum antibody being important where the virus has to pass through the bloodstream before reaching its target organ and local antibody being essential where the target

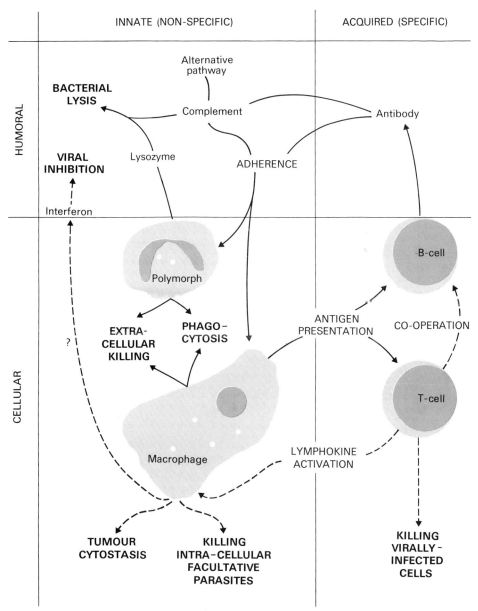

FIGURE 7.18. Simplified scheme to emphasize the interactions between natural and specific immunity mechanisms. Reactions influenced by T-cells are indicated by a broken line. (Developed from Playfair J.H.L. (1974) *Brit. Med. Bull.*, **30**, 24.)

organ is the same as the portal for entry (e.g. influenza); however, interferon may be more effective in the *recovery* from these infections. Cells infected with non-cytopathic viruses which 'bud', have altered surface antigens and can be destroyed by cytotoxic T-cells. Free 'budded' viral particles can be destroyed by antibody but the other route of intercellular virus spread can only be stopped by macrophages (recruited and activated by lymphokines from viral stimulated specific T-cells) which inhibit intercellular bridges and make local cells resistant to infection by bathing them in interferon.

Generally speaking, the acquired response operates to amplify and enhance innate immune mechanisms; the inter-actions are summarized in figure 7.18.

Immunity can be acquired passively, from the mother or by injection of preformed antibody, or induced actively either by natural infection or vaccination using killed or live attenuated organisms and toxoids. Live replicating vaccines provide a larger and more potent stimulus in the tissues relevant to the natural infection. Attenuated viral strains are being produced by genetic recombination. The efficiency of non-living antigens may be enhanced by adjuvants which act as antigen depots and activate macrophages. The risk of complications attendant upon vaccination must be weighed against the chance of contracting the disease.

Primary immunodeficiency states affecting the complement system, phagocytic cells or antibody synthesis lead to infection by pyogenic bacteria. Children with T-cell deficiency cannot deal adequately with 'budding' viruses (e.g. pox type) and fungi. Severe combined immunodeficiency occurs where there is a failure in differentiation of lymphoid stem cells. In many instances replacement therapy is possible: Ig for B-cell, thymus graft for T-cell and bone marrow (stem cells) or adenosine deaminase for severe combined immunodeficiency. The deficiency may arise secondarily as a consequence of mal-nutrition, viral and other infection, cytotoxic drugs, or lymphoproliferative disorders.

Further reading

Bergsma D., Good R.A., Finstad J. & Paul N.W. (eds) (1975) *Immunodeficiency in Man and Animals*. Birth Defects Series, vol. 11, no. 1. National Founda-tion, March of Dimes, New York.

Cohen S. & Sadun E. (eds) (1976) *Immunology of Parasitic Infections*. Blackwell Scientific Publications, Oxford.

Davis B.D., Dulbecco R., Eisen H.N., Ginsberg H.S. & Wood W.B. (1973) *Microbiology* (Including Immunology), 2nd edn. Harper International.

Dick G. (1978) *Immunisation*. Update Books, London.

Fougereau M. & Dausset J. (eds) (1980) *Progress in Immunology IV*. Academic Press, London.

van Furth R. (ed.) (1975) *Mononuclear Phagocytes in Immunity, Infection and Pathology*. Blackwell Scientific Publications, Oxford.

Lachmann P.J. & Peters D.K. (eds) (1982) *Clinical Aspects of Immunology*, 4th edn. Blackwell Scientific Publications, Oxford. See chapters on immunity to infection and immunoprophylaxis.

Gray A.R. (1969) Antigenic variation in trypanosomes. *Bull.WHO*, **41**, 805.

Mims C.A. (1976) *The Pathogenesis of Infectious Disease*. Academic Press, London.

Notkins A.L. (ed.) (1975) *Viral Immunology and Immunopathology*. Academic Press, New York.

Porter R. & Knight J. (1974) *Parasites in the Immunized Host*. Ciba Foundation Symposium. Elsevier, Amsterdam.

Shvartsman Ya.S & Zykov M.P. (1976) Secretory anti-influenza immunity. *Adv.Immunol.*, **22**, 291.

Taussig M.J. (1979) *Processes in Pathology*. Blackwell Scientific Publications, Oxford.

Wheelock E.F. & Toy S.T. (1973) Participation of lymphocytes in viral infections. *Adv. Immun.*, **16**, 124.

Wilson G.S. (1967) *The Hazards of Immunization*. Athlone Press, London.

Wilson G.S. (1973) *Cell Mediated Immunity and Resistance to Infection*. WHO Technical Report Series, Geneva.

8 Hypersensitivity

When an individual has been immunologically primed, further contact with antigen leads to secondary boosting of the immune response. However, the reaction may be excessive and lead to gross tissue damage (*hypersensitivity*) if the antigen is present in relatively large amounts or if the humoral and cellular immune state is at a heightened level. It should be emphasized that the mechanisms underlying these excessive reactions are those normally employed by the body in combating infection as discussed in chapter 7. We speak of *hypersensitivity reactions* and a state of *hypersensitivity*. Coombs and Gell defined four types of hypersensitivity, to which can be added a fifth, viz. 'stimulatory', which they mention. Types I, II, III and V depend on the interaction of antigen with humoral antibody and tend to be called 'immediate' type reactions although some are more immediate than others! Type IV involves receptors bound to the lymphocyte surface and because of the longer time course this has in the past been referred to as 'delayed-type sensitivity'. The essential basis of these reactions is summarized below and then each considered separately in more detail.

TYPE I—ANAPHYLACTIC SENSITIVITY

The antigen reacts with antibody bound to mast cells or circulating basophils through a specialized region of the Fc piece. This leads to degranulation of the mast cells and release of vasoactive amines (figure 8.1). These antibodies are termed homocytotropic (also referred to as reagins).

TYPE II—ANTIBODY-DEPENDENT
CYTOTOXIC HYPERSENSITIVITY

Antibodies binding to an antigen on the cell surface cause: (a) phagocytosis of the cell through opsonic (Fc) or immune (C3) adherence, (b) non-phagocytic extracellular cytoxicity by killer cells with receptors for IgFc, and (c) lysis through the operation of the full complement system up to C8, 9 (figure 8.2).

185

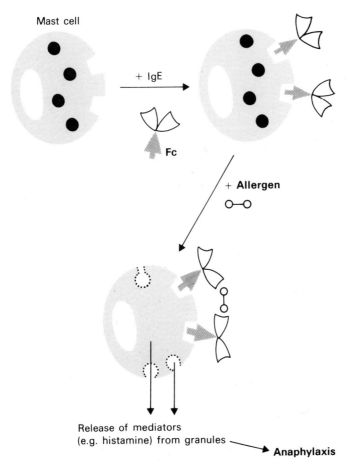

Mast cell

+ IgE

Fc

+ **Allergen**

Release of mediators
(e.g. histamine) from granules
→ **Anaphylaxis**

FIGURE 8.1. Type I—anaphylactic hypersensitivity. Mast-cell degranulation following interaction of antigen with bound homocytotropic (reaginic) antibodies.

TYPE III—COMPLEX-MEDIATED HYPERSENSITIVITY

The formation of complexes between antigen and humoral antibody can lead to activation of the complement system and to the aggregation of platelets with the consequences listed in figure 8.3.

TYPE IV—CELL-MEDIATED
(DELAYED-TYPE) HYPERSENSITIVITY

Thymic derived T-lymphocytes bearing specific receptors on their surface are stimulated by contact with macrophage-bound antigen to release lymphokines (cf. p. 70) which mediate delayed-type hypersensitivity (e.g. Mantoux test for tuberculin

186

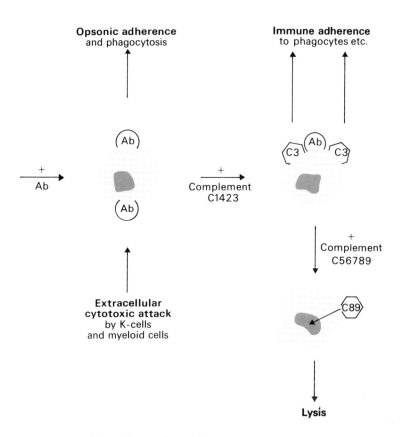

FIGURE 8.2. Type II—antibody-dependent cytotoxic hypersensitivity. Antibodies directed against cell surface antigens cause cell death not only by C-dependent lysis but also by adherence reactions leading to phagocytosis or, through non-phagocytic extracellular killing by certain lymphoreticular cells (antibody-dependent cell-mediated cytotoxicity).

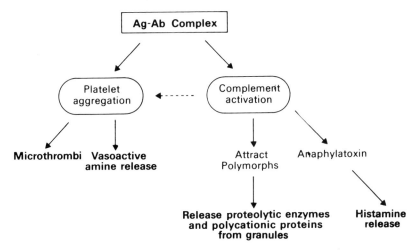

FIGURE 8.3. Type III—complex-mediated hypersensitivity.

sensitivity); in the reaction against virally infected cells or transplants, the stimulated lymphocytes transform into blast-like cells capable of killing target cells bearing the sensitizing antigens. Failure to eliminate the antigen will cause an accumulation of macrophages and the formation of a granuloma (figure 8.4).

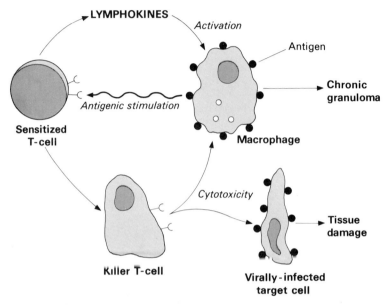

FIGURE 8.4. Type IV—cell-mediated (delayed type) hypersensitivity.

TYPE V—STIMULATORY
HYPERSENSITIVITY

Non-complement fixing antibodies directed against certain cell surface components may actually stimulate rather than destroy the cell (figure 8.5). Theoretically stimulation could also occur through the development of antibodies to naturally occurring mitotic inhibitors in the circulation.

Type I—anaphylactic sensitivity

SYSTEMIC ANAPHYLAXIS

A single injection of 1 mg of an antigen such as egg albumin into a guinea-pig has no obvioius effect. However, if the injection is repeated two or three weeks later, the sensitized animal reacts very dramatically with the symptoms of generalized anaphylaxis; almost immediately the guinea-pig begins to

188

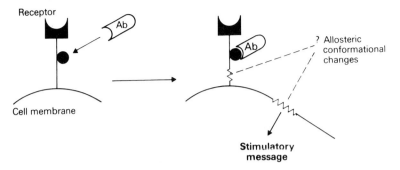

Receptor

Cell membrane

? Allosteric
conformational
changes

**Stimulatory
message**

FIGURE 8.5. Type V—stimulatory hypersensitivity.

wheeze and within a few minutes dies from asphyxia. Examination shows intense constriction of the bronchioles and bronchi and generally there is: (a) contraction of smooth muscle; and (b) dilatation of capillaries.

Similar reactions can occur in human subjects and have been observed following insect bites or injections of penicillin in appropriately sensitive individuals. In many instances only a timely intravenous injection of adrenaline to counter the smooth muscle contraction and capillary dilatation can prevent death.

MECHANISM OF ANAPHYLAXIS

Sir Henry Dale recognized that histamine mimics the systemic changes of anaphylaxis and furthermore that the uterus from a sensitized guinea-pig releases histamine and contracts on exposure to antigen (Schultz–Dale technique). Serum from such an animal can passively sensitize the uterus from a normal guinea-pig so that it, too, will contract on addition of the specific antigen. Contraction is associated with an explosive degranulation of the mast cells (figure 8.6a & b) which is responsible for the release of histamine and, in certain species, of another mediator of anaphylaxis, 5-hydroxytryptamine (serotonin). Other mediators which are released include a slow reacting substance (SRS-A) capable of inducing a prolonged contraction of certain smooth muscles, platelet activating factor (PAF), heparin and chemotactic factors for both neutrophils and eosinophils. The eosinophils are thus attracted to the site of mast cell degranulation where they proceed to neutralize the effects of the released mediators; histamine is defused by histaminase and PAF by phospholipase D. In this way eosinophils modulate the reactions consequent upon mast cell activation (figure 8.7).

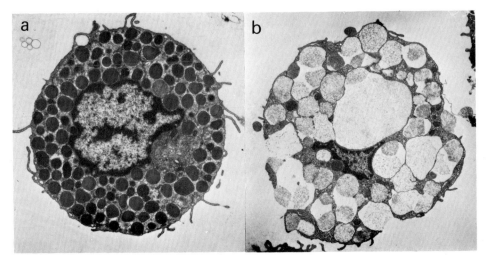

FIGURE 8.6. The mast cell. (a) An unreleased cell containing many membrane-bound, histamine-containing granules (×5400). (b) A mast cell degranulated by treatment with anti-Ig for 30 sec. at 37°. Note that the granules have released their histamine and are morphologically altered, being larger and less electron dense. Although most of the altered granules remain within the circumference of the cell, they are open to the extracellular space (×5400). (By courtesy of Drs D. Lawson, C. Fewtrell, B. Gomperts & M. Raff: from *J.Exp.Med.*, (1975) **142**, 391.)

It seems clear that the mast cells become coated by a particular type of antibody whose Fc region can bind specifically to sites on the mast cell surface. The most effective homocytotropic antibodies belong to the IgE class but it is clear that IgG antibodies can also act as reagins although the extent of their contribution to the allergic state in the human is not yet resolved. The technique of *passive cutaneous anaphylaxis* (PCA) introduced by Ovary utilizes this dermal reaction as a highly sensitive indicator for reaginic antibodies. For example, high dilutions of guinea-pig serum containing γ_1-globulin antibodies may be injected into the skin of a normal animal and following the intravenous injection of antigen with a dye such as Evans' Blue, the anaphylactic reaction in the skin will lead to release of vasoactive amines and hence a local 'blueing'.

Degranulation of the mast cell occurs when the bound homocytotropic antibodies are cross-linked either by specific antigen (figure 8.1) or by the corresponding divalent anti-immunoglobulin (e.g. anti-IgE or anti-light chain); univalent (Fab) anti-IgE will not cause degranulation. This cross-linking reaction induces a membrane signal which causes an increase in cAMP and an influx of calcium ions which leads to release of preformed mediators. Changes in cyclic nucleotides associated

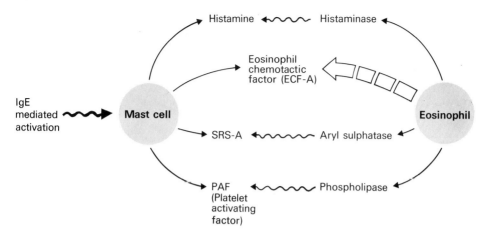

FIGURE 8.7. The mast cell response and its modulation by eosinophils. SRS-A, now known to be a mixture of leukotrienes C_4 and D_4, is produced optimally in collaboration with accessory cells.

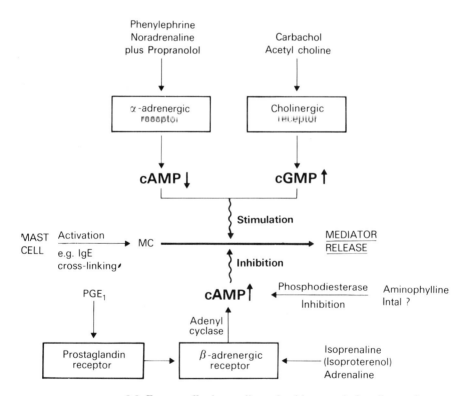

FIGURE 8.8. Factors affecting cyclic nucleotide control of mediator release from mast cells. Release of preformed mediators triggered by mast cell activation is associated with an increase in cAMP concentration in a compartment or pool which is separate from the cyclic nucleotide pools linked to the hormone receptors indicated. (After Austen F.)

with hormone receptors on the mast cell influence mediator release as summarized in figure 8.8.

ATOPIC ALLERGY

Nearly 10% of the population suffer to a greater or lesser degree with allergies involving localized anaphylactic reactions to extrinsic allergens such as grass pollens, animal danders, mites in house dust and so on. Contact of the allergen with cell-bound IgE in the bronchial tree, the nasal mucosa and the conjunctival tissues releases mediators of anaphylaxis and produces the symptoms of asthma or hay fever as the case may be. For those unfortunates sensitized to foods such as the strawberry, the price of indulgence may be a generalized urticaria caused by reaction in the skin to materials absorbed from the gut into the blood stream. Acute anaphylaxis although rare may occur in highly sensitive subjects after an insect bite or injections of penicillin or procaine.

Sensitivity is normally assessed by the response to intra-dermal challenge with antigen. The release of histamine and other mediators rapidly produces a wheal and erythema (figure 8.13a), maximal within 30 minutes and then subsiding. The responsible IgE antibodies can be demonstrated by the ability of patient's serum to passively sensitize the skin of normal humans (Praüsnitz–Küstner or 'P K' test) or preferably of monkeys. This passive sensitization of human skin can be blocked most effectively by prior injection of a myeloma of IgE rather than of any other class. The interpretation is that the specialized sites on the skin mast cells become fully saturated by binding to the Fc regions of the IgE myeloma globulin which blocks the subsequent attachment of specific IgE antibodies. In some instances, intranasal challenge with allergen provokes a response even though skin tests and the radioallergosorbent test (RAST, p. 126) for specific serum IgE are negative, a phenomenon attributable to local synthesis of IgE antibodies.

The lymphocytes from patients with atopic allergy undergo blast-cell transformation and release a migration inhibition factor on contact with allergen. These are thought to be indi-cators of cell-mediated immunity, and delayed-type hyper-sensitivity reactions (see below) have been elicited in some patients in whom the immediate response had been suppressed with anti-histamines.

The symptoms of atopic allergy are largely but not always completely controllable by anti-histamines. Other effective drugs such as Isoprenaline and disodium cromoglycate (Intal) probably act by stabilizing the adenyl cyclase–cyclic-AMP system to prevent vasoactive amine release. Attempts to desensitize patients immunologically by repeated treatment with allergen have at least the merit of a long history and in a significant but as yet unpredictable proportion of patients can lead to worthwhile improvement. It has generally been assumed that the purpose of these inoculations was to boost the synthesis of 'blocking' IgG antibody whose function was to divert the allergen from contact with tissue-bound IgE. This would be of unquestioned value were the increase in protective antibody (? particularly IgA) to occur locally at the sites vulnerable to allergen exposure. However, if T-lymphocyte co-operation is important for IgE synthesis, the beneficial effects of antigen injection may also be mediated through induction of tolerant or even suppressor T-cells.

There is a strong familial predisposition to the development of these disorders but although this is linked to inheritance of a given HL-A haplotype within any one family, no association with specific HL-A types has so far come to light. Curiously, it is said that patients with allergy are less likely than their non-atopic counterparts to develop tumours.

Type II—antibody-dependent cytotoxic hypersensitivity

Where an antigen is present on the surface of a cell, combination with antibody will encourage the demise of that cell by promoting contact with phagocytes either by reduction in surface charge, by opsonic adherence directly through the Fc, or by immune adherence through bound C3. Cell death may also occur through activation of the full complement system up to C8 and C9 producing direct membrane damage. Although in the case of haemolytic antibodies, the generation of a single active complement site is enough to cause erythrocyte lysis, other cells appear to have repair mechanisms and it is likely that several complement sites need to be recruited in order to overwhelm the cell's defences.

The operation of a quite distinct cytotoxic mechanism is suggested by Perlmann's finding that target cells coated with low concentrations of IgG antibody can be killed 'non-specifically' through an extracellular non-phagocytic mechanism involving nonsensitized lymphoreticular cells which bind to the target by their specific receptors for IgG Fc (figure 8.9). This so-called antibody-dependent cell-mediated cytotoxicity (ADCC) may be exhibited by both phagocytic and

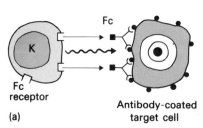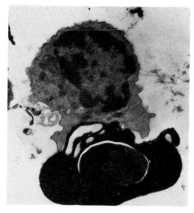

FIGURE 8.9. Killing of antibody-coated target by antibody-dependent cell-mediated cytotoxicity (ADCC). The surface receptors for the If Fc region bind the effector cell to the target which is then killed by an extracellular mechanism. Several different cell types may display ADCC activity.
(a) Diagram of effector and target cells. (b) Electron micrograph of attack on antibody-coated chick red cell by a mouse K-cell showing close apposition of effector and target and vacuolation in the cytoplasm of the latter (courtesy of P. Penfold).

nonphagocytic myeloid cells (polymorphs and monocytes) and by a weakly glass-adherent cell with Fc receptors dubbed the 'K-cell'. Although morphologically similar to a fairly small lymphocyte, the precise lineage of the K-cell is still uncertain. A proportion of human effector cells bear T-markers and therefore belong to the T_G sub-population. The remainder are 'null' cells in the sense that they lack the presently employed surface markers of mature B- or T-lymphocytes and it will be of interest to see whether they represent stages in the differentiation of lymphoid (or myeloid) lines or belong to an entirely distinct cell type.

Contact between the effector and target cells is essential and activity is inhibited by cytochalasin B which interferes with cell movement, and aggregated IgG which binds firmly to the Fc receptors and blocks their ability to interact with antibody on the surface of the target. ADCC is not affected by inhibitors of protein synthesis and the presence of complement components has not so far been found to be mandatory although nature would have shown a certain tidiness had the complement system been utilized to provide the cytotoxic effector molecule.

So far, ADCC has been studied exclusively as a phenomenon *in vitro*; to give examples, human K-cells have been shown to be strikingly unpleasant to chicken red cells coated with rabbit antibody, Chang liver cells coated with human antibody and human lymphocytes bearing anti-HLA. Whether ADCC is

194

merely a curiosity of the laboratory test-tube or plays a positive role *in vivo* remains an open question.

Transfusion reactions

Of the many different polymorphic constituents of the human red cell membrane, ABO blood groups form the dominant system. The antigenic groups A and B are derived from H substance (figure 8.10) by the action of glycosyl transferases encoded by A or B genes respectively. Individuals with both genes (group AB) have the two antigens on their red cells while those lacking these genes (group O) synthesize H substance only. Antibodies to A or to B occur when the antigen is absent from the red cell surface; thus a person of blood group A will possess anti-B and so on. These *isohaemagglutinins* are usually IgM and are thought to arise through immunization against antigens of the gut flora which are similar to the blood group substances so that the antibodies formed cross-react with the appropriate red cell type. If an individual is blood group A, he will be tolerant to antigens closely similar to A and will only form cross-reacting antibodies capable of agglutinating B red cells; similarly an O individual will make anti-A and anti-B. On transfusion, mismatched red cells will be coated by the isohaemagglutinins and cause severe reactions.

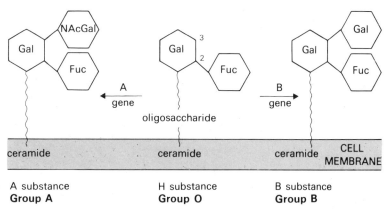

| A substance | H substance | B substance |
| **Group A** | **Group O** | **Group B** |

FIGURE 8.10. The ABO system. The allelic genes A and B code for transferases which add either N-acetylgalactosamine or galactose respectively to H substance. The oligosaccharide is anchored to the cell membrane by coupling to a sphingomyelin called ceramide. 85% of the population secrete blood group substances in the saliva where the oligosaccharides are present as soluble polypeptide conjugates formed under the action of a secretor (se) gene.

Rhesus incompatibility

The Rhesus (Rh) blood groups form the other major antigenic system, the RhD antigen being of the most consequence for isoimmune reactions. A mother with an RhD negative blood group can readily be sensitized by red cells from a baby carrying RhD antigens. This occurs most often at the birth of the first child when a placental bleed can release a large number of the baby's erythrocytes into the mother. The antibodies formed are predominantly of the IgG class and are able to cross the placenta in any subsequent pregnancy. Reaction with the D-antigen on the fetal red cells leads to their destruction through opsonic adherence giving haemolytic disease of the newborn (figure 8.11).

These anti-D antibodies fail to agglutinate RhD+red cells *in vitro* ('incomplete antibodies') because the low density of antigenic sites does not allow sufficient antibody bridges to be formed between the negatively charged erthrocytes to overcome the electrostatic repulsive forces. Erythrocytes coated with anti-D can be made to agglutinate by addition of albumin or of an anti-immunoglobulin serum (Coombs' reagent).

If a mother has natural isohaemagglutinins which can react with any fetal erythrocytes reaching her circulation, sensitization to the D antigens is less likely due to 'deviation' of the red cells away from the antigen sensitive cells. For example, a group O Rh−ve mother with a group A Rh+ve baby would destroy any fetal erythrocytes with her anti-A before they could immunize to produce anti-D. In an extension of this principle, Rh−ve mothers are now treated prophylactically with small

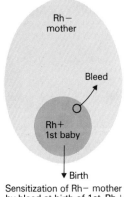

Sensitization of Rh− mother by bleed at birth of 1st Rh+ baby leading to synthesis of anti-D.

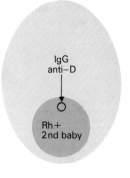

D+ erythrocytes in 2nd child affected by IgG anti-D crossing the placenta.

FIGURE 8.11. Haemolytic disease of the newborn due to rhesus incompatibility.

amounts of avid IgG anti-D at the time of birth of the first child, and this greatly reduces the risk of sensitization.

Organ transplants

A long-standing homograft which has withstood the first onslaught of the cell-mediated reaction can evoke humoral antibodies in the host directed against surface transplantation antigens on the graft. These may be directly cytotoxic, or cause adherence of phagocytic cells or 'non-specific' attack by K cells (cf. figure 8.2). They may also lead to platelet adherence when they combine with antigens on the surface of the vascular endothelium.

AUTOIMMUNE REACTIONS

Autoantibodies to the patient's own red cells are produced in autoimmune haemolytic anaemia. Red cells coated with these antibodies have a shortened half-life largely through their adherence to phagocytic cells.

The sera of patients with Hashimoto's thyroiditis contain antibodies which in the presence of complement are directly cytotoxic for isolated human thyroid cells in culture. In Goodpasture's syndrome (included here for convenience), antibodies to kidney glomerular basement membrane are present. Biopsies show these antibodies together with complement components bound to the basement membranes where the action of the full complement system leads to serious damage (figure 8.12a).

DRUG REACTIONS

This subject is very complicated. Drugs may become coupled to body components and thereby undergo conversion from a hapten to a full antigen which will sensitize certain individuals (we do not know which). If IgE antibodies are produced, anaphylactic reactions can result. In some circumstances, particularly with topically applied ointments, cell-mediated hypersensitivity may be induced. In other cases where coupling to serum proteins occurs, the possibility of type III complex-mediated reactions may arise. In the present context we are concerned with those instances where the drug appears to form an antigenic complex with the surface of a formed element of the blood and evokes the production of antibodies which are cytotoxic for the cell-drug complex. When the drug is

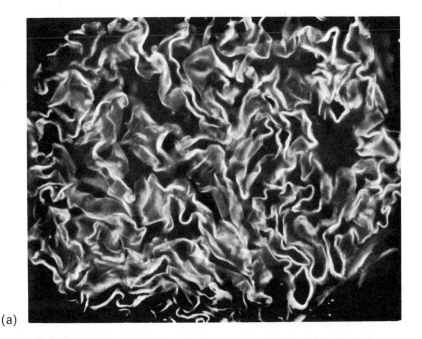

(a)

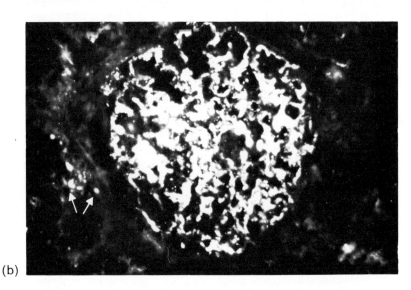

(b)

FIGURE 8.12. Glomerulonephritis: (a) due to linear deposition of antibody to glomerular basement membranes here visualized by staining the human kidney biopsy with a fluorescent anti-IgG (courtesy of Dr F.J. Dixon) and (b) due to deposition of antigen–antibody complexes which can be seen as discrete masses lining the glomerular basement membrane following immunofluorescent staining with anti-IgG; patches of blue autofluorescence are present in the extraglomerular tissue arrowed) (courtesy of Dr D. Doniach). Similar patterns to these are obtained with a fluorescent anti-C3.

198

withdrawn, the sensitivity is no longer evident. Examples of this mechanism have been seen in the *haemolytic anaemia* sometimes associated with continued administration of chlorpromazine or phenacetin, in the *agranulocytosis* associated with the taking of amidopyrine or of quinidine, and the classic situation of *thrombocytopenic purpura* which may be produced by Sedormid. In the latter case, freshly drawn serum from the patient will lyse platelets in the presence but not in the absence of Sedormid; inactivation of complement by preheating the serum at 56°C for 30 minutes abrogates this effect.

Type III—complex-mediated hypersensitivity

The union of soluble antigens and antibodies within the body give rise to an acute inflammatory reaction (cf. figure 8.3). If complement is fixed, anaphylatoxins will be released as split products of C3 and C5 and these will cause histamine release with vascular permeability changes. The chemotactic factors also produced will lead to an influx of polymorphonuclear leucocytes which begin the phagocytosis of the immune complexes; this in turn results in the extracellular release from the polymorph granules of proteolytic enzymes (including neutral proteinases and collagenase), kinin-forming enzymes and polycationic proteins which increase vascular permeability through both mastocytolytic and histamine-independent mechanisms. These will damage local tissues and intensify the inflammatory responses. Further damage may be mediated by reactive lysis in which activated C567 becomes attached to the surface of nearby cells and binds C8,9. Under appropriate conditions, platelets may be aggregated with two consequences: they provide yet a further source of vasoactive amines and may also form microthrombi which can lead to local ischaemia. (The discerning reader will appreciate the need for the complex system of inhibitors present in the body.)

The outcome of the formation of immune complexes *in vivo* depends not only on the absolute amounts of antigen and antibody, which determine the intensity of the reaction, but also on their *relative* proportions which govern the nature of the complexes (cf. precipitin curve, p. 8) and hence their distribution within the body. Between *antibody excess* and *mild antigen excess*, the complexes are rapidly precipitated and tend to be localized to the site of introduction of antigen, whereas in *moderate* to *gross antigen excess*, soluble complexes are formed which circulate and may cause systemic reactions and be widely deposited in the kidneys, joints and skin.

Maurice Arthus found that injection of soluble antigen intradermally into hyperimmunized rabbits with high levels of precipitating antibody produced an erythematous and oedematous reaction reaching a peak at 3–8 hours and then usually resolving. The lesion was characterized by an intense infiltration with polymorphonuclear leucocytes (figure 8.14a). The injected antigen precipitates with antibody often within the venule and the complex binds complement; using the appropriate fluorescent reagents, antigen, immunoglobulin and complement components can all be demonstrated in this lesion. Anaphylatoxin is soon generated and causes histamine liberation. Local intravascular complexes will cause platelet aggregation and vasoactive amine release. The formation of chemotactic factors leads to the influx of polymorphs and, as a result, erythema and oedema increase. The Arthus reaction can be blocked by depletion of complement or of the neutrophil polymorphs (by nitrogen mustard or specific antipolymorph sera).

Intrapulmonary Arthus-type reactions to exogenous inhaled antigen appear to be responsible for a number of hypersensitivity disorders in man such as Farmer's lung which occurs within 6–8 hours of exposure to the dust from mouldy hay.

Injection of relatively large doses of foreign serum (e.g. horse anti-diphtheria) used to be employed for various therapeutic purposes. It was not uncommon for a condition known as 'serum sickness' to arise some eight days after the injection. A rise in temperature, swollen lymph nodes, a generalized urticarial rash and painful swollen joints associated with a low serum complement and transient albuminuria could be encounterd. These result from the deposition of soluble antigen-antibody complexes formed in antigen excess.

The deposition of complexes is a dynamic affair and long lasting disease is only seen when the antigen is persistent as in chronic infections and autoimmune diseases. Experimentally, Dixon produced chronic glomerular lesions by repeated administration of foreign proteins to rabbits. Not all animals showed the lesion and perhaps only those genetically capable of producing low affinity antibody (Soothill & Steward) or antibodies to a restricted number of determinants (Christian) formed soluble complexes in the right size range. The smallest complexes reach the epithelial side but progressively larger complexes are retained in or on the endothelial side of the glomerular basement membrane.

Many cases of glomerulonephritis are associated with circulating complexes and biopsies give a fluorescent staining pattern similar to that of figure 8.12b which depicts DNA/anti-DNA/complement deposits in the kidney of a patient with systemic lupus erythematosus (cf. p. 266). Well known is the disease which can follow infection with certain strains of so-called 'nephritogenic' streptococci and the nephrotic syndrome of Nigerian children associated with quartan malaria where complexes with antigens of the infecting organism have been implicated.

DETECTION OF IMMUNE COMPLEX FORMATION

Tissue-bound complexes are usually visualized by the immunofluorescent staining of biopsies with conjugated anti-immunoglobulins and anti-C3 (cf. figure 8.12b).

Many techniques for the detection of circulating complexes have been described and because of variations in the size, complement-fixing ability and Ig class of different complexes, it is useful to apply more than one method. In our laboratory we tend to prefer:

(1) precipitation of complexed IgG from serum at concentrations of polyethylene glycol which do not bring down significant amounts of IgG monomer, followed by estimation of IgG in the precipitate by single radial diffusion or laser nephelometry; and

(2) binding of serum complexes to plastic tubes coated with C1q and estimation of the amount and class of Ig in the complex with radio- or enzyme-labelled class-specific anti-Ig (cf. method used for determination of antibody-binding capacity, p. 126).

TREATMENT

The avoidance of exogenous inhaled antigens inducing type III reactions is obvious. Elimination of micro-organisms associated with immune complex disease by chemotherapy may provide a further reaction due to copious release of antigen. Suppression of the accessory factors thought to be necessary for deposition of complexes would seem logical; for example, the development of serum sickness is prevented by histamine and 5HT antagonists. Disodium cromoglycate, heparin and salicylates are often used, the latter being an effective platelet stabilizer as well as a potent anti-inflammatory agent. Corticosteroids are particularly powerful inhibitors of inflammation and are immunosuppressive. In many cases, particularly those involving auto-immunity, conventional immunosuppressive agents may be justified. Where type III hypersensitivity is thought to arise from an inadequate immune response, the more aggressive approach of immunopotentiation to boost avidity is being advocated, but that is a path that will be trod gently.

Type IV—cell-mediated (delayed-type) hypersensitivity

This form of hypersensitivity is encountered in many allergic reactions to bacteria, viruses and fungi, in the contact dermatitis resulting from sensitization to certain simple chemicals and in the rejection of transplanted tissues. Perhaps the best known example is the Mantoux reaction obtained by injection of tuberculin into the skin of an individual in whom previous infection with the mycobacterium had induced a state of cell-mediated immunity (CMI). The reaction is characterized by erythema and induration (figure 8.13b) which appears only after several hours (hence the term 'delayed') and reaches a maximum at 24–48 hours, thereafter subsiding. Histologically the earliest phase of the reaction is seen as a perivacular cuffing with mononuclear cells followed by a more extensive exudation of mono- and polymorphonuclear cells. The latter soon migrate out of the lesion leaving behind a predominantly mononuclear cell infiltrate consisting of lymphocytes and cells of the monocyte-macrophage series (figure 8.14b). This contrasts with the essentially 'polymorph' character of the Arthus reaction (figure 8.14a).

Comparable reactions to soluble proteins are obtained when sensitization is induced by incorporation of the antigen into complete Freund's adjuvant (p. 170). In some but not all cases, if animals are primed with antigen alone or in incomplete Freund's adjuvant (which lacks the mycobacteria), the delayed hypersensitivity state is of shorter duration and the dermal response more transient. This is known as 'Jones–Mote' sensitivity but has recently been termed cutaneous basophil

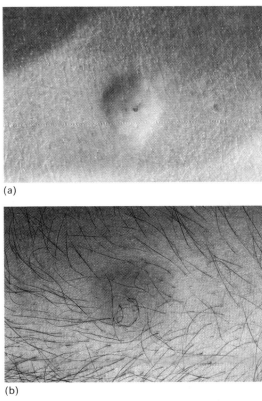

(a)

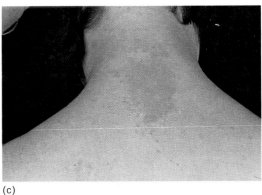

(b)

(c)

FIGURE 8.13. Hypersensitivity reactions. (a) Type 1 anaphylactic intradermal reaction to pollen allergen showing a well-developed wheal and a degree of erythema (flare).

(b) Type IV cell-mediated hypersensitivity reaction to tuberculin, characterized by induration and erythema.

(c) Type IV contact hypersensitivity reaction to nickel caused by the clasp of a necklace.

((a & b) kindly provided by Dr J. Brostoff, photographed by Mr B.N. Rice; (c) reproduced from British Society of Immunology teaching slides with permission of the Society and Dermatology Department, London Hospital.)

203

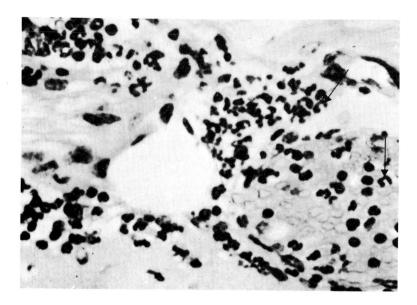

(a)

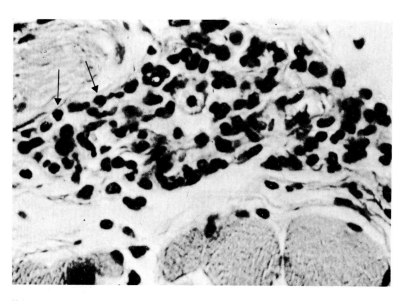

(b)

FIGURE 8.14. Histology of intradermal hypersensitivity reactions. (a) Acute inflammatory response in Arthus reaction (type III) in rabbit skin with predominance of polymorphs (arrows). (b) Type IV cell-mediated (delayed type) hypersensitivity reaction to intradermal antigen revealing the mononuclear cell infiltration (arrows).

204

hypersensitivity on account of the high proportion of basophils infiltrating the skin lesion.

Unlike the other forms of hypersensitivity which we have discussed, delayed-type reactivity cannot be transferred from a sensitive to a non-sensitized individual with serum antibody; lymphoid cells, in particular the T-lymphocytes, are required. Thus a guinea-pig with negative skin reactions to tuberculin gives a positive response after injection of peritoneal exudate cells (containing lymphocytes and macrophages), lymph node cells, or peripheral blood cells from a donor previously sensitized to the tubercle bacillus provided donor and recipient share major histocompatibility antigens in the I region. Transfer of delayed hypersensitivity has also been achieved in the human using viable blood white cells and interestingly, by a low molecular weight material extracted from them (Lawrence's transfer factor). The nature of this substance is, however, a mystery. It appears to be capable of stimulating precommitted T-cells mediating delayed hypersensitivity, but its role as an informational molecule conferring antigen-specific reactivity is still a highly contentious issue.

It cannot be stressed too often that the hypersensitivity lesion results from an exaggerated interaction between antigen and the *normal* cell-mediated immune mechanisms (cf. p. 67). Following earlier priming, memory T-cells recognize the antigen together with I-region molecules on a macrophage and are stimulated into blast cell transformation and proliferation. A proportion of the stimulated T-cells release a number of soluble factors which function as mediators of the ensuing hypersensitivity response while a separate population develops cytotoxic powers.

IN VITRO TESTS FOR CELL-MEDIATED HYPERSENSITIVITY

Migration inhibition tests

The production of macrophage migration inhibition factor (MIF) by peritoneal exudate cells from sensitized guinea-pigs on incubation with antigen is widely accepted as an *in vitro* correlate of cell-mediated hypersensitivity. The cells are packed into capillary tubes which are placed in small tissue culture chambers. On incubation the macrophages migrate out to form a fan of cells on the bottom of the chamber. If specific antigen is present in the medium, MIF is produced and the migration is inhibited. The degree of inhibition is assessed from the area of the macrophage fan obtained in the presence of antigen expressed as a percentage of that in the control chambers lacking antigen (figure 8.15) and this correlates with the intensity of the delayed hypersensitivity state.

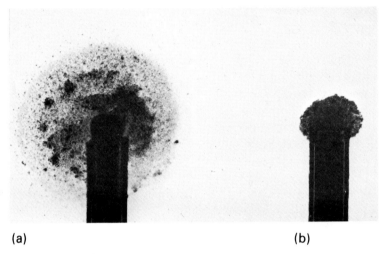

(a)   (b)

FIGURE 8.15. Migration inhibition as an *in vitro* test for cell-mediated hypersensitivity. Migration of peritoneal exudate cells from a sensitized guinea-pig: (a) control in absence of antigen and (b) in the presence of antigen. (Courtesy of Dr J. Brostoff.)

The macrophages act as non-specific indicators of the reaction between antigen and specifically sensitized lymphocytes. Thus a purified small lymphocyte population isolated from the peritoneal exudate of a sensitized pig is able to induce migration inhibition in the presence of antigen when mixed with as many as 50 times its number of macrophages taken from unsensitized animals; purified macrophages from the sensitized animal however are unable to produce MIF when mixed with lymphocytes from normal donors and incubated with antigen.

Greater difficulties have been encountered in attempting migration inhibition tests in the human. One variant is to incubate blood lymphocytes with antigen for several days and then to assay for MIF in the supernatant by addition to guinea-pig macrophages. Inhibitory tests involving migration of buffy coat cells are potentially most useful but the conditions required to define when this represents a direct expression of T-cell reactivity have yet to be rigidly established.

Transformation

The proliferation of sensitized cells on contact with specific antigen and their change in morphology to larger blast-like cells with paler staining nuclei and basophilic cytoplasm (figure 3.6c, p. 57) has frequently been used as an *in vitro* test for cell-mediated hypersensitivity and several studies have shown reasonable correlation with *in vivo* results. The degree of stimulation is assessed either by the percentage of blast-like cells surviving in the culture or by the incorporation of labelled thymidine into newly synthesized DNA. The test is complicated by the possibility of recruitment into division of non-sensitized lymphocytes through release of a mitogenic factor from stimulated cells and also by the fact that B-lymphocytes may also be transformed.

Comparable changes can be induced in lymphocytes by certain plant mitogens of which the best known are phytohaemagglutinin (PHA) and concanavalin A (conA). These are termed polyclonal activators because they react with the cell surface non-specifically (i.e. not as an antigen) and produce the same series of cellular events as does antigen locking on to its specific surface receptor. Unlike the situation with antigen stimulation where only a small fraction of the cells are sensitive, PHA transforms a major proportion of the T-cells. Additionally, some B-cells are affected although their response appears to be T-cell dependent. The picture is emerging that helper T-cells are preferentially stimulated by PHA and suppressors by conA. Pokeweed activates both T- and B-lymphocytes while lipopolysaccharide (in the mouse at least) is a B-cell mitogen.

Cytotoxicity

The degree of cytolysis produced by cytotoxic cells is assessed by measuring the release of radioactive chromium from pre-labelled target cells into the supernatant fluid at varying ratios of effector to target cells. The T-cell dependence of the phenomenon can be established by depletion with anti-Thy 1 plus complement in the mouse, or by rosetting with sheep red cells in the human.

TISSUE DAMAGE

Infection

The development of a state of cell-mediated hypersensitivity to bacterial products is probably responsible for the lesions associated with bacterial allergy such as the cavitation, caseation and general toxaemia seen in human tuberculosis and the granulomatous skin lesions found in patients with the tuberculoid form of leprosy. When the battle between the replicating bacteria and the body defences fails to be resolved in favour of the host, persisting antigen provokes a chronic local delayed hypersensitivity reaction. Continual release of lymphokines from sensitized T-lymphocytes leads to the accumulation of large numbers of macrophages, many of which give rise to arrays of epithelioid cells, while others fuse to form giant cells. Macrophages bearing bacterial antigen on their surface become targets for killer T-cells and are destroyed. Further tissue damage will occur as a result of indiscriminate cytotoxicity by lymphokine activated macrophages (and NK cells?) and perhaps lymphotoxin itself. Morphologically, this combination of cell types with proliferating lymphocytes and fibroblasts associated with areas of fibrosis and necrosis is termed a *chronic granuloma* and represents an attempt by the body to wall off a site of persistent infection.

The skin rashes in smallpox and measles and the lesions of herpes simplex may be largely attributed to delayed type allergic reactions with extensive damage to virally infected cells by cytotoxic T-lymphocytes. Cell-mediated hypersensitivity has also been demonstrated in the fungal disease candidiasis.

Contact dermatitis

The dermal route of inoculation tends to favour the development of a T-cell response through processing by Langerhans'

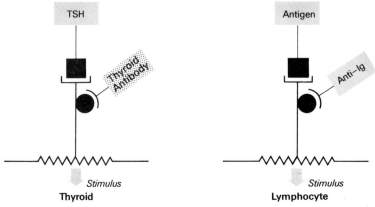

FIGURE 8.16. Stimulation of thyroid cell and of lymphocyte by a physiological agent or by antibody both of which cause comparable membrane changes leading to cell activation by reacting with surface receptors.

cells which migrate to the lymph nodes and present antigen to T-lymphocytes (p. 60). Thus, delayed-type reactions in the skin are often produced by foreign materials capable of binding to body constituents, possibly surface molecules of the Langerhans cell, to form new antigens. Thus contact hypersensitivity can occur in people who become sensitized while working with chemicals such as picryl chloride and chromates, or who repeatedly come into contact with the substance urushiol from the poison ivy plant. *p*-Phenylene diamine in certain hair dyes, neomycin in topically applied ointments and nickel salts formed from articles such as nickel suspenders can provoke similar reactions (figure 8.13).

Other examples

Delayed hypersensitivity contributes significantly to the prolonged reactions which result from insect bites. The possible implication of homograft rejection by cytotoxic T-cells as a mechanism for the control of cancer cells is discussed in chapter 9. The contribution made by cell-mediated hypersensitivity reactions to different autoimmune diseases is even now rather uncertain (cf. p. 270).

Type V—stimulatory hypersensitivity

Many cells receive instruction by agents such as hormones through surface receptors which specifically bind the external agent presumably through complementarity of structure. This combination may lead to allosteric changes in configuration of the receptor or of adjacent molecules which become activated and transmit a signal to the cell interior. For example, when thyroid stimulating hormone (TSH) of pituitary origin binds to the thyroid cell receptors there appears to be an activation of adenyl cyclase in the membrane which generates cyclic-AMP from ATP and this substance acts to stimulate activity in the thyroid cell. The thyroid stimulating antibody present in the sera of thyrotoxic patients (cf. p. 263) is an autoantibody directed against an antigen on the thyroid surface which stimulates the cell and produces the same changes as TSH, similarly utilizing the cyclic-AMP pathway. It is likely that the antibody combines with a site on the TSH receptor or an adjacent molecule to produce the allosteric change required for adenyl cyclase activation. The situation is analogous to lymphocyte stimulation; B-lymphocytes with immunoglobulin surface receptors can be stimulated by changes induced through the receptor molecules either by binding of specific antigen or by an antibody to the immunoglobulin (even anti-Fc) as shown in figure 8.16.

Summary

The normal effector mechanisms for cell-mediated and humoral immunity are dependent upon the activation of T- and B-cells respectively (figure 8.17). Inappropriate stimulation of these effector mechanisms by antigen in a sensitized host can lead to tissue damage and we speak of hypersensitivity reactions of which five main types can be distinguished.

Type I—anaphylactic hypersensitivity depends upon the reaction of antigen with specific IgE antibody bound through its Fc to the mast cell, leading to release from the granules of the mediators histamine, slow reacting substance-A and platelet activating factor, plus an eosinophil chemotactic factor. Eosinophils neutralize the mast cell mediators. Hay fever and extrinsic asthma represent the most common atopic allergic disorders. The offending antigen is identified by intradermal prick tests giving immediate wheal and erythema reactions or by provocation testing. Symptomatic treatment involves the use of mediator antagonists or agents which maintain intracellular cAMP and thereby stabilize the mast cell granules. Courses of antigen injection may desensitize by formation of blocking IgG or IgA antibodies or by turning off IgE production.

Type II—antibody-dependent cytotoxic hypersensitivity involves the death of cells bearing antibody attached to a surface antigen. The cells may be taken up by phagocytic cells to which they adhere through their coating of IgG or C3b or lysed by the operation of the full complement system. Cells bearing IgG may also be killed by myeloid cells (polymorphs and macrophages) or by non-adherent lymphoid K cells through an extracellular mechanism (antibody-dependent cell-mediated cytotoxicity). Examples are: transfusion reactions, haemolytic disease of the newborn through Rhesus incompatibility, antibody mediated graft destruction, autoimmune reactions directed against the formed elements of the blood and kidney glomerular basement membranes, and hypersensitivity resulting from the coating of erythrocytes or platelets by a drug.

Type III—complex-mediated hypersensitivity results from the effects of antigen–antibody complexes through: (a) activation of com-

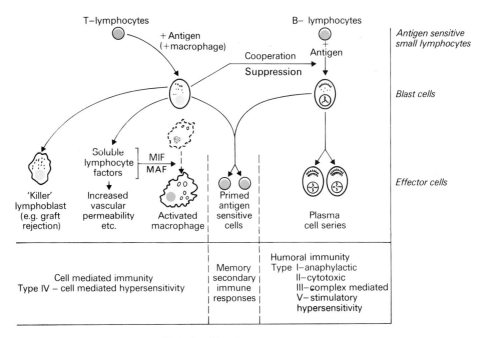

FIGURE 8.17. Relationship of B- and T-cell activity to different forms of hypersensitivity and immunity. Different T-cell functions are mediated by distinct sub-populations.

plement and attraction of polymorphonuclear leucocytes which release tissue damaging enzymes on contact with the complex and: (b) aggregation of platelets to cause microthrombi and vasoactive amine release. Where circulating antibody levels are high, the antigen is precipitated near the site of entry into the body. The reaction in the skin is characterized by polymorph infiltration, oedema and erythema maximal at 3–8 hours (Arthus reaction). Examples are Farmer's lung, pigeon fancier's disease and pulmonary aspergillosis where inhaled antigens provoke high antibody levels, reactions to an abrupt increase in antigen caused by microbial cell death during chemotherapy for leprosy or syphilis, and an element of the synovial lesion in rheumatoid arthritis. In relative *antigen excess*, soluble complexes are formed which circulate and are deposited under circumstances of increased vascular permeability at certain preferred sites, the kidney glomerulus, the joints, the skin and the choroid plexus. Complexes can be detected in tissue biopsies by immunoflorescence and in serum by precipitation with polyethylene glycol, reaction with C1q, changes in C3 and C3c, and binding to the C3 receptor on the Raji cell line. Examples are: serum sickness following injection of large quantities of foreign protein, glomerulonephritis associated

211

with systemic lupus or infections with streptococci, malaria and other parasites, neurological disturbances in systemic lupus and subacute sclerosing panencephalitis, polyarteritis nodosa linked to hepatitis B virus, and haemorrhagic shock in dengue viral infection.

Type IV—cell-mediated or delayed-type hypersensitivity is based upon the interaction of antigen with primed T-cells. A number of soluble mediators (lymphokines) are released which account for the events which occur in a typical delayed hypersensitivity response such as the Mantoux reaction to tuberculin, namely, the delayed appearance of an indurated and erythematous reaction which reaches a maximum at 24−48 hours and is characterized histologically by infiltration first with poly-morphs and subsequently with mononuclear phagocytes and lymphocytes. The lymphokines include: macrophage migration inhibition (MIF), macrophage activation (MAF), mono-nuclear chemotactic, skin reactive, lymphocyte mitogenic, and cytostatic (lymphotoxin) factors. Interferon is also generated. Another sub-population of T-cells are activated by major histocompatibility antigens to become directly cytotoxic to target cells bearing the appropriate antigen; they also react to viral determinants on the surface of infected cells which are recognized in association with these MHC antigens. *In vitro* tests for cell-mediated hypersensitivity include macrophage migration inhibition, assessement of blast cell transformation and direct cytotoxicity. Examples are: tissue damage occurring in bacterial (tuberculosis, leprosy), viral (smallpox, measles, herpes), fungal (candidiasis, histoplasmosis) and parasitic (leishmaniasis, schistosomiasis) infections, contact dermatitis from exposure to chromates and poison ivy, and insect bites. Continuing provocation of delayed hypersensitivity by per-sisting antigen leads to formation of chronic granulomata. ·

Type V—stimulatory hypersensitivity where the antibody reacts with a key surface component such as a hormone receptor and 'switches on' the cell. An example is the thyroid hyper-reactivity in Graves' disease due to a thyroid stimulating autoantibody.

Features of the five types of hypersensitivity are compared in Table 8.1.

TABLE 8.1. Comparison of different types of hypersensitivity

	I Anaphylactic	II Cytotoxic	III Complex-mediated	IV Cell-mediated	V Stimulatory
Antibody mediating reaction	Homocytotropic Ab Mast-cell binding	Humoral Ab ±CF*	Humoral Ab ±CF	Receptor on T-lymphocyte	Humoral Ab Non-CF
Antigen	Usually exogenous (e.g. grass pollen)	Cell surface	Extracellular	Associated with MHC antigens on macrophage or target cell	Cell surface
Response to intradermal antigen:					
Max. reaction	30 min	—	3–8 h	24–48 h	—
Appearance	Wheal and flare	—	Erythema and oedema	Erythema and induration	—
Histology	Degranulated mast cells; oedema; eosinophils	—	Acute inflammatory reaction; predominant polymorphs	Perivascular inflammation: polymorphs migrate out leaving predominantly mononuclear cells	—
Transfer sensitivity to normal subject	Serum antibody ―――――――――――――――――			→ Lymphoid cells Transfer factor	Serum antibody
Examples:	Atopic allergy, e.g. hay fever	Haemolytic disease of newborn (Rh)	Complex glomerulonephritis Farmer's lung	Mantoux reaction to TB Killing virally infected cells Contact sensitivity	Thyrotoxicosis

*CF = complement fixation.

Further reading

Brostoff J. (1973) Atopic allergy. *Brit.J.Hosp.Med.*, **9,** 29.

Cochrane C.G. & Koffler D. (1973) Immune complex disease in experimental animals and man. *Adv. Immun.*, **16,** 186.

Fudenberg H.H., Stites D.P., Caldwell J.L. & Wells J.V. (1978) *Basic and Clinical Immunology*, 2nd edn. Lange Medical Publications, Los Altos, California.

Lachmann R. & Peters D.K. (eds) (1982) *Clinical Aspects of Immunology*, 4th edn, section IV. Blackwell Scientific Publications, Oxford.

Ling N.R. (1975) *Lymphocyte Stimulation*, 2nd edn. North-Holland, Amsterdam.

Maini R.N. & Holborrow E.J. (eds) (1977) Detection and measurement of circulating soluble antigen–antibody complexes and anti-DNA antibodies. *Ann.Rheum.Dis.*, **36,** suppl. no. 1.

Mollison P.L. (1970) Red cell destruction. *Brit.J.Haematol.*, **18,** 249.

O'Regan S., Smith M. & Drumond K.N. (1976) Antigens in human immune complex nephritis. *Clin.Nephrol.*, **6,** 417.

Pepys J. (1969) *Hypersensitivity Diseases of the Lungs due to Fungi and Organic Dusts.* Karger, Basle.

Roitt I.M., Shen L. & Greenberg A.H. (1976) Antibody-dependent cell-mediated cytotoxicity. In *The Role of Immunological Factors in Infectious, Allergic and Autoimmune Processes.* Beers R.F. & Bassett E.G. (eds). Raven Press, New York.

Rose N.R. & Friedman H. (1976) *Manual of Clinical Immunology.* American Society of Microbiology, Washington, D.C.

Stanworth D.S. (1973) *Immediate Hypersensitivity.* North-Holland, Amsterdam.

Turk J.L. (1975) *Delayed Hypersensitivity*, 2nd edn. North-Holland, Amsterdam.

Turk J.L. (1978) *Immunology in Clinical Medicine*, 3rd edn. Heinemann, London.

9 Transplantation

The replacement of diseased organs by a transplant of healthy tissue has long been an objective in medicine but has been frustrated to no mean degree by the unco-operative attempts by the body to reject grafts from other individuals. Before discussing the nature and implications of this rejection phenomenon, it would be helpful to define the terms used for transplants between individuals and species:

Autograft—tissue grafted back onto the original donor.

Isograft—graft between syngeneic individuals (i.e. of identical genetic constitution) such as identical twins or mice of the same pure line strain.

Allograft (old term, homograft)—graft between allogeneic individuals (i.e. members of the same species but different genetic constitution), e.g. man to man and one mouse strain to another.

Xenograft (heterograft)—graft between xenogeneic individuals (i.e. of different species), e.g. pig to man.

It is with the allograft reaction that we have been most concerned although it should one day be possible to use grafts from other species. The most common allografting procedure is probably blood transfusion where the unfortunate consequences of mismatching are well known. Considerable attention has been paid to the rejection of solid grafts such as skin and the sequence of events is worth describing. In mice, for example, the skin allograft settles down and becomes vascularized within a few days. Between 3 and 9 days the circulation gradually diminishes and there is increasing infiltration of the graft bed with lymphocytes and monocytes but very few plasma cells. Necrosis begins to be visible macroscopically and within a day or so the graft is sloughed completely (figure 9.1).

Evidence that rejection is immunological

First and second set reactions

It would be expected if the reaction has an immunological basis, that the second contact with antigen would represent a

215

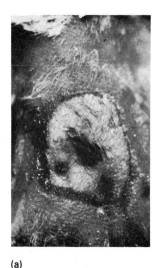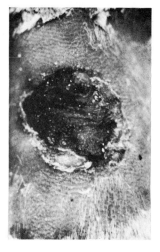

(a)   (b)

FIGURE 9.1. Rejection of CBA skin graft by strain A mouse. (a) Ten days after transplantation; the discoloured areas are caused by destruction of epithelium and drying of the exposed dermis. (b) Thirteen days after transplantation; the scabby surface indicates total destruction of the graft. (Courtesy of Professor L. Brent.)

more explosive event than the first and indeed the rejection of a second graft from the same donor is much accelerated. The initial vascularization is poor and may not occur at all. There is a very rapid invasion by polymorphonuclear leucocytes and lymphoid cells including plasma cells. Thrombosis and acute cell destruction can be seen by three to four days.

Specificity

Second set rejection is not the fate of all subsequent allografts but only of those derived from the original donor or a related strain. Grafts from unrelated donors are rejected as first set reactions.

Role of the lymphocyte

Neonatally thymectomized animals have difficulty in rejecting skin grafts but their capacity is restored by injection of lymphocytes from a syngeneic normal donor, suggesting that T-cells are implicated. The recipient of lymphoid cells from a donor which has already rejected a graft will give accelerated rejection of a further graft of the same type (figure 9.2) showing that the lymphoid cells are primed and retain memory of the first contact with graft antigens.

216

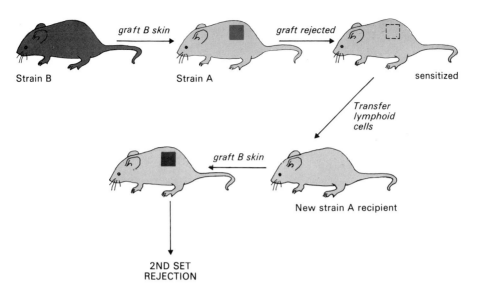

Strain B

graft B skin

Strain A

graft rejected

sensitized

Transfer lymphoid cells

graft B skin

New strain A recipient

2ND SET
REJECTION

FIGURE 9.2. Transfer of ability to give accelerated graft rejection with lymphoid cells from a sensitized animal.

Production of antibodies

After rejection, humoral antibodies with specificity for the graft donor may be recognized. In the mouse where the erythrocytes carry transplantation antigens, haemagglutination tests become positive; in the human, lymphocytotoxins are found. A Jerne plaque test using donor strain thymocytes in place of sheep erythrocytes will often demonstrate the presence of antibody-forming cells in the lymphoid tissues of grafted animals.

Transplantation antigens

GENETICS

The specificity of the antigens involved in graft rejection is under genetic control. Genetically identical individuals such as mice of a pure strain or uniovular twins have identical transplantation antigens and grafts can be freely exchanged between them. The Mendelian segregation of the genes controlling these antigens has been revealed by interbreeding experiments between mice of different pure strains. Since these mice breed true within a given strain and always accept grafts from each other, they must be homozygous for the 'transplantation' genes. Consider two such strains, A and B, with allelic genes differing at one locus. In each case paternal and maternal genes will be

217

identical and they will have a genetic constitution of, say, AA and BB respectively. Crossing strains A and B gives first familial generation (F1) of constitution AB. These accept grafts from either parent; they must therefore be tolerant to the antigens expressed by both A and B genes and in fact these genes are codominant, i.e. individual cells carry both types of transplantation antigen (figure 9.3) as may be shown by immunofluorescent studies. By intercrossing the F1 generation, it will be seen from figure 9.3 that three out of four of the F2 generation accept parental strain grafts. Extending the analysis, if instead of one locus with a pair of allelic genes, there were n loci, the fraction of the F2 generation accepting parental strain grafts would be $(3/4)^n$. In this way an estimate of the number of loci controlling transplantation antigens can be made.

In the mouse at least 20 such loci have been established, but of these, one complex locus termed H-2 predominates in the sense that it controls the 'strong' transplantation antigens which provoke intense allograft reactions that are the most difficult to suppress. This H-2 locus constitutes the *major histocompatibility complex* (MHC), and it is a feature of all the vertebrate species so far studied that each possesses a single MHC which dominates allo-transplantation reactivity.

THE MAJOR HISTOCOMPATIBILITY COMPLEX IN MICE

Classical transplantation (type I) antigens

Although the H-2 locus appeared to be a single entity, it is now

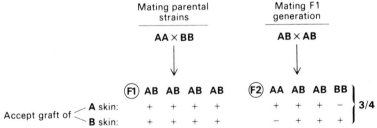

FIGURE 9.3. Inheritance of genes controlling transplantation antigens. A represents a gene expressing the 'A' antigen and B the corresponding allelic gene at the same genetic locus. The pure strains are homozygous for AA and BB respectively. Since the genes are codominant, an animal with an AB genome will express both antigens, become tolerant to them and therefore accept grafts from either A or B donors. The illustration shows that for each gene controlling a transplantation antigen specificity, three-quarters of the F2 generation will accept a graft of parental skin. For n genes the fraction is $(3/4)^n$.

seen to be far more complicated and may be broken down into regions which are separable by genetic recombination (i.e. by chromosomal crossing over between the subregions). Allo-antisera obtained by grafting or immunization between different mouse strains identify two major regions K and D (figure 9.4) each defined by a major genetic locus (with numerous alleles) which encodes a single 'strong' trans-plantation antigen. Each chromosome therefore controls the synthesis of an H-2K and an H-2D antigenic specificity. Because they are the most potent antigens of the H-2 complex in provoking an antibody response, they were the first to be recognized by sera from allografted animals and the term classical transplantation antigens is appropriate, and as it turns out, useful. A third locus codes for H-2L, a minor series of polymorphic antigens structurally similar to H-2D/K. All lymphoid cells are rich in H-2D/K antigens; liver, lung and kidney have moderate amounts whereas brain and skeletal

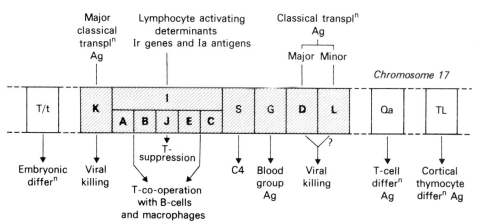

FIGURE 9.4. The H-2 major histocompatibility gene complex (▨) and its subregions in the mouse (bold letters encode antigens concerned in transplantation reactions; differ^n, differentiation; Ag, antigen). The complex spans 0.5 centimorgans equivalent to a recombination frequency between the D and K ends of 0.5%. The genes making up a given H-2 complex are termed a haplotype, usually represented by a superscript, e.g. DBA has the H-2^d haplotype. Because the genes are close together, the haplotype appears to segregate as a single Mendelian trait, the complexity only being revealed by recombination through crossing over. Each H-2K and D molecule possesses several antigenic specificities corresponding with a number of different antigenic determinants and these are classed as: (a) private specificities unique for a given haplotype; (b) public specificities shared between different haplotypes but unique for K or D regions; and (c) public specificities shared between K and D regions. The H-2K product provokes a more powerful transplantation reaction than H-2D. Other genes within the H-2 complex control levels of C2, C3 and Factor B.

219

muscle have relatively little. The antigens are evidently on the cell surface since lymphocytes are readily lysed by antibody in the presence of complement. Capping experiments and SDS-polyacrylamide gel analysis of immunoprecipitates of radio-labelled, detergent-solubilized H-2 show the K and D specificities to be associated with separate molecules. They are located on peptides of molecular weight 43,000 which are associated non-covalently with β_2-microglobulin (cf. HLA-A, figure 9.7). Both β_2-microglobulin and the H-2D/K peptides show a high degree of homology with the immunoglobulin constant region domains and appear to adopt a similar tertiary configuration suggesting a common evolutionary origin. There is evidence that in the absence of β_2-microglobulin, the classical transplantation antigens fail to be expressed on the cell surface. These antigens are transmembrane glycoproteins and the sero-logical specificity lies in the amino acid sequence rather than the carbohydrate moiety.

Lymphocyte activating determinants (type II antigens)

Mixed lymphocyte reaction (MLR). When lymphocytes from genetically dissimilar mice are cultured together, blast cell transformation and mitosis occurs (MLR), each population of lymphocytes reacting against 'foreign' determinants on the surface of the other population. For the 'one-way MLR', the stimulator cells are made unresponsive by treatment with mitomycin C or X-rays and then added to the responder lymphocytes from the other donor. The responding cells belong predominantly to a subpopulation of Ly1 positive T-lympho-cytes and they are stimulated by lymphocyte activating deter-minants (Lad) present mostly on B-cells and macrophages, the genes which code for them lying within the I region (figure 9.4). Antisera to I region antigens (anti-Ia) block the Lad of the stimulator cells and thereby inhibit the MLR, suggesting that the Lad are present on Ia molecules. It will be recalled that the Ia antigens are concerned in T help and T suppression. Cells bearing I-J evoke suppressors and T-lymphocytes positive for I-A and I-E/C mediate delayed sensitivity and B-cell help. I-A and I-E/C are transmembrane glycoproteins each consisting of an α- and a β-polypeptide, both of which are polymorphic (cf. figure 9.7).

Graft vs. host (g.v.h.) reaction. When competent lymphoid cells are transferred from a donor to a recipient which is incapable of rejecting them, the grafted cells survive and have time to recognize the host antigens and react immunologically against them. Instead of the normal transplantation reaction of host against graft, we have the reverse, the so-called graft vs. host reaction. In the young rodent there can be inhibition of growth (runting), spleen enlargement and haemolytic anaemia (due to production of red cell antibodies). In the human, fever, anaemia, weight loss, rash, diarrhoea and splenomegaly are observed. The 'stronger' the transplantation antigen difference, the more severe the reaction. Where donor and recipient differ at HLA or H-2 loci, the reaction can be fatal.

Two possible situations leading to g.v.h. reactions are illustrated in figure 9.5. In the human this may arise in immunologically anergic subjects receiving bone marrow grafts, e.g. for combined immunodeficiency (p. 177), for red cell aplasia after radiation accidents or as a possible form of cancer therapy. Competent lymphoid cells in blood or present in grafted organs given to immunosuppressed patients may give g.v.h. reactions; so could maternal cells which adventitiously cross the placenta, although in this case there is as yet no evidence of diseases caused by such a mechanism in the human.

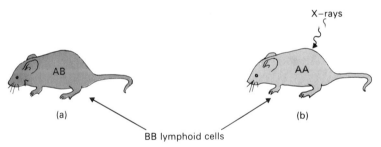

FIGURE 9.5. Graft vs. host reaction. When competent lymphoid cells are inoculated into a host incapable of reacting against them, the grafted cells are free to react against the antigens on the host's cells which they recognize as foreign. The ensuing reaction may be fatal. Two of many possible situations are illustrated: (a) the hybrid AB receives cells from one parent (BB) which are tolerated but react against the A antigen on host cells; (b) an X-irradiated AA recipient restored immunologically with BB cells cannot react against the graft and a g.v.h. reaction will result.

THE MAJOR HISTOCOMPATIBILITY
COMPLEX IN MAN

In man, as in the mouse, there is also one dominant group of antigens which provokes strong reactions—the HLA system. In addition, the ABO group provides strong transplantation antigens.

Of the four principal HLA loci identified, HLA-A and HLA B probably represent the counterpart of the murine sero-logically defined antigens H-2K and H-2D in that they most readily evoke the formation of complement-fixing cytotoxic antibodies which can be used for tissue typing. Operationally mono-specific sera are selected from patients transfused with whole blood and multigravidas who often become immunized with fetal antigens with specificities defined by paternally derived genes absent from the mother's genome. An individual is typed by setting up their lymphocytes against a panel of such sera in the presence of complement, cell death normally being

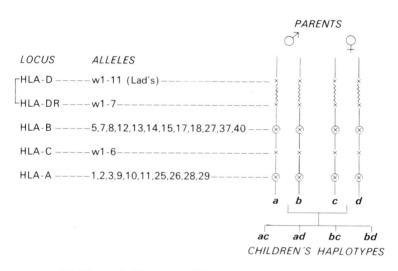

FIGURE 9.6. The major histocompatibility complex in man (HLA) and its inheritance. The four loci lie on chromosome 6, the D locus being closest to the centromere. ⊗, Major loci originally defined by serological tissue typing which parallel the murine H-2K and H-2D classical transplantation loci; there are several more specificities at each locus but only the most solidly established are given. A further locus with just two alleles, HLA-Bw4 and Bw6 (formerly 4a/4b), is intimately linked to HLA-B. Specificities at the D locus (Lad's) are defined by their mixed lymphocyte reactions against homozygous typing cells, but closely related (HLA-DR), if not sometimes identical, antigens are also being characterized using cytotoxic antibodies. The small 'w' before a number stands for 'workshop' and indicates that the specificity concerned has not yet been characterized sufficiently for upgrading to full HLA-status.

Since there are several possible alleles at each locus, the probability of a random pair of subjects from the general population having identical HLA specificities is low. However, there is a 1:4 chance that two *siblings* will be identical in this respect because each group of specificities on a single chromosome forms a haplotype which will be inherited *en bloc* giving four possible combinations of paternal and maternal chromosomes. Parent and offspring can only be identical (1:2 chance) if the mother and father have one haplotype in common.

judged by the inability to exclude trypan blue. Antigens arbitrarily assigned the specificities 1, 2, 3, 9, 10, 11, 28 and 29 by this means are negatively associated with each other in population studies; no individual has more than two of these antigens and not more than one is transmitted to an offspring from each parent: they therefore form an allelic series referred to as the HLA-A locus (figure 9.6). HLA-B5, 7, 8, 12, 13, 14, 18 and 27 constitute a second locus. Thus, an individual heterozygous at each locus must express four *major* serologically defined HLA specificities, two from maternally derived and two from the paternally derived chromosomes (figure 9.6). Serologically defined antigens encoded by a third locus, HLA-C, induce a somewhat weaker response.

The major lymphocyte activating determinants are controlled by alleles at a fourth locus, HLA-D. Typing is carried out by looking for non-reactivity in the MLR against a

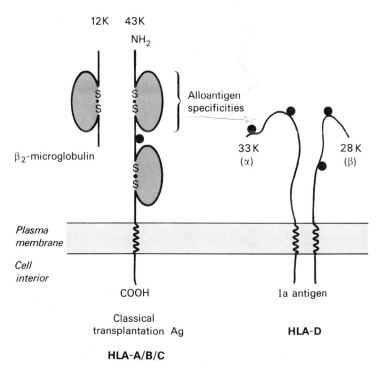

FIGURE 9.7. Structure of major HLA molecules. They are transmembrane glycoproteins (●, carbohydrate) with hydrophobic segments (〜〜〜) inserted into the plasma membrane. Regions with homology for Ig domains are shaded (▦). The molecular weight of each peptide in thousands is shown. (After Barnstable C.J., Jones E.A. & Crumpton M.J. (1978) *Brit. med. Bull.*, **34**, 241. Based on structures suggested by Strominger, Snarg & colleagues.)

homozygous stimulating cell. Such typing cells may be obtained from the children of first cousin marriages (where there is a 1 : 16 chance of homozygosity) or from patients with a disease known to be strongly associated with certain D alleles, e.g. multiple sclerosis and HLA-Dw2. Another approach is to use spermatozoa as stimulators since they only carry one haplotype; spermatozoa expressing the other paternal haplotype can be eliminated by appropriate cytotoxic antisera directed against A or B locus antigens. Closely related, if not identical antigens are also being characterized by cytotoxic antibodies. These HLA-D related serologically defined specificities (HLA-DR) are most abundant on B-lymphocytes and are often termed B-cell alloantigens; however, they are also present on macrophages and are probably the equivalent of murine Ia antigens. The structures of the different HLA molecules are represented in figure 9.7.

Rejection mechanisms

LYMPHOCYTE-MEDIATED REJECTION

A great deal of the work on allograft rejection has involved transplants of skin or solid tumours because their fate is relatively easy to follow. In these cases there is little support for the view that humoral antibodies are instrumental in destruction of the graft although as we shall see later this is not necessarily so with transplants of other organs such as the kidney. Whereas passive transfer of *serum* from an animal which has rejected a skin allograft cannot usually accelerate the rejection of a similar graft on the recipient animal, injection of *lymphoid cells* (particularly recirculating small lymphocytes) is effective in shortening graft survival (cf. figure 9.2). Tissue culture studies have shown that such lymphoid cells taken from animals sensitized by a graft which they have rejected are able to kill target cells possessing the same transplantation antigens as the original graft. The sensitized lymphocytes recognize the target cells through specific surface receptors and this combination with antigen leads to surface membrane changes responsible for the cytotoxic potential of the lymphocytes.

A primary role of lymphoid cells in first set rejection would be consistent with the histology of the early reaction showing infiltration by mononuclear cells with very few polymorphs or plasma cells. The dramatic effect of neonatal thymectomy in prolonging skin transplants, as mentioned earlier, and the long survival of grafts on children with thymic deficiencies implicate the T-lymphocytes in these reactions. In the chicken, homograft rejection and g.v.h. reactivity are influenced by neonatal thymectomy but not bursectomy. More direct evidence has come from *in vitro* studies showing that the sensitized mouse lymphocytes responsible for killing certain target allograft in tissue culture bear the Thy 1 marker on their surface (see p. 55) and are therefore T-lymphocytes.

Lymphoid cells sensitized to a graft can release macrophage migration inhibition factor (MIF); see 205) when confronted with the appropriate histocompatibility antigens and it is possible that this test will give an early indication of sensitization in a grafted individual.

THE ROLE OF HUMORAL ANTIBODY

It has long been recognized that isolated allogeneic cells such as lymphocytes can be destroyed by cytotoxic (type II) reactions involving humoral antibody. However, although earlier experience with skin and solid tumour-grafts suggested that they were not readily susceptible to the action of cytotoxic antibodies, it is now clear that this does not hold for all types of organ transplants. Consideration of the different ways in which kidney allografts can be rejected illustrates the point:

(1) *Hyperacute rejection* within minutes of transplantation, characterized by sludging of red cells and microthrombi in the glomeruli, occurs in individuals with pre-existing humoral antibodies—either due to blood group incompatibility or presensitization through blood transfusion.

(2) *Acute early rejection* occurring up to 10 days or so after transplantation is characterized by dense cellular infiltration and rupture of peritubular capillaries and appears to be a cell-mediated hypersensitivity reaction involving T-lymphocytes.

(3) *Acute late rejection*, which occurs from 11 days onwards in patients suppressed with prednisone and azathioprine, is probably caused by the binding of immunoglobulin (presumably antibody) and complement to the arterioles and glomerular capillaries where they can be visualized by immuno-fluorescent techniques. These immunoglobulin deposits on the vessel walls induce platelet aggregation in the glomerular capillaries leading to acute renal shutdown. The possibility of damage to antibody-coated cells through antibody-dependent cell-mediated cytotoxicity must also be considered.

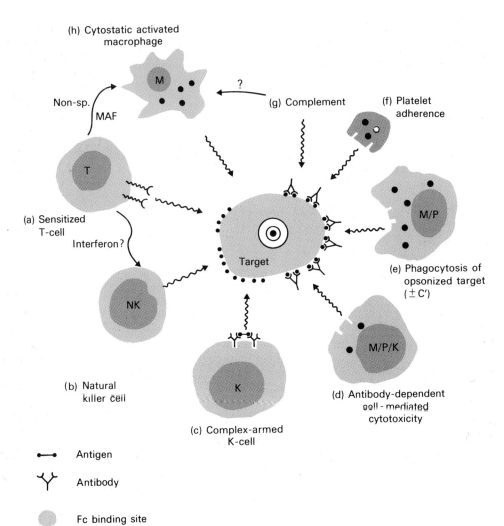

(h) Cytostatic activated
macrophage

M

Non-sp.
MAF

(g) Complement

?

(f) Platelet
adherence

T

M/P

(a) Sensitized
T-cell

Interferon?

Target

(e) Phagocytosis of
opsonized target
($\pm$ C')

NK

(b) Natural
killer cell

K

M/P/K

(c) Complex-armed
K-cell

(d) Antibody-dependent
cell-mediated
cytotoxicity

•—•   Antigen

Y   Antibody

    Fc binding site

FIGURE 9.8. Mechanisms of target cell destruction. M, macrophage; P, polymorph; K, K cell. (a) Direct killing by sensitized T cells binding through specific surface receptors. In addition a non-specific soluble toxin is released. (b) Killing by NK cells (p. 239) enhanced by interferon. (c) Specific killing by an immune-complex-armed K cell which recognizes the target through free antibody valencies in the complex. (d) Attack by antibody-dependent cell-mediated cytotoxicity (in a–d the killing is extra-cellular). (e) Phagocytosis of target coated with antibody (heightened by bound C3). (f) Sticking of platelets to antibody bound to the surface of graft vascular endothelium leading to formation of microthrombi. (g) Complement mediated cytotoxicity. (h) Macrophages activated non-specifically by agents such as BCG, endotoxin, poly-I:C, T-cell non-specific macrophage activating factor and (?) C3b are cytostatic and sometimes cytotoxic for dividing tumour cells perhaps through extracellular action of peroxide and O_2^- derived radicals generated at the cell surface (p. 150). In some situations *in vitro*, sensitized B cells secrete antibody which coats the target rendering it susceptible to attack by ADCC.

(4) *Insidious and late* rejection associated with subendothelial deposits of immunoglobulin and C3 on the glomerular basement membranes which may sometimes be an expression of an underlying immune complex disorder (originally necessitating the transplant) or possibly complex formation with soluble antigens derived from the grafted kidney.

The complexity of the action and interaction of cellular and humoral factors in graft rejection is therefore considerable and an attempt to summarize the postulated mechanisms involved is presented in figure 9.8.

There are also circumstances when antibodies may actually *protect* a graft from destruction and this important phenomenon of *enhancement* will be considered further below.

Prevention of graft rejection

TISSUE MATCHING

Based upon experience of matching blood for transfusion and of transplantation between mice of similar specificities it could reasonably be expected that the chances of rejection in the human would be minimized by matching donor and recipient at the HLA loci. Indeed in the case of human kidney transplantation, the data based upon typing for HLA-A and -B specificities indicate that the closer the match, the better the survival of the graft. This is especially true with matched siblings (figure 9.9) but it would be wrong to conclude that full matching at A and B loci is all that is necessary since grafts between unrelated individuals who fulfil this condition are markedly less successful than those between siblings. Now we have seen that matched siblings have the same haplotypes (figure 9.6) and are therefore identical at all *four* loci, and if we further note that the generation of T helpers for cytotoxicity (and antibody?) is largely dependent upon D locus differences, it seems likely that matching the D antigens will prove to be a major factor in improving graft survival.

Because of the many thousands of different HLA phenotypes possible (figure 9.6), it is usual to work with a large pool of potential recipients on a continental basis so that when graft material becomes available the best possible match can be made. The position will be improved when the pool of available organs can be increased through the development of long-term tissue storage banks but techniques are not good enough for this at present except in the case of bone marrow cells which can be kept viable even after freezing and thawing. With a paired organ such as the kidney, living donors may be used; siblings provide the best chance of a good match (cf. figure 9.6). However, the use of living donors poses difficult ethical problems and the objective must be to perfect the use of cadaver material (? or animal organs—or mechanical substitutes!).

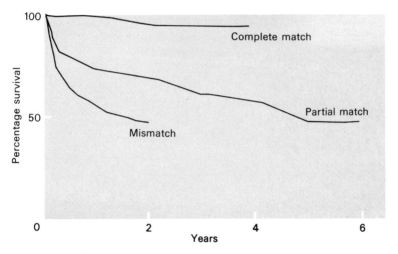

FIGURE 9.9. Survival of kidney transplants in relation to the degree of matching at HLA-A and -B loci. Complete match (siblings) = all antigens identical; partial match (siblings and parent to child) = only antigens on one chromosome (haplotype) identical; mismatch (unrelated) = all antigens different. (Data taken from Dausset J. & Hors J. (1973), *Transpl. Proc.*, **V**, 223.)

GENERAL IMMUNOSUPPRESSION

Graft rejection can be held at bay by the use of agents which non-specifically interfere with the induction or expression of the immune response. Because these agents are non-specific, patients on immunosuppressive therapy tend to be susceptible to infections; they are also more prone to develop lympho-reticular cancers.

Lymphoid cell ablation

Thymectomy, splenectomy and lymphadenectomy in adult recipients do not appear to help, although extra-corporeal irradiation of blood, injections of anti-lymphocyte globulin (ALG) and thoracic duct cannulation have proved beneficial. Total lymphoid irradiation would appear somewhat Draconian but has been shown to prolong skin grafts in mice when given in divided doses over an extended period. The most striking feature of this work is that allogeneic bone marrow cells given at

228

the end of this treatment schedule are fully accepted without the development of g.v.h. reactions (Strober & Slavin).

Perhaps the most commonly used drug in this field is *azathioprine* which has a preferential effect on T-cell mediated reactions. It is broken down in the body first to 6-mercaptopurine and then converted to the active agent, the ribotide. Because of the similarity in shape (figure 9.10), this competes with inosinic acid for enzymes concerned in the synthesis of guanylic and adenylic acids; it also inhibits the synthesis of 5-phosphoribosylamine, a precursor of inosinic acid, by a feedback mechanism. The net result is inhibition of nucleic acid synthesis. Another drug, methotrexate, through its action as a folic acid antagonist also inhibits synthesis of nucleic acid. The N-mustard derivative cyclophosphamide probably attacks DNA by alkylation and cross-linking so preventing correct duplication during cell division. These agents appear to exert their damaging effects on cells during mitosis and for this reason are most powerful when administered after presentation of antigen at a time when the antigen-sensitive cells are dividing. Cyclosporin A, a rather insoluble fungal metabolite, is of particular interest since not only will it act on these antigen-sensitive dividing cells and spare the resting cells which carry the vital memory for immunity to microbial infections, but it seems to be differentially toxic to dividing lymphocytes as compared with other active cells in the gut and bone marrow. Whether or not Cyclosporin itself proves to be of permanent clinical value, it does seem to offer a new pathway towards the development of agents with selective action against dividing lymphocytes.

Steroids such as prednisone intervene at many points in the immune response, affecting lymphocyte recirculation and the generation of cytotoxic effector cells for example; in addition, their outstanding anti-inflammatory potency rests on features such as inhibition of neutrophil adherence to vascular

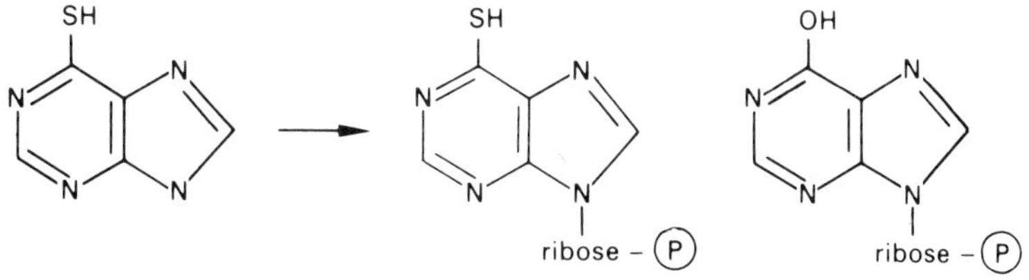

6 – Mercaptopurine

6 – Mercaptopurine riboside

Inosinic acid

FIGURE 9.10. Metabolic conversion of azathioprine through 6-mercaptopurine to the ribotide: similarity to inosinic acid with which it competes.

endothelium in an inflammatory area and suppression of monocyte/macrophage functions such as microbicidal activity and response to lymphikines. The combination of azathioprine and prednisone is commonly employed in the long-term management of kidney grafts.

Immunological tolerance

If the disadvantages of blanket immunosuppression are to be avoided, we must aim at knocking out only the reactivity of the host to the antigens of the graft leaving the remainder of the immunological apparatus intact. One approach is through the induction of tolerance in the patient. Through selective action on antigen-sensitive dividing cells, Cyclosporin A may induce clonal abortion. Total lymph node irradiation plus bone marrow (see above) is thought to induce specific T-suppression, and grafts of skin and heart from the same donor enjoy prolonged survival. As purified histocompatibility antigens become available it should ultimately not be beyond the wit of *Homo sapiens* to juggle the relative timing and dosages of antigen and various immunosuppressants to produce a specific hyporesponsive state.

Enhancement

There is another possible solution which may be easier to achieve and that is deliberate immunization with these antigens to evoke antibodies which protect rather than destroy the graft. It has long been recognized that such *enhancing* sera are responsible for the prolonged survival of tumour allografts after prior immunization with irradiated tumour cells. The precise mechanism has still to be revealed but explanations usually fall under two headings, masking by antibody and blocking by antigen (figure 9.11).

Successful enhancement of kidney and bone-marrow grafts have been reported in isolated instances and one supposes this will inevitably be extended. There are indications that serum enhancing factors may inhibit tumour destruction by cell-mediated mechanisms in some cancer patients as will be discussed later.

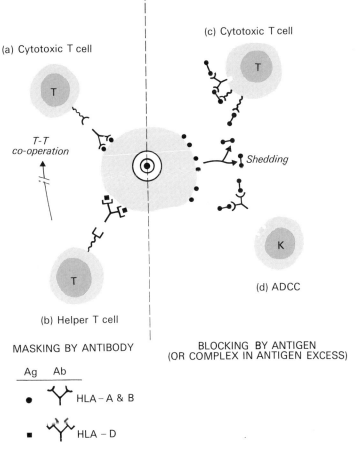

(a) Cytotoxic T cell

(c) Cytotoxic T cell

T-T
co-operation

Shedding

(b) Helper T cell

(d) ADCC

MASKING BY ANTIBODY

BLOCKING BY ANTIGEN
(OR COMPLEX IN ANTIGEN EXCESS)

Ag   Ab

HLA – A & B

HLA – D

FIGURE 9.11. Enhancement: possible mechanisms. *Block by antibody*—(a) Masking the HLA-A or B antigens on the target surface inhibits attack by cytotoxic T-cells. (b) Masking of Ia on the target prevents the induction of T-helpers and hence of cytotoxic T-cells. There is evidence that tolerance may be induced if classical transplantation antigens are presented in the absence of Ia-induced T-helpers (cf. the idea that one signal tolerizes and two signals trigger a B-cell).

Block by antigen—Sufficient antigen shed from the surface of the target, either free or as a complex in antigen excess, can (c) block the receptors on cytotoxic T-cells and possibly tolerize their precursors or (d) block the antibody involved in antibody dependent cell-mediated cytotoxicity.

It has also been suggested that antibody could opsonize antigen-sensitive cells which had bound antigen to their surface, so causing their elimination.

Clinical experience in grafting

Privileged sites

Corneal grafts survive without the need for immuno-suppression. Because they are avascular they do not sensitize the recipient although they become cloudy if the individual has been presensitized. Grafts of cartilage are successful in the same

231

way but an additional factor is the protection afforded the chondrocytes by the matrix. With bone and artery it doesn't really matter if the grafts die because they can still provide a framework for host cells to colonize.

Kidney

Thousands of kidneys have been transplanted and with improvement in patient management there is a high survival rate (figure 9.9). Patients are partially immunosuppressed at the time of transplantation because uraemia causes a degree of immunological anergy. Recipients sharing three or four of the A and B locus antigens with the donor show improved results if they have previously been transfused with blood; will this prove to be a case of serendipitous enhancement through production of Ia antibodies? Unquestionably the importance of D-locus matching is widely recognized. If kidney function is poor during a rejection crisis renal dialysis can be used.

Heart

Something like 40–50% of transplant patients survive by one year. The results have not been as good as with kidney grafting but special factors should be taken into account. The recipient patients were in irreversible cardiac failure with wasting and advanced secondary changes of passive congestion, and the clinical urgency made it difficult to find well-matched donor organs. Aside from the rejection problem it is likely that the number of patients who would benefit from cardiac replacement is much greater than the number dying with adequately healthy hearts. More attention will have to be given to the possibility of xenogeneic grafts and mechanical substitutes.

Biological significance of the major histocompatibility complex

POLYMORPHISM

With four loci on each of two chromosomes and several alleles at each locus, there are literally millions of different possible phenotypes; in other words the MHC is an extraordinarily polymorphic system. That this holds for widely divergent species like man, mouse and chicken implies that the maintenance of such polymorphism confers a survival advantage in evolutionary terms. One suggestion is that a polymorphic system provides a defence against microbial molecular mimicry in which a whole species might be put at risk by its inability to recognize as foreign an organism which displayed determinants similar in structure to those of the host. It is also possible that in some way the existence of a high degree of polymorphism helps to maintain the diversity of antigenic recognition within the lymphoid system of a given species.

One consequence of this multi-allelic complex is that it ensures *heterozygosity*, with its connotation of 'hybrid vigour' (yet another phenomenon whose mechanisms remain obscure but could involve almost anything from fertilization onwards).

IMMUNOLOGICAL RELATIONSHIP
OF MOTHER AND FETUS

A further consequence of polymorphism in an outbred population is that mother and fetus will almost certainly have different MHCs. Some examples of selection for heterozygotes (where maternally and paternally derived haplotypes are different) over homozygotes (both fetal haplotypes identical with the mother's) in viviparous animals suggest that this is beneficial.

The threat posed to the fetus as a potential graft due to the possession of paternal transplantation antigens so intrigued Lewis Thomas that he was moved to suggest that rejection of the fetus might initiate parturition, although it would be difficult to account for the normal birth of female offspring to pure strain mating pairs where fetus and mother would have identical histocompatibility antigens without further postulating a placenta-specific surface antigen.

Nonetheless, in the human haemochorial placenta, maternal blood with immunocompetent lymphocytes does circulate in contact with the fetal trophoblast and the fetus probably avoids allograft rejection through the low density or absence of classical transplantation antigens on the syncytiotrophoblast cells and the protection of the trophoblast cells against cytotoxic lymphocytes by a surrounding barrier (admittedly incomplete) of sialic acid-rich mucopolysaccharide.

RECOGNITION SYSTEMS

It is becoming increasingly clear that the major transplantation antigens subserve an intercellular recognition function. We do not known whether they are involved in phenomena like the reassortment of dispersed kidney cells in culture which

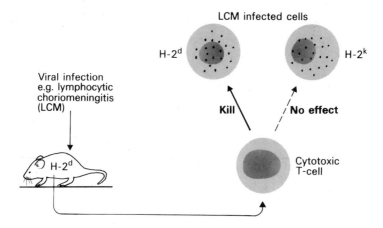

LCM infected cells

Viral infection
e.g. lymphocytic
choriomeningitis
(LCM)

H-2^d

Kill   No effect

Cytotoxic
T-cell

(a) MHC RESTRICTED CYTOTOXICITY OF T-CELLS FOR VIRALLY
INFECTED TARGETS IN VITRO

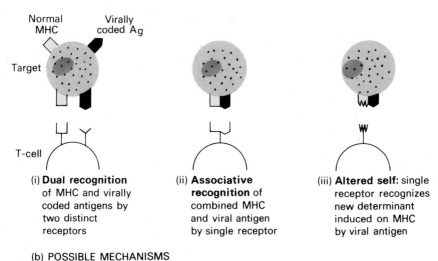

Normal   Virally
MHC   coded Ag

Target

T-cell

(i) **Dual recognition**
of MHC and virally
coded antigens by
two distinct
receptors

(ii) **Associative
recognition** of
combined MHC
and viral antigen
by single receptor

(iii) **Altered self:** single
receptor recognizes
new determinant
induced on MHC
by viral antigen

(b) POSSIBLE MECHANISMS

FIGURE 9.12. The Doherty and Zinkernagel phenomenon of haplotype
restriction in recognition of virally infected targets by cytotoxic T-cells. The
same mechanisms apply to the recognition of H-2 linked minor
transplantation antigens such as the male (Y) antigen and to the response to
Ia associated antigen on the macrophage surface.

A consequence of the altered self model is that there must be as many new
determinants inducible on the MHC molecule as there are distinct cytotoxic
T-cell specificities. Both dual and associative models involve recognition of
self MHC + viral antigen; whether it is stereochemically likely that
determinants on MHC and a separate surface antigen, even in a fluid
membrane, can become sufficiently closely apposed to fit into a single receptor
has not been established. I have proposed a two receptor model, each a single
peptide using the V_H genes and a constant region gene characteristic for
T-cells, there being no need for allelic exclusion as in B-cells. If many V_H

234

preferentially reaggregate with each other despite admixture with hepatocytes but they do undoubtedly play a central role in directing T-cell interactions.

Haplotype restriction

Of dramatic significance has been the revelation that the MHC is intimately involved in the T-cell recognition of macrophage-processed antigens (cf. p. 88), collaboration with B-cells (p. 88) and killing of virally infected cells (cf. p. 163). In essence, T-cells recognize antigen in association with one of the products of the MHC complex. Memory T-cells are most effectively triggered by exposure to antigen in association with the MHC haplotype used for priming.

Let us look at an example of this phenomenon of so-called 'haplotype restriction' in more detail. If I may be permitted to refresh your mind, dear reader, cytotoxic T-cells provoked by a virus infection will only kill target cells infected with that virus *in vitro* if they share the same classical transplantation antigens as the original host. Thus cytotoxic T-cells arising in a mouse of H-2^d haplotype infected with lymphocytic choriomeningitis virus (LCM) will kill LCM infected cells of H-2^d but not H-2^k haplotype (figure 9.12a). By using target cells from strains derived by genetic recombination within the H-2 complex, the relevant MHC molecule recognized by the T-cell has been pinpointed as H-2D. With certain other viruses such as vaccinia, the target cell shows H-2K restriction. Various models have been proposed for these recognition processes: (a) two distinct receptors combine with self H-2D (or H-2K) and virally coded antigen respectively, (b) a single receptor recognizes a determinant formed by association of H-2D/K and viral antigen, or (c) the virus modifies the synthesis or configuration of the H-2D/K molecule to produce a new 'altered self' determinant. These are discussed further in the legend to figure 9.12b.

---

segments have specificity for the constant regions (framework) of the MHC, random combination with D and J segments (p. 115) would generate a diversity of receptors enabling at least some T-cells to recognize almost any MHC private specificity. Cells which recognize self MHC with receptor will be selected for and amplified probably by the thymus or perhaps by the MHC on the body cells which prime T-lymphocytes; thus the majority of differentiated T-cells will have one receptor able to recognize self and the other, randomly selected from the V_H repertoire, able to combine with virus, minor transplantation antigens, etc.

When a cell is first infected with virus, there is an eclipse phase during which the machinery of the cell is being switched for viral replication and the only marker of the complete microbe is the viral antigen on the cell surface. At this stage, killing of the cell by a cytotoxic T-cell will prevent viral replication.

How does the killer T-cell know when it has reached its target? It has to recognize two features before striking: one is the presence of viral antigen and the other is its location on the surface of a body cell. The microbial antigen is recognized by the specific T-receptor and the cell through its marker, the classical transplantation antigens which are present on nearly every cell in the body. Thus, the killer cell in the mouse for example, operates on the basis that:

$$\text{viral antigen} + \text{H-2D/K} = \text{virally infected cell}$$

and that is why its receptor(s) has to see both antigens. The human utilizes the HLA-A and B (and probably C) loci in the same way.

The situation is quite different with intracellular bacteria and protozoa which do not go through an eclipse phase after phagocytosis by macrophages but are held as infectious entities; lysis by cytotoxic T-cells will merely release the organisms, not kill them. A separate strategy utilizing the delayed-type hypersensitivity T-cell population is required and, in this case, the effector T-lymphocyte recognizes the infected macrophage by the presence of microbial antigen on the surface in association with an I-region molecule. This interaction triggers the release of lymphokines which enable the macrophage to kill the intracellular parasites (p. 159). Similarly, in T-B co-operation, the B-cell is recognized by an Ia molecule associated with the foreign antigen while I-J is used as a marker for T-cells mediating suppression. In summary, each T-lymphocyte

TABLE 9.1. Guidance of T sub-populations to appropriate target cell by MHC molecules

Function	Cell interaction	MHC marker on target cell
T-help	T-B	I
T-proliferation	T-macrophage	I
T-delayed sensitivity	T-macrophage	I
T-suppression	T-T	I(J)
T-cytotoxic	T-infected cell	D/K

236

subset has to communicate with a particular cell type in order to make the *appropriate* immune response and it does so by recognizing not only foreign antigen (or idiotype, cf. p. 92), but also the particular MHC molecule used as a marker of that cell (table 9.1).

The ability to reject transplants of tissue may be traced back a long way down the evolutionary tree—back even as far as annelid worms. Long before the studies on the involvement of self-MHC in immunological responses, Lewis Thomas suggested that the allograft rejection mechanism represented a means by which the body's cells could be kept under *immunological surveillance* so that altered cells with a neoplastic potential could be identified and summarily eliminated. For this to operate, cancer cells must display a new surface antigen which can be recognized by the lymphoid cells and examples have been discovered.

Tumour surface antigens (figure 9.13)

(1) *Virally controlled.* Cells infected with oncogenic viruses usually display two new antigens on their surface, one (V) identical with an antigen on the isolated virion and the other (T), also a product of the viral genome, present only on infected cells; the latter represents a strong transplantation antigen and generates haplotype restricted cytotoxic T cells. All syngeneic tumours induced by a given virus carry the same surface antigen, irrespective of their cellular origin, so that immunization with any one of these tumours confers resistance to subsequent challenge with the others.

(2) *Embryonic.* Tumours derived from the same cell type often express a common differentiation antigen also present on embryonic cells (so-called oncofetal antigens). Examples would be α-fetoprotein in hepatic carcinoma and carcinoembryonic antigen (CEA) in cancer of the intestine.

(3) *Division.* The carbohydrate moiety of surface membrane glycoproteins may change during cell division. For example, Thomas found that the density of surface sugar determinants with blood group H specificity fell as murine mastocytoma cells moved into the G_1 phase of the division cycle while reciprocally, group B determinants increased; it was postulated that the

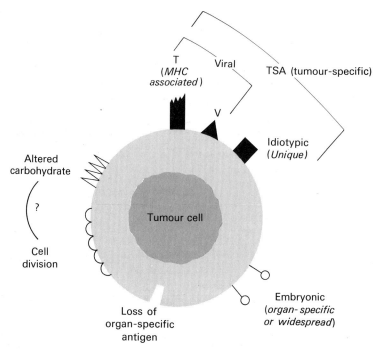

FIGURE 9.13. Tumour associated antigens. Even virally induced tumours may possess idiotypic specificities. If the tumour is cycling, surface components associated with mitosis may be detected and could be responsible for the lectin-binding carbohydrates thought at one time to be characteristic of transformed tumour cells.

continued expression of this latter component was related to a commitment to further division.

(4) *Idiotypic.* Tumours induced by chemical agents, benzopyrene for example, also possess specific transplantation antigens, but each tumour produced by a given chemical carcinogen has its own individual idiotypic antigen; even when a carcinogen produces two different primary tumours in the same animal, they do not exhibit the same antigenic specificities and do not confer cross-resistance by immunization.

Immune response to tumours

These tumour antigens can provoke immune responses in experimental animals which lead to resistance against tumour growth but they vary tremendously in their efficiency. Powerful antigens associated with tumours induced by oncogenic viruses or ultraviolet light generate strong resistance while chemically induced tumours are weaker and somewhat variable; disappointingly, tumours which arise spontaneously in animals produce little or no response. This would seem to reason against the immune surveillance theory, although it might be argued that most tumours were silenced at their inception by immunological control and that only the very few which lacked a provocative surface component were 'successful'. However, athymic nude mice have a normal incidence of spontaneous tumours and this makes a single, exclusively T-cell surveillance system most unlikely. Furthermore, the only increase in cancer reported in immunosuppressed patients was related to the lympho-reticular system which could have been the direct target for the drugs employed; one exception was the considerable increase in skin cancer in immunosuppressed patients living in high sunshine regions north of Brisbane and we have already noted the 'antigen strength' of such tumours provoked in experimental animals.

Perhaps in speaking of immunity to tumours, one too readily thinks in terms of acquired responses whereas it is possible that innate mechanisms will prove to be of greater significance. Macrophages taken from BCG-infected animals, or activated by a diversity of factors, bacterial lipopolysaccharide, double-stranded RNA, T-cell lymphokine and so forth, will inhibit the division of tumour cells in tissue culture. There is an uncommon flurry of interest in the natural killer (NK) cell which is similar in many ways to the K cell of ADDC fame (p. 194). NK cells are spontaneously cytolytic for certain, but by no means all, tumour lines in culture as well as for cells infected with herpes and mumps viruses or *Listeria monocytogenes*. The target molecule might be a surface membrane glycoprotein with altered carbohydrate and the blocking of cytotoxicity by anti-Ly5 sera tentatively suggests that this differentiation antigen could be the NK receptor. Interferon markedly enhances the activity of NK cells and at the same time, increases the resistance of *normal* cells to lysis. Agents such as BCG and *C. parvum* which stimulate macrophages also increase NK activity.

Immunotherapy

On one point all are agreed, if immunotherapy is to succeed, it is essential that the tumour load should first be reduced by surgery, irradiation or chemotherapy, since not only is it unreasonable to expect the immune system to cope with a large tumour mass, but considerable amounts of antigen released by shedding would prevent the generation of any significant response. This leaves the small secondary deposits as the proper target for immunotherapy.

For active immunization we need antigen. Based on the not unreasonable belief that certain forms of cancer (e.g. lymphoma) are caused by oncogenic viruses, attempts are being made to isolate the virus and prepare a suitable vaccine from it. In fact, large-scale protection of chickens against the development of Marek's disease lymphoma has been successfully achieved by vaccination with another herpes virus native to turkeys. In the human, patients with Burkitt's lymphoma develop antibodies which react with antigens on cells of their own and other Burkitt tumours which are controlled by a herpes group organism, the Epstein-Barr (EB) virus. The unique idiotype on monoclonal B-cell tumours with surface Ig also offers a potentially feasible target for immunotherapy.

Despite reports of cytotoxic antibodies in a proportion of patients with malignant melanoma and cytotoxic leukocytes from patients with neuroblastoma or bladder cancer, which indicate that some form of immunological response to tumour antigens is possible, it must be said that attempts to control human cancer by injection of tumours with adjuvants have had very mixed and in many ways somewhat disappointing results. Perhaps we have to devise new ways of boosting the inherently weak autoantigenicity of the oncofetal antigens when present, to generate an appropriate response? There have also been numerous, not very successful, attempts to boost 'non-specific' effector mechanisms mediated by macrophages and NK cells through the injection of BCG, *Corynebacterium parvum* and interferon. Intimate contact of the adjuvant with the tumour itself can produce dramatic results and one hopeful study records the beneficial effects of intrathoracic BCG in lung cancer.

Immunodiagnosis

Analysis of blood for the oncofetal antigens α-fetoprotein in hepatoma and carcinoembryonic antigen in tumours of the colon has provided valuable diagnostic information, but enthusiasm has been slightly curtailed by the knowledge that there is a high incidence of so-called 'false positives'.

ASSOCIATION WITH DISEASE

An impressive body of data is accumulating which links specific HLA antigens with particular disease states in the human (table 9.2). Because of *linkage disequilibrium* (a state where

240

TABLE 9.2. Association of HLA with disease

Disease	HLA	Estimated relative risk*
Ankylosing spondylitis	B27	81
Reiter's disease	B27	48
Psoriatic arthritis ⎱ when spine involved Juvenile RA ⎰	B27	5·4
Acute anterior uveitis	B27	16·9
Psoriasis vulgaris	B13	4·3
Dermatitis herpetiformis	B8	4·3
Insulin dependent diabetes	B8	2·3
	Dw3	3·8
	Dw4	3·5
Addison's disease	B8	3·9
	Dw3	8·8
Thyrotoxicosis	B8	2·3
	Dw3	4·4
Myasthenia gravis	B8	4·4
	Dw3	2·3
Sjögren with Sicca syndrome	B8	3·2
Chronic active hepatitis	B8	2·9
	Dw3	6·8
Coeliac disease	B8	9·5
Rheumatoid arthritis	Dw4 ⎱ DRw4 ⎰	6·0
Behcet's disease	B5	4·6
Multiple sclerosis	B7	1·5
	Dw2	5·0
Subacute thyroiditis	Bw35	14
Ragweed hay fever	Haplotype linkage	
Hodgkin's disease	A1	1·4
	B5	1·6
	B8	1·3
	B18	1·9

No deviations from normal found in: rheumatoid arthritis; gout; non-insulin dependent diabetes; childhood asthma; leprosy; TB; *H.influenza* and infectious mononucleosis infection; ulcerative colitis and Crohn's; other liver disorders; sarcoidosis; SLE; rheumatic fever; essential hypertension; asbestosis; schizophrenia; pernicious anaemia; mammary carcinoma with respect to HLA-A and -B antigens. There is strong linkage disequilibrium between B7 and Dw2 and between B8 and Dw3.

*Increased chance of contracting the disease for individuals bearing the antigen relative to those lacking it.
Much of the data is taken from Ryder L.P. & Svejgaard A. (1976) *Associations between HLA and Disease*. Published by the authors, State University Hospital, Copenhagen.

closely linked genes on a chromosome tend to remain associated rather than undergo genetic randomization in a given population) which is often a feature of this region of the chromosome, the associations seen may be even more directly linked with a gene other than that coding for the HLA antigen in question. For example, in multiple sclerosis an association with the B7 allele was first established but when patients were typed for the D locus, a much stronger correlation with Dw2 emerged. The initial correlation with B7 resulted from linkage disequilibrium between B7 and Dw2. Carrying the argument a stage further, one cannot exclude the possibility of finding an even greater association with another closely linked gene.

The association with HLA in ankylosing spondylitis is quite extraordinary; up to 95% of patients are of B27 phenotype as compared with around 5% in controls. The incidence of B27 is also markedly raised in other conditions when accompanied by sacro-iliitis, e.g. Reiter's disease, acute anterior uveitis, psoriasis and other forms of infective sacro-iliitis such as yersinia, gonococcal and salmonella arthritis. The very close association with B27 makes it unlikely that as good a correlation with any other gene will be found. The involvement of infective agents may provide a clue: does molecular similarity to B27 imply a tolerance to certain microbial antigens, or is there some more subtle interaction with microbial products? Reports by Ebringer and colleagues of a cross-reaction of B27 with *Klebsiella pneumoniae* and a higher faecal carriage rate for these organisms in patients with active disease are certainly provocative in this respect.

The B8-Dw3 axis is found with undue frequency in auto-immune diseases where cell surface antigens are prime targets. In Graves' disease and myasthenia gravis these have been identified as TSH and ACh receptors respectively and the question of some link between Dw3 and these receptors has been mooted. HLA antigens might also affect the susceptibility of a cell to viral attachment or infection, thereby influencing the development of autoimmunity to associated surface components.

Summary

Graft rejection is an immunological reaction: it shows specificity, the second set response is brisk, it is mediated by lymphocytes, and antibodies specific for the graft are formed. In each vertebrate species there is a major histocompatibility complex (MHC) which is responsible for provoking the most intense graft reactions. MHC antigens inherited from mother and father are codominantly expressed on the cell surface. The MHC in the mouse (H-2) is a complex region with two loci encoding major classical transplantation antigens, H-2K and H-2D, each with many polymorphic specificities defined by the antibodies they so readily evoke. The molecules contain two peptides, one of H-2 specificity and the other β_2-microglobulin. Another major region, I, codes for lymphocyte activating determinants (Lad) which provoke a mixed lymphocyte reaction of proliferation and blast transformation when genetically dissimilar lymphocytes interact; this reaction stimulates the formation of helper T-cells required for the generation of cytotoxic T-cells directed against H-2D/K determinants (cf. T-B co-operation with carrier-hapten), the process being termed cell-mediated lympholysis. Lad (Ia) differences are responsible for the reaction of tolerated grafted lymphocytes against host antigens (g.v.h.). The genes in the whole MHC being closely linked tend to be inherited *en bloc* and are referred to as a haplotype. The MHC in man (HLA) consists of three loci (HLA-A, B & C) for classical transplantation antigens and one (HLA-D) for the major Lad. Individuals are typed by cytotoxic antisera and by the mixed lymphocyte reaction. Siblings have a 1:4 chance of identity with respect to MHC.

Grafts are rejected either by cytotoxic T-cells or by antibody inducing platelet aggregation or type II hypersensitivity reactions (e.g. antibody-dependent cell-mediated cytotoxicity). Rejection may be prevented by: (a) tissue matching including the D-locus, (b) anti-mitotic drugs (e.g. azathioprine), anti-inflammatory steroids and anti-lymphocyte globulin which produce general immunosuppression, or (c) antigen-specific depression through tolerance induction or enhancement by deliberate immunization.

Cornea and cartilage grafts are avascular and comparatively well tolerated. Kidney grafting has been the most widespread although immunosuppression must normally be continuous. Bone marrow grafts for immunodeficiency and aplastic anaemia are accepted from matched siblings but it is difficult to avoid g.v.h. disease with allogeneic marrow.

The very high degree of polymorphism of the MHC may protect a species from molecular mimicry by parasites, maintain diversity of antigenic recognition and ensure heterozygosity ('hybrid vigour'). Differences between MHC of mother and fetus may be beneficial to the fetus but as a potential graft it must be protected against transplantation attack by the mother; suggested defence mechanisms are: (a) lack of classical transplantation antigens on syncytiotrophoblast, (b) mucopolysaccharide coat around trophoblast, and (c) local production of immunosuppressant.

The MHC subserves recognition functions. The immune response (Ir) genes code for molecules (Ia) which in association with carrier determinants optimally regulate priming of T-cells by macrophage-processed antigen and interactions between T- and B-cells. Other MHC antigens are involved in the generation of cytotoxic T-cells in response to viral infection. Thus *the MHC would appear to be part of a system for signalling changes in 'self'* which enables the T-cells to make the appropriate immune response. Each cell in the body bears H-2D/K determinants so the cytotoxic T-cells use these to recognize a virally infected cell. The antigens of organisms such as TB, leishmania and toxoplasma which live within macrophages are processed to form an association with Ia on the macrophage surface which can stimulate 'delayed hypersensitivity' T-cells; these release factors enabling the macrophages to kill their intracellular parasites.

The immune surveillance theory of cancer postulates that changes in the surface of the neoplastic cell are recognized by the immune system and eliminated. However, although virally coded, idiotypic and oncofetal antigens may be detected on experimentally induced tumour cells together with components linked to cell division, the incidence of spontaneous cancers in immunosuppressed individuals is not generally higher than normal. Examples of immune responses to tumours in human cancer are known but attempts at control by immunization with tumour plus adjuvant have not been encouraging. Other strategies involve non-specific activation of macrophages and NK cells by adjuvants such as BCG, *C. parvum* and lecithin analogues. Oncofetal antigens may be useful in diagnosis (e.g. α-fetoprotein in primary hepatoma).

Genes controlling C3 and its complementary proteins map in the MHC. HLA specificities are often associated with particular diseases, e.g. HLA-B27 with ankylosing spondylitis, B8 with myasthenia gravis, Dw4 with rheumatoid arthritis and Dw2 with multiple sclerosis.

Further reading

Albert E. *et al.* (1978) Nomenclature for factors of the HLA system, 1977. *Bull. W.H.O.*, **56**, 461.
Billingham R. & Silvers W. (1971) *The Immunobiology of Transplantation.* Foundations of Immunology Series. Prentice-Hall, New Jersey.

Bodmer W.F. (ed.) (1978) The HLA System. *Brit. Med. Bull.*, **34**, No. 3.

Castro J.E. (ed.) (1978) *Immunological Aspects of Cancer*. M.T.P., Lancaster.

Dausset J. & Hors J. (1973) Statistics of 416 consecutive kidney transplants in the France-Transplant organization. *Transpl. Proc.*, **5**, 223.

Doherty P.C. & Zinkernagel R.M. (1975) A biological role for the major histocompatibility antigens. *Lancet*, **i**, 1406.

Festenstein H. & Demant P. (1978) *Immunogenetics of the Major Histocompatibility System*. Edward Arnold, London.

Fougerean M. & Dausset J. (eds) (1980) *Progress in Immunology IV*. Academic Press, London.

Kiesling R. & Haller O. (1978) Natural killer cells in mice. *Contemporary Topics in Immunobiology*, **8**, 171. Plenum, New York.

Lance E.M., Medawar P.B. & Taub R.N. (1973) Antilymphocyte serum. *Adv. Immun.*, **17**, 2.

Mitchison N.A. (1980) Protective immunity (to tumours) *in vivo*. In *Clinical Aspects of Immunology*, 4th edn. Peters K. & Lachmann P. (eds). Blackwell Scientific Publications, Oxford.

Möller G. (ed.) (1979) Natural killer cells. *Immunol. Rev.*, **44**.

Munro A. & Bright S. (1976) Products of the major histocompatibility complex and their relationship to the immune response. *Nature*, **264**, 145.

Rose N.R., Bigazzi P.E. & Warner N.L. (eds) (1978) *Genetic Control of Auto-immune Disease*. Elsevier North-Holland, New York.

Skinner M.D. & Schwartz R.S. (1972) Immunosuppressive therapy. *N.Eng.J.Med.*,,**287**, 221 and 281.

Smith R.T. & Landy M. (1975) *Immunobiology of the Tumour–Host Relationship*. Academic Press, New York.

Zinkernagel R.M. & Doherty P.C. (1979) MHC-restricted cytotoxic T-cells: studies on the biological role of polymorphic major transplantation antigens determining T-cell restriction–specificity, function and responsiveness. *Adv. Immunol.*, **27**, 51.

10 Autoimmunity

There are in the body appropriate mechanisms to prevent the recognition of 'self' components as antigens by the lymphoid system but, as with all machinery, there is always a chance that these mechanisms might break down, and the older the individual, the greater the chance of a breakdown. When this happens autoantibodies (i.e. antibodies capable of reacting with 'self' components) are produced. Grabar is of the opinion that autoantibodies have a biological function to act as 'transporting' agents for cellular breakdown products thereby aiding their disposal. While antibodies can act in this way, we are here concerned more with autoimmune phenomena which appear in relation to certain defined human diseases. Ideally we wish to apply the term 'autoimmune disease' to those cases where it can be shown that the autoimmune process contributes to the pathogenesis of the disease rather than situations where apparently harmless autoantibodies are formed following tissue damage, e.g. heart antibodies appearing after a myocardial infarction. Yet the role of autoimmunity in many disorders is still not clearly defined, and it is as a matter of convenience that we will refer to all maladies firmly associated with auto-antibody formation as 'autoimmune diseases', except where it can be shown that the immunological phenomena are purely secondary findings.

The spectrum of antoimmune diseases

These disorders may be looked upon as forming a spectrum. At one end we have 'organ-specific diseases' with organ-specific auto-antibodies. Hashimoto's disease of the thyroid is an example: there is a specific lesion in the thyroid involving infiltration by mononuclear cells (lymphocytes, histiocytes and plasma cells), destruction of follicular cells and germinal centre formation, accompanied, as we showed originally, by the production of circulating antibodies with absolute specificity for certain thyroid constituents (Roitt, Doniach & Campbell).

Moving towards the centre of the spectrum are those disorders where the lesion tends to be localized to a single organ

247

TABLE 10.1. Spectrum of autoimmune diseases

Organ specific ←				→ Non-organ specific
Hashimoto's thyroiditis Primary myxoedema	Goodpasture's syndrome Myasthenia gravis	Autoimmune haemolytic anaemia Idiopathic thrombocytopenic purpura	Primary biliary cirrhosis Active chronic hepatitis HB_s-ve	Systemic lupus erythematosus (SLE) Discoid LE
Thyrotoxicosis Pernicious anaemia Autoimmune atrophic gastritis Addison's disease Premature meno-pause (few cases) Male infertility (few cases)	Juvenile diabetes Pemphigus vulgaris Pemphigoid Sympathetic ophthalmia Phacogenic uveitis (?? Multiple sclerosis ??)	Idiopathic leucopenia	Cryptogenic cirrhosis (some cases) Ulcerative colitis Sjögren's syndrome	Dermatomyositis Scleroderma Rheumatoid arthritis

but the antibodies are non-organ specific. A typical example would be primary biliary cirrhosis where the small bile ductule is the main target of inflammatory cell infiltration but the serum antibodies present—mainly mitochondrial—are not liver specific.

At the other end of the spectrum are the 'non-organ specific diseases' exemplified by systemic lupus erythematosus (SLE) where both lesions and autoantibodies are not confined to any one organ. Pathological changes are widespread and are primarily lesions of connective tissue with fibrinoid necrosis. They are seen in the skin (the 'lupus' butterfly rash on the face is characteristic), kidney glomeruli, joints, serous membranes and blood vessels. In addition the formed elements of the blood are often affected. A bizarre collection of autoantibodies are found some of which react with the DNA and other nuclear constituents of all cells in the body.

An attempt to fit the major diseases considered to be associated with autoimmunity into this spectrum is shown in table 10.1.

Autoantibodies in human disease

At this stage in the discussion it may be of value to have a more precise account of the major autoantibodies detected in the different diseases to provide a framework for reference. Table 10.2 documents a list of these antibodies and the methods employed in their detection. The notes following the table amplify specific points while some of the tests are illustrated in figures 10.1–10.3, 6.13 and 6.14.

248

TABLE 10.2. Autoantibodies in human disease (IFT, Immunofluorescent test; CFT, complement fixation test.)

Disease	Antigen	Detection of antibody
Hashimoto's thyroiditis ⎫ Primary myxoedema ⎭	Thyroglobulin	Precipitins; passive haemaggln.
	2nd colloid Ag (CA2)	IFT on fixed thyroid
	Cytoplasmic microsomes	IFT on unfixed thyroid; passive haemaggln.
	Cell surface	IFT on viable thyroid cells; C′-mediated cytotoxicity
Thyrotoxicosis	Cell surface TSH receptors	Bioassay—stimulation of mouse thyroid *in vivo*; blocking combination TSH with receptors; stimulation adenyl cyclase
Pernicious anaemia [1]	Intrinsic factor	Neutralization; blocking combination with vit-B$_{12}$; binding to Int.Fact-B$_{12}$ by copptn.
	Parietal cell microsomes	IFT on unfixed gastric mucosa
Addison's disease	Cytoplasm adrenal cells	IFT on unfixed adrenal cortex
Premature onset of menopause [2]	Cytoplasm steroid producing cells	IFT on adrenal and interstitial cells of ovary and testis
Male infertility (some) [3]	Spermatozoa	Sperm agglutination in ejaculate
Juvenile diabetes [4]	Cytoplasm of islet cells Cell surface	IFT on unfixed human pancreas Leucocyte cytotoxicity
(Multiple sclerosis)	Brain	Cytotoxic effects on cerebellar cultures by serum and lymphocytes (? secondary to disease)
Goodpasture's syndrome	Glomerular and lung basement membrane	Linear staining by IFT of kidney biopsy with fluorescent anti-IgG
Pemphigus vulgaris	Desmosomes between prickle cells in epidermis	IFT on skin
Pemphigoid	Basement membrane	IFT on skin
Phacogenic uveitis	Lens	Passive haemaggln.
Sympathetic ophthalmia	Uvea	(Delayed skin reaction to uveal extract)
Myasthenia gravis	Skeletal and heart muscle Acetyl choline receptor	IFT on skeletal muscle Blocking or binding radioassay with α-bungarotoxin
Autoimmune haemolytic anaemia [5]	Erythrocytes	Coombs' antiglobulin test
Idiopathic thrombocytopenic purpura	Platelets	Shortened platelet survival *in vivo*
Primary biliary cirrhosis	Mitochondria (mainly)	IFT on mitochondria rich cells (e.g. distal tubules of kidney)

249

Table 10.2 (*contd.*)

Disease	Antigen	Detection of antibody
Active chronic hepatitis	Smooth muscle, nuclei	IFT (e.g. on gastric mucosa)
	Cell surface lipoprotein	Leucocyte cytotoxicity
Ulcerative colitis	Colon 'lipopoly-saccharide'	IFT; passive haemaggln. (cytotoxic action of lymphocytes on colon cells)
Sjögren's syndrome[6]	Ducts, mitochondria, nuclei, thyroid,	IFT
	IgG	Antiglobulin tests
Rheumatoid arthritis[7]	IgG	Antiglobulin tests: latex aggln., sheep red cell aggln. test (SCAT) & radioassay
	RANA[8]	IFT on EB-transformed cell line
	Collagen	Passive haemaggln.
Discoid lupus erythematosus ⎫ Dermatomyositis ⎬ Scleroderma[9] ⎭	Nuclear IgG	IFT Antiglobulin tests
Mixed connective tissue disease[10]	Extractable nuclear	IFT; countercurrent electrophoresis
Systemic lupus erythematosus	DNA	Radioassay[11]; pptn; CFT
	Nucleoprotein	IFT; latex aggln. L.E. cells[12]
	Cytoplasmic sol.Ag	'Non-organ sp.CFT'
	Array of other Ag incl. formed elements of blood, clotting factors, IgG	
	and Wasserman antigen	'Biological false positive' CFT

1. Two major types of antibody to intrinsic factor are detected, viz. blocking and binding (figure 10.1). Binding antibody combines with preformed Int.Fact.–radioactive B_{12}(*B_{12}) complex which can then be precipitated at 50% ammonium sulphate (cf. Farr test–salt copptn., p. 125) and the radioactivity in the precipitate counted. Blocking antibody prevents binding of *B_{12} to Int.Fact. and the uncombined *B_{12} can then be adsorbed to charcoal and counted.

2. Antibodies occur in the minority of patients with associated Addison's disease.

3. Only a small percentage show agglutinins. Spermatozoa may be agglutinated head to head, tail to tail or joined through their mid-piece. They are seen also in a small percentage of infertile women.

4. Most if not all juvenile (insulin dependent) diabetics have islet cell antibodies at some stage during the first year of onset. In contrast, islet cell antibodies in diabetic patients with an associated autoimmune polyendocrinopathy persist for many years.

5. The Coombs' test involves the demonstration of bound antibody on the washed red cell by agglutination with an antiglobulin. Erythrocyte autoantibodies, which bind well over the temperature range 0–37°C ('warm' Ab), are mostly IgG; approximately 60% of cases are primary, the remainder being

associated with other autoimmune disorders, e.g. SLE, ulcerative colitis. 'Cold' Ab, which react best over the range 0–20°C, are mostly IgM and red cells coated with this Ab can often be agglutinated by anti-complement sera; approximately half are primary, the others being associated with *Mycoplasma pneumoniae* infection or generalized neoplastic disease of the lymphoreticular tissues.

6. Antibodies specifically reacting with the epithelium of salivary gland excretory ducts are demonstrable by immunofluorescence in up to half the cases.

7. The main antiglobulin factors react with the Fc portion of IgG which is usually adsorbed onto latex particles (human IgG) or present in an antigen–antibody complex (sheep red cells coated with a subagglutinating dose of rabbit antibody). In the radioassay test, rabbit IgG is bound to a plastic tube, the patient's serum added and the antiglobulin bound assessed by subsequent binding of labelled anti-human IgG or IgM (cf. p. 126).

8. The rheumatoid arthritis nuclear antigen (RANA) is revealed as speckled staining by IFT using cells transformed by EB virus; normal cells are negative.

9. In scleroderma (progressive systemic sclerosis) antinucleolar antibodies are frequently found.

10. This syndrome combines features of scleroderma, rheumatoid arthritis, SLE and dermatomyositis. The antigen is an extractable nuclear antigen which gives speckled fluorescence and RNase-sensitive precipitation by countercurrent electrophoresis.

11. Antibodies to single or double-stranded DNA are assayed by the Farr test (cf. p. 125) using labelled Ag, or by a DNA-coated tube test similar to the radioassay for antiglobulins (note 7 above).

12. When blood from an SLE patient is incubated at 37°C, some white cells are damaged and allow the entry of antibodies. Certain of the antibodies combining with the nuclear surface bind complement and attract polymorphs which strip away the cytoplasm and engulf the nucleus. The polymorph containing the engulfed homogenized nucleus is called an LE-cell (figure 10.3).

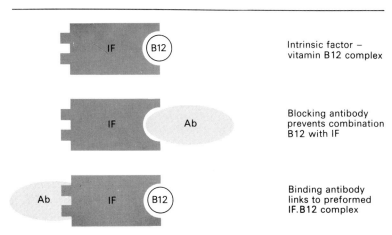

FIGURE 10.1. Intrinsic factor autoantibodies: sites of determinants for binding and blocking. (After Roitt I.M., Doniach D. & Shapland C. (1964) *Lancet*, **ii,** 469.)

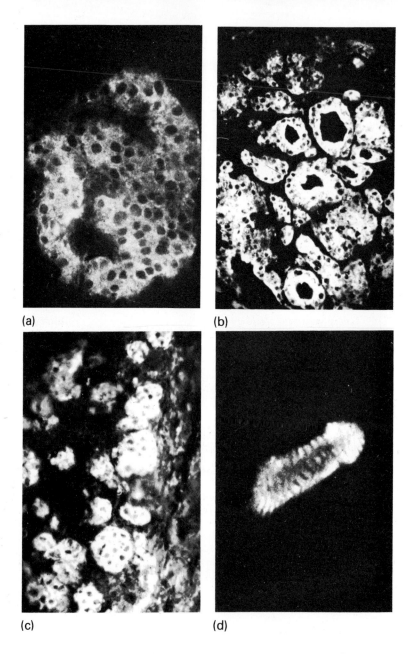

(a) (b)

(c) (d)

FIGURE 10.2. Autoantibodies demonstrable by indirect immunofluorescent test (section treated with one patient's serum, washed, then stained with fluorescein-conjugate of anti-human Ig, cf. p. 128): (a) fluorescence of cells in the pancreatic islets of Langerhans after treatment with serum from an insulin-dependent 'juvenile' diabetic; (b) thyroid microsomal antibodies staining the cytoplasm of acinar cells; (c) serum of a patient with Addison's disease staining cytoplasm of adrenal cells; (d) striated muscle antibodies in serum of a patient with myasthenia gravis reacting with 'myoid' cell in human thymus; (e) fluorescence of distal tubular cells of the kidney after reaction with

FIGURE 10.2 (contd.)

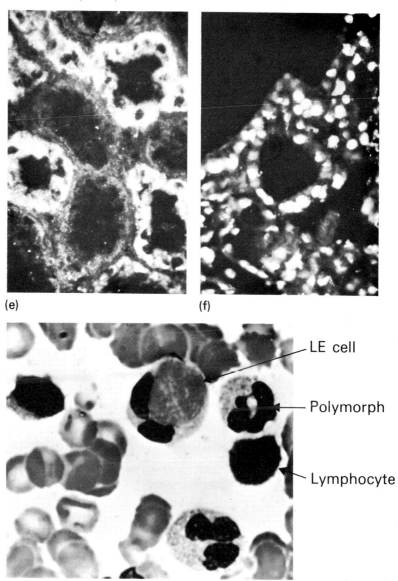

(e)   (f)

LE cell

Polymorph

Lymphocyte

FIGURE 10.3. LE-cell in preparation from peripheral blood of an SLE patient. The homogeneous nucleus lies within the polymorph which engulfed it by phagocytosis. Two normal polymorphs and two small lymphocytes are also present. (Photographed from material kindly provided by Professor J.W. Stewart.)

FIGURE 10.2 (contd.).
mitochondrial autoantibodies; (f) diffuse nuclear staining obtained with nucleoprotein antibodies on a thyroid section. ((a) Kindly provided by Dr F. Bottazzo, (d) by Dr T.E.W. Feltkamp, the others by courtesy of Dr D. Doniach.)

Overlap of autoimmune disorders

There is a tendency for more than one autoimmune disorder to occur in the same individual and when this happens the association is often between diseases within the same region of the autoimmune spectrum (cf. table 10.1). Thus patients with autoimmune thyroiditis (Hashimoto's disease or primary myxoedema) have a much higher incidence of pernicious anaemia than would be expected in a random population matched for age and sex (10% as against 0.2%). Conversely both thyroiditis and thyrotoxicosis are diagnosed in pernicious anaemia patients with an unexpectedly high frequency. Other associations are seen between Addison's disease and autoimmune thyroid disease and in the rare cases of juveniles with pernicious anaemia and polyendocrinopathy which includes Addison's disease, hypoparathyroidism, diabetes and thyroiditis.

There is an even greater overlap in serological findings. Thirty per cent of patients with autoimmune thyroid disease have concomitant parietal cell antibodies in their serum. Conversely, thyroid antibodies have been demonstrated in up to 50% of pernicious anaemia patients. It should be stressed that these are not cross-reacting antibodies. The thyroid specific antibodies will not react with stomach and vice versa. When a serum reacts with both organs it means that two populations of antibodies are present, one with specificity for thyroid and the other for stomach.

At the non-organic-specific end of the spectrum, SLE is clinically associated with rheumatoid arthritis and several

TABLE 10.3. Organ-specific and non-organ-specific serological interrelationships in human disease

Disease	% positive reactions for antibodies to				
	Thyroid*	Stomach*	Nuclei*	Non-organ-specific antigen**	IgG†
Hashimoto's thyroiditis	99.9	32	8	5	2
Pernicious anaemia	55	89	11	7	
Sjögren's syndrome	45	14	56	19	75
Rheumatoid arthritis	11	16	50	10	75
SLE	2	2	99	66	35
Controls‡	0–15	0–16	0–19	0–10	2–5

* Immunofluorescence test.   ** CFT with kidney.   † Rheumatoid factor classical tests
‡ Incidence increases with age and females > males.

other diseases which are themselves uncommon: haemolytic anaemia, idiopathic leucopenia and thrombocytopenic purpura, dermatomyositis and Sjögren's syndrome. Antinuclear antibodies, non-organ-specific complement fixation reactions, and antiglobulin (rheumatoid) factors are a general feature of these disorders.

Sjögren's syndrome occupies an interesting position (table 10.3); aside from the clinical and serological features associated with non-organ-specific disease mentioned above, characteristics of an organ-specific disorder are evident. Antibodies reacting with salivary ducts are demonstrable and there is an abnormally high incidence of thyroid autoantibodies; histologically the affected lacrimal and salivary glands reveal changes of a similar nature to those seen in Hashimoto's disease, namely a replacement of the glandular elements by patchy lymphocytic and plasma cell granulomatous tissue. Associations between diseases at the two ends of the spectrum have been reported, but, as might be predicted from the serological data (table 10.3), they are not common.

There is still no entirely satisfactory explanation to account for the rare tendency to develop hypogammaglobulinaemia and the increased incidence of certain cancers occurring in autoimmune disease. Patients with organ specific disorders are slightly more prone to develop cancer in the affected organ whereas generalized lymphoreticular neoplasia shows up with uncommon frequency in non-organ-specific disease.

Genetic factors in autoimmune disease

Autoimmune phenomena tend to aggregate in certain families. For example, the first degree relatives (sibs, parents and children) of patients with Hashimoto's disease show a high incidence of thyroid autoantibodies and of overt and subclinical thyroiditis. Interestingly there is also an increased frequency of 'non-immunological' thyroid disorders, such as non-toxic nodular goitre. The proportion with autoantibodies is higher in those families where more than one member is clinically affected. Parallel studies have disclosed similar relationships in the families of pernicious anaemia patients in that gastric pariental cell antibodies are prevalent in the relatives who are wont to develop achlorhydria and atrophic gastritis.

These familial relationships could be ascribed to environmental factors such as an infective micro-organism, but there is evidence that one or more genetic components must be given serious consideration. In the first place, when thyrotoxicosis occurs in twins there is a greater concordance rate (i.e. both twins affected) in identical than in non-identical twins. Furthermore, there are strong associations between several autoimmune diseases and particular HLA specificities, e.g. B8-Dw3 in Addison's disease and Dw4 in rheumatoid arthritis (Table 9.2, p. 241). Since only very restricted determinants on the autoantigenic molecules evoke autoantibodies (e.g. thyroglobulin of molecular weight 650,000, has a valency of 4), one is tempted to think in terms of Ir genes, it being precisely under such conditions that Ir genes can be recognized.

It is also intriguing to note that lines of animals have been bred which spontaneously develop autoimmune disease. In other words, the autoimmunity is genetically programmed. There is an obese line of chickens with autoimmune thyroiditis and the New Zealand Black (NZB) mouse with autoimmune haemolytic anaemia. The hybrid of NZB with another strain the New Zealand White (B × W hybrid) actually develops LE-cells, antinuclear antibodies and a fatal immune complex induced glomerulonephritis. Suitable intercross and backcross breeding of these mice has established that a *minimum* of three genes determines the expression of autoimmunity and that the production of both red cell and nuclear antibodies may be under separate genetic control, i.e. there may be different factors predisposing to autoimmunity on the one hand, and to the selection of antigen on the other.

Autoantibodies are demonstrable in comparatively low titre

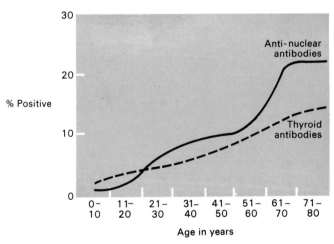

FIGURE 10.4. Incidence of autoantibodies in the general population. A serum was considered positive for thyroid antibodies if it reacted at a dilution of 1/10 in the tanned red cell test or neat in the immunofluorescent test and positive for antinuclear antibodies if it reacted at a dilution of 1/4 by immunofluorescence.

256

in the general population and the incidence of positive results increases steadily with age (figure 10.4) up to around 60–70 years. In the case of the thyroid and stomach at least, biopsy has indicated that the presence of antibody is almost invariably associated with minor thyroiditis or gastritis lesions (as the case may be), and it is of interest that post mortem examination has identified 10% of middle-aged women with significant degrees of lymph-adenoid change in the thyroid similar in essence to that characteristic of Hashimoto's disease.

The point should also be made here that, in general, auto-antibodies and autoimmune diseases are found more frequently in women than in men.

Aetiology of autoimmune response

How do autoantibodies arise? Our earliest view, with respect to organ specific antibodies at least, was that the antigens were sequestered within the organ and through lack of contact with the lymphoreticular system failed to establish immunological tolerance. Any mishap which caused a release of the antigen would then provide an opportunity for auto-antibody formation. For a few body constituents this holds true and in the case of sperm, lens and heart for example, release of certain components directly into the circulation can provoke autoantibodies. But in general, the experience has been that injection of *unmodified* extracts of those tissues concerned in the organ-specific autoimmune disorders does not elicit antibody formation. Indeed detailed investigation of the thyroid auto-antigen, thyroglobulin, has disclosed that it is not completely sequestered within the gland but gains access to the extra-cellular fluid around the follicles and leaves via the thyroid lymphatics (figure 10.5) reaching the serum in normal human subjects at concentrations of approximately $0.01-0.05 \mu g/ml$.

Concentrations of this order produce 'low zone tolerance' in mice by affecting the T-lymphocytes, probably through suppressors. Extrapolating to man, we are presumably dealing with a situation in which T-cells are tolerant to thyroglobulin and B-cells are not. Indeed a small proportion of the B-cells in normal individuals bind human thyroglobulin through their surface Ig receptors.

It is worth noting that anti-idiotypic responses are also essentially auto-immune in nature. The message then is that we are all sitting on a minefield of potentially self-reactive cells, but since autoimmune disease is more the exception than the rule, the body must have homeostatic mechanisms to prevent them

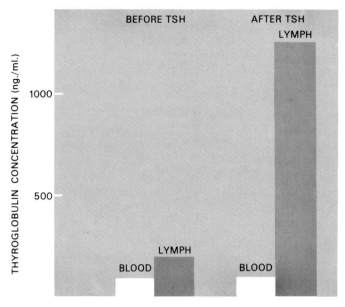

FIGURE 10.5. Thyroglobulin in the cervical lymph draining the thyroid in the rat. The concentration of thyroglobulin is increased after injection of pituitary thyroid stimulating hormone (TSH) suggesting that the release from thyroid follicles is linked to the physiological activity of the acinar cells. (From Daniel P.N., Pratt O.E., Roitt I.M. & Torrigiani G. (1967) *Quart.J.exp.Physiol.* **52**, 101.)

being triggered under normal circumstances. We are now ready to examine ways in which these mechanisms may be circumvented to allow autoimmunity to develop.

PROVISION OF NEW CARRIER DETERMINANT

If, as discussed above, auto-reactive T-cells are rendered helpless through self-tolerance (cf. p. 257), then T-B collaboration to generate autoantibodies (reaction 1, figure 10.6) is not possible. Using this model, Allison and Weigle argued independently that provision of new carrier determinants to which no self-tolerance had been established would bypass this mechanism and lead to autoantibody production (reaction 2, figure 10.6).

Modification of the molecule

A new carrier could arise through some modification to the molecule, for example, by defects in synthesis or by an abnormality in lysosomal breakdown yielding a split product exposing some new groupings. Experimentally it has been

258

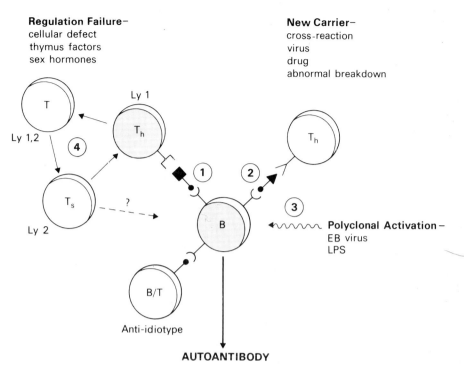

Regulation Failure–
cellular defect
thymus factors
sex hormones

New Carrier–
cross-reaction
virus
drug
abnormal breakdown

FIGURE 10.6. Mechanisms of autoantibody formation to non-sequestered body components. T-B co-operation in the response to an autoantigen ① is normally held in check by immunoregulatory mechanisms ④. This may be circumvented by association of the autoantigen with a new carrier ②, by polyclonal activators ③ or by a failure in regulation ④. —● Autoantigenic determinant (hapten) recognized by B-cell. ■— Autoantigenic determinant (carrier) recognized by T-cell. ◀— New carrier determinant. Shaded lymphocytes react with autoantigen. (After Drs A. Cooke & P.M. Lydyard.)

found that large proteolytic fragments of thyroglobulin are autoantigenic when injected alone but no evidence for such a mechanism has yet been uncovered in man; where antibodies to a split product such as the F(ab′)₂ fragment of IgG have been detected, they have not reacted with the whole molecules.

Incorporation into Freund's complete adjuvant frequently endows these molecules with autoantigenic properties and as we shall see later this enables us to induce many autoallergic diseases in laboratory animals. It is conceivable that the physical constraints on the proteins at the water–oil interface of the emulsion provide the required alteration in configuration of the 'carrier portions' of the molecules.

Modification can also be achieved through combination with a drug. The autoimmune haemolytic anaemia associ-

259

ated with administration of a α-methyl dopa might be attributable to modification of the red-cell surface. Myasthenia gravis and symptoms of pemphigus have been described in some patients on penicillamine. It is not clear in every case whether the drug provides carrier help through direct modification of the autoantigen or of some independent molecule concerned in associative recognition.

Associative recognition

This term applies to the phenomenon in which one membrane component may provide help for the immune response to another. In the context of autoimmunity, a new helper determinant may arise through drug modification as mentioned above, or through the insertion of viral antigen into the membrane of an infected cell. That this can promote a reaction to a pre-existing cell component is clear from the studies in which infection of a tumour with influenza virus elicited resistance to uninfected tumour cells.

Cross-reactions

Many examples are known in which potential autoantigenic determinants are present on an exogenous cross-reacting antigen which provides the new carrier to provoke auto-antibody formation. Some micro-organisms carry determinants which cross-react with the human and this may prove to be an important way of inducing autoimmunity. In rheumatic fever antibodies produced to the streptococcus also react with heart, and the sera of 50% of children with the disease who develop Sydenham's chorea give neuronal immunofluorescent staining which can be absorbed out with streptococcal membranes. Colon antibodies present in ulcerative colitis have been found to cross-react with *Escherichia coli* 014.

POLYCLONAL ACTIVATION

Microbes often display adjuvant properties through their possession of polyclonal lymphocyte activators such as bacterial endotoxins which may act by providing the second (non-specific) inductive signal for B-cell stimulation (p. 65), so bypassing the need for specific T-cell help. This can occur by direct interaction with the B-lymphocyte or indirectly through stimulating the secretion of non-specific factors from T-cells or macrophages. A good example is the thymus-dependent production of autoantibodies by injection of mice with thyroglobulin and endotoxin (LPS). The variety of autoantibodies detected in cases with infectious mononucleosis must surely be attributable to the polyclonal activation of B-cells by EB virus.

Body constituents circulating in high concentration are thought to induce tolerance through clonal abortion, whereas unresponsiveness to other molecules present at low levels is probably controlled through some form of T-suppression (p. 98 and figure 10.6). If this regulation mechanism were to fail, then autoreactive lymphocytes would be triggered. In accord with this view, manipulations which reduce T-suppressors encourage the development of autoantibodies. Irradiated mice reconstituted with spleen cells deprived of Ly2 positive T-cells produce antibodies to thyroglobulin, nuclei and lymphocytes. When rats were thymectomized at a few weeks of age and given divided doses of X-rays, they developed thyroglobulin auto-antibodies and thyroiditis. Neonatal thymectomy which greatly depletes the T-suppressor population, induces or exacerbates spontaneous autoimmune states in susceptible animals, e.g. autoimmune haemolytic anaemia in NZB mice.

Less is known of regulatory circuits in man although there is increasing evidence that non-specific T suppressor function in SLE may be poorly regulated. B-lymphocytes from patients with active disease secrete larger amounts of Ig when cultured *in vitro* than normal B-cells. Concanavalin A-induced non-specific suppressors are reduced or absent and T_G cells which suppress pokeweed mitogen-stimulated lymphocytes (p. 92) are low, the defect being greater the more active the disease. The thymic factor FTS is also depressed in these patients.

The origins of such defects are obscure. They might be the consequence of some subtle viral infection of the lymphoid system; the shedding of tremendous amounts of a C type oncornavirus from NZB T-cell lines may be of relevance to this. Or one may be dealing with some ageing process affecting the thymus or the lymphoid stem cells. Sex hormones may also contribute to the increased frequency of autoimmunity in females. Thus, oopherectomy and testosterone treatment alleviate the disease in female (NZB × NZW)FI hybrids.

These considerations apply in general to non-specific suppressor mechanisms, yet the different autoimmune states are usually associated with specific autoantigens. If idiotype network interactions are involved in these T-cell control circuits, this could provide one explanation for antigen-specific defects. Furthermore, anti-idiotype may provide a persistent *stimulus* to autoantibody production even when the circumstances initiating synthesis are only temporary (e.g. virus infection).

Pathogenic mechanisms in autoimmune disease

We have mentioned that despite certain exceptions as, for instance, myocardial infarction or damage to the testis, traumatic release of organ constituents does not in general elicit antibody formation. Destruction of thyroid tissue by therapeutic doses of radio-iodine does not initiate thyroid autoimmunity nor does damage to the liver in alcoholic cirrhosis result in the synthesis of mitochondrial antibodies, to give but two examples. We should now look at the evidence which bears directly on the issue of whether autoimmunity, however it arises, plays a *primary* pathogenic role in the production of tissue lesions in the group of diseases labelled as 'autoimmune'.

EFFECTS OF HUMORAL ANTIBODY

Blood

The erythrocyte antibodies play a role in the destruction of red cells in autoimmune haemolytic anaemia. Normal red cells coated with autoantibody eluted from Coombs' positive erythrocytes have a shortened half-life after reinjection into the normal subject. Normal red cells also have a shortened survival when infused into patients with haemolytic anaemia, but only if they possess the antigens against which the patient's autoantibodies are directed showing that the destructive process must be linked to the autoimmune response. Platelet antibodies are apparently responsible for idiopathic thrombocytopenic purpura (ITP). IgG from a patient's serum when given to a normal individual causes a depression of platelet counts and the active principle can be absorbed out with platelets. The transient neonatal thrombocytopenia which may be seen in infants of mothers with ITP is explicable in terms of transplacental passage of IgG antibodies to the child.

Thyroid

Cytotoxic antibodies. The serum of patients with Hashimoto's disease is cytotoxic for human thyroid cells growing in monolayer culture after dispersal by trypsin. This is a typical complement-mediated antibody reaction directed against cell surface antigens but it is still difficult to assess the extent to which this can operate *in vivo*.

Thyroid stimulating antibodies. Under certain circumstances antibodies to the surface of a cell may stimulate rather than destroy (cf. type V sensitivity; chapter 8). This would seem to be the case in thyrotoxicosis (Graves' or Basedow's disease). There has long been indirect evidence suggesting a link between autoimmune processes and this disease: thyroid antibodies are detectable in up to 85% of thyrotoxic patients and histologically the majority of the glands removed at operation show varying degrees of thyroiditis and local antibody formation in addition to the characteristic acinar cell hyperplasia (figure 10.7); thyrotoxicosis is found with undue frequency in the families of Hashimoto patients; there is

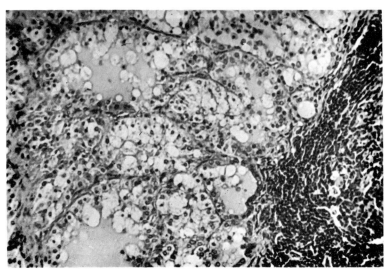

FIGURE 10.7. Lymphoid follicle adjacent to hyperactive thyroid cells in gland taken from patient with thyrotoxicosis.

an association with gastric autoimmunity in that 30% have gastric antibodies and up to 10% pernicious anaemia. The direct link came with the discovery by Adams and Purves of thyroid stimulating activity in the serum of thyrotoxic patients.

Intrinsic factor

Autoantibodies to this product of gastric mucosal secretion were first demonstrated in pernicious anaemia patients by oral administration of intrinsic factor, vitamin B_{12} and the serum from a patient with this disease. The serum was found to prevent intrinsic factor from mediating the absorption of B_{12} into the body, and further studies showed the active principle to be an antibody. Circulating antibody does not seem to be capable of neutralizing the physiological activity of intrinsic factor; a patient immunized parenterally with hog intrinsic factor in complete Freund's adjuvant had high serum antibody levels and good cell-mediated skin responses but still absorbed B_{12} well when fed with hog intrinsic factor. These data imply that the antibodies have to be present within the lumen of the gastrointestinal tract to be biologically effective, and indeed they can be identified in the gastric juice of these patients, synthesized by plasma cells in the gastritic lesion.

Glomerular basement membrane (gbm)

With immunological kidney disease the experimental models preceded the finding of parallel lesions in the human. Injection of cross-reacting heterologous gbm preparations in complete Freund's adjuvant produces glomerulonephritis in sheep and other experimental animals. Antibodies to gbm can be picked up by immunofluorescent staining of biopsies from nephritic animals with anti-IgG. The antibodies are largely if not completely absorbed out by the kidney *in vivo* but they appear in the serum on nephrectomy and can passively transfer the disease to another animal of the same species.

An entirely analogous situation occurs in man in certain cases of glomerulonephritis, particularly those associated with lung haemorrhage (Goodpasture's syndrome). Kidney biopsy from the patient shows *linear* deposition of IgG and C3 along the basement membrane of the glomerular capillaries (figure 8.12a). After nephrectomy, gbm antibodies can be detected in the serum. Dixon and his colleagues eluted the gbm antibody

264

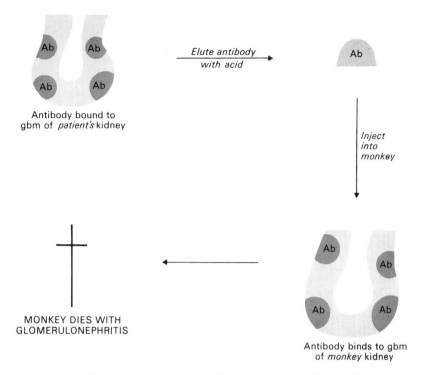

Antibody bound to
gbm of *patient's* kidney

*Elute antibody
with acid*

Ab

*Inject
into
monkey*

MONKEY DIES WITH
GLOMERULONEPHRITIS

Antibody binds to gbm
of *monkey* kidney

FIGURE 10.8. Passive transfer of glomerulonephritis to a squirrel monkey
by injection of antiglomerular basement membrane (anti-gbm)
antibodies isolated by acid elution from the kidney of a patient with
Goodpasture's syndrome. (After Lerner R.A., Glassock R.J. & Dixon F.J.
(1967) *J.exp.Med.*, **126,** 989.)

from a diseased kidney and injected it into a squirrel monkey.
The antibody rapidly fixed to the gbm of the recipient animal
and produced a fatal nephritis (figure 10.8). It is hard to escape
the conclusion that the lesion in the human was the direct result
of attack on the gbm by these complement-fixing antibodies.
The lung changes in Goodpasture's syndrome may be
attributable to cross-reaction with some of the gbm antibodies.

Muscle

The transient muscle weakness seen in babies born to mothers
with myasthenia gravis calls to mind neonatal thrombo-
cytopaenia and hyperthyroidism and would certainly be
compatible with the transplacental passage of an IgG capable
of inhibiting neuromuscular transmission. Strong support for
this view is afforded by the consistent finding of antibodies to
muscle acetyl choline receptors in myasthenics and the
depletion of these receptors within the motor end plates.

265

TABLE 10.4. Direct pathogenic effects of humoral antibodies

Disease	Autoantigen	Lesion
Autoimmune haemolytic anaemia	Red cell	Erythrocyte destruction
Lymphopenia (some cases)	Lymphocyte	Lymphocyte destruction
Idiopathic thrombocytopenic purpura	Platelet	Platelet destruction
Male infertility (some cases)	Sperm	Agglutination of spermatozoa
Pernicious anaemia	Intrinsic factor	Neutralization of ability to mediate B_{12} absorption
Hashimoto's disease	Thyroid surface antigen	Cytotoxic effect on thyroid cells in culture
Thyrotoxicosis	TSH receptors	Stimulation of thyroid cells
Goodpasture's syndrome	Glomerular basement membrane	Complement mediated damage to basement membrane
Myasthenia gravis	Acetyl choline receptor	Blocking and destruction of receptors
Acanthosis nigricans (type B) & ataxia telangiectasia with insulin resistance	Insulin receptor	Blocking of receptors

Table 10.4 summarizes these direct pathogenic effects of humoral autoantibodies.

EFFECTS OF COMPLEXES

Systemic lupus erythematosus (SLE)

Where autoantibodies are formed against soluble components to which they have continual access, complexes may be formed which can give rise to lesions similar to those occurring in serum sickness (cf. p. 202). In SLE, complexes of DNA and other nuclear antigens, and possibly C-type viral components, together with immunoglobulin and complement can be detected by immunofluorescent staining of kidney biopsies from patients with evidence of renal dysfunction. The staining pattern with a fluorescent anti-IgG or anti-C3 is punctate or 'lumpy-bumpy' as some would describe it (figure 8.12b). During the active phase of the disease, serum complement levels fall as components are affected by immune aggregates in the kidney and circulation.

Immunofluorescent studies on skin biopsies from patients

with the related disease discoid lupus erythematosus also reveal the presence of immune complexes.

Rheumatoid arthritis

A strong case can be made for the fairly straightforward proposition that an autoimmune response to the Fc portion of IgG gives rise to complexes which are ultimately responsible for the pathological changes characteristic of the rheumatoid joint. Virtually all patients with rheumatoid arthritis have demonstrable antibodies to IgG—the so-called rheumatoid or anti-globulin factors. The majority have IgM antiglobulins which react in the classical latex and sheep cell agglutination tests (table 10.2, note 7) and both they and the 'seronegative' patients who fail to react in these tests can be shown to have elevated levels of IgG antiglobulins detectable by tube absorption techniques (cf. p. 126) (figure 10.9). Sensitization to self IgG is therefore an almost universal feature of the disease.

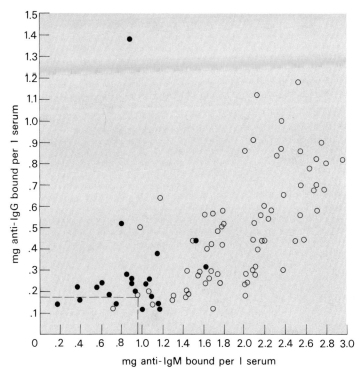

FIGURE 10.9. IgM and IgG antiglobulins determined by tube radioassay in patients with seropositive (o) and seronegative (•) rheumatoid arthritis. The dotted lines indicate the 95% confidence limits (mean + 2 S.D.) of the normal group. (From Nineham L., Hay F.C. & Roitt I.M. (1976) *J. clin. Path.*, **29,** 1121.)

The synovium typically is very heavily infiltrated with mono-nuclear cells often aggregated in the form of lymphoid follicles; there are many plasma cells and it has been estimated that the synthesis of IgG can be as high as that of a stimulated lymph node. If IgG is the main antigen responsible for evoking this response, most of the plasma cells should be synthesizing anti-globulins, yet ony a minority (say 10–20%) bind fluo-resceinated IgE, either in the form of heat-aggregated material or immune complexes (rheumatoid factor is a low affinity anti-body and good binding is only seen when multivalent IgG is used as antigen). However, we must take into account a strange and unique feature of IgG antiglobulins; because they are both antigen and antibody at the same time, they are capable of self-association (figure 10.10b) and this hides the majority of free antiglobulin valencies. Cleverly realizing that destruction of the Fc regions by pepsin would liberate these hidden binding sites (figure 10.10c), Munthe & Natvig observed that as many as 40–70% of the plasma cells in the synovium displayed an anti-IgG specificity following treatment with this enzyme.

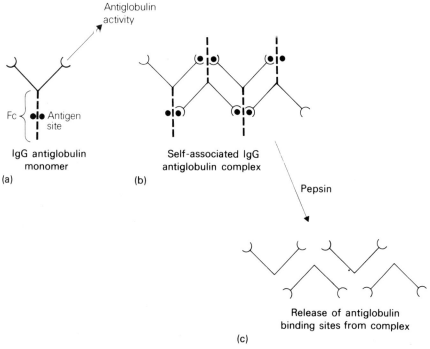

FIGURE 10.10. Self-associated complexes of IgG antiglobulins and the exposure of 'hidden' binding sites by pepsin. Such complexes in the joint may be stabilized by IgM antiglobulin and C1q which have polyvalent binding sites for IgG.

268

IgG aggregates, presumably products of these plasma cells, can be regularly detected in the synovial tissues and fluid. Analysis shows them to consist almost exclusively of immunoglobulins and complement while a major proportion of the IgG is present as self-associated antiglobulin as shown by binding to an Fcγ immunosorbent after treatment with pepsin. The complexes can mediate cartilage breakdown through different pathways (figure 10.11). In the joint space itself they initiate an Arthus reaction leading to an influx of polymorphs with which they react to release lysosomal enzymes. These include neutral proteinases and collagenase which can damage the articular cartilage by breaking down proteoglycans and collagen fibrils. More damage results if the complexes are adherent to the cartilage since the polymorph binds but is unable to internalize them ('frustrated phagocytosis'); as a result the lysosomal hydrolases are released extracellularly into the space between the cell and the cartilage where they are protected from enzyme inhibitors such as α_2-macroglobulin.

The aggregates may also stimulate the macrophage-like cells of the synovial lining, either directly through their surface receptors or indirectly through the release of lymphokines from

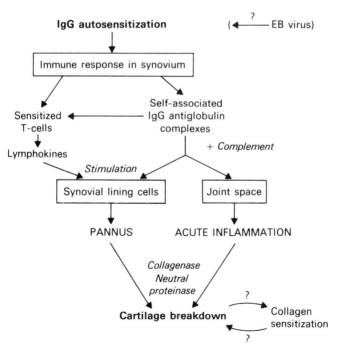

FIGURE 10.11. Hypothetical scheme showing how initial autosensitization to IgG can lead to the pathogenetic changes characteristic of rheumatoid arthritis.

269

sensitized T-cells. The activated synovial cells grow out as a malignant pannus (cover) over the cartilage and at the margin of this advancing granulation tissue, breakdown can be seen, almost certainly as a result of enzyme release. Activated macrophages also secrete plasminogen activator and the plasmin formed as a consequence activates a latent collagenase produced by synovial cells. Sensitization to partially degraded collagen may occur and this could lead secondarily to amplification of the lesion. Prostaglandin E_2, another product of the stimulated macrophage, can bring about bone resorption which is a further complication of severe disease. Subcutaneous nodules are granulomata possibly formed through local production of insolubilized self-associating antiglobulins.

CELLULAR HYPERSENSITIVITY

The inflammatory infiltrate in organ specific autoimmune disease is usually essentially mononuclear in character and, although not an infallible guide, this has been taken as an expression of cell-mediated hypersensitivity. Direct evidence is still thin. At the time of writing, skin reactions to autoantigens have proved difficult to assess and *in vitro* leucocyte inhibition tests have not been unequivocally accepted although for example in autoimmune thyroiditis and thyrotoxicosis there is a consistent finding of inhibition of leucocyte migration by thyroid microsomes. The killing of colon cells in culture by lymphocytes from patients with ulcerative colitis is encouraging and it has been reported that long-term culture of thyroid target cells with Hashimoto leucocytes leads to significant failure in the metabolic handling of iodine. Firm evidence for a direct participation of T-lymphocytes in any of these reactions has yet to be provided. There is more inclination to think in terms of K-cell killing, either by pre-armed cells or of targets coated with antibody secreted into the cultures by the effector cell population.

The nature of the cellular attack in organ-specific disorders is still not resolved but it is not improbable that cell-mediated hypersensitivity, direct antibody cytotoxicity and inflammatory reactions due to immune complexes may operate alone or in concert.

EXPERIMENTAL MODELS OF
AUTOIMMUNE DISEASE

If autoimmune processes are pathogenic in human diseases we

270

would expect that the production of autoimmunity should lead to comparable lesions in experimental animals.

Experimental autoallergic disease

When animals are injected with extracts of certain organs emulsified in oil containing killed turbercle bacilli (i.e. in complete Freund's adjuvant), autoantibodies and destructive inflammatory lesions specific to the organ used for immunization result. Thus, Rose and Witebsky found that rabbits receiving rabbit thyroglobulin in Freund's adjuvant developed antibodies to thyroglobulin and thyroiditis involving invasion of the gland by mononuclear cells of lymphocytic and histiocytic types with destruction of the normal follicular architecture.

Diagnostic value of autoantibody tests

Serum autoantibodies frequently provide valuable diagnostic markers. The most useful routine test is screening of the serum by immunofluorescence on a frozen section prepared from a composite block of unfixed human thyroid and stomach, and rat kidney and liver. This is supplemented by agglutination tests for rheumatoid factors and for thyroglobulin, thyroid microsome and red cell antibodies and by radioassay for antibodies to intrinsic factor, DNA and IgG (see table 10.2). The salient information is summarized in table 10.5.

The tests will also prove of value in screening for people at risk, e.g. relatives of patients with autoimmune disease, thyroiditis patients (for gastric autoimmunity and *vice versa*) and ultimately the general population.

Treatment of autoimmune disorders

The majority of approaches to treatment, not unnaturally, involve manipulation of immunological responses (figure 10.12). However, in many organ-specific diseases, metabolic control is usually sufficient, e.g. thyroxine replacement in primary myoedema, insulin in juvenile diabetes, vitamin B12 in pernicious anaemia, anti-thyroid drugs for Graves' disease and so forth. Anticholinesterase drugs are commonly used for long-term therapy in myasthenia gravis. Thymectomy is of benefit in most cases and it is conceivable that the gland contains ACh receptors in a particular antigenic form.

Patients with severe myasthenic symptoms respond well to

TABLE 10.5. Autoantibody tests and diagnosis

Disease	Antibody	Comment
Hashimoto's thyroiditis	Thyroid	Distinction from colloid goitre, thyroid cancer and subacute thyroiditis Thyroidectomy usually unnecessary in Hashimoto goitre
Primary myxoedema	Thyroid	Tests +ve in 99% of cases. If suspected hyputhyroidism, assess 'thyroid reserve' by TRH stimulation test
Thyrotoxicosis	Thyroid	High titres of cytoplasmic Ab indicate active thyroiditis and tendency to post-operative myxeodema: anti-thyroid drugs treatment of choice although HLA-B8 patients have high chance of relapse
Pernicious anaemia	Stomach	Help in diagnosis of latent PA, in differential diagnosis of non-auto-immune megaloblastic anaemia and in suspected subacute combined degeneration of the cord
Idiopathic adrenal atrophy	Adrenal	Distinction from tuberculous form
Myasthenia gravis	Muscle ACh receptor	When positive suggests associated thymoma (more likely if HLA-B12) Positive in > 80%
Pemphigus vulgaris and pemphigoid	Skin	Different fluorescent patterns in the two diseases
Autoimmune haemolytic anaemia	Erythrocyte (Coombs' test)	Distinction from other forms of anaemia
Sjögren's syndrome	Salivary duct cells	
Primary biliary cirrhosis (PBC)	Mitochondrial	Distinction from other forms of obstructive jaundice where test rarely +ve Recognize subgroup within cryptogenic cirrhosis related to PBC with +ve mitochondrial Ab
Active chronic hepatitis	Smooth muscle anti-nuclear and 20% mitochondrial	Smooth muscle Ab distinguish from SLE
Rheumatoid arthritis	Antiglobulin, e.g. SCAT and latex fixation	High titre indicative of bad prognosis
SLE	High titre antinuclear, DNA; LE-cells	DNA antibodies present in active phase Ab to double-stranded DNA characteristic
Scleroderma	Nucleolar	
Other 'collagenoses'	Nuclear	

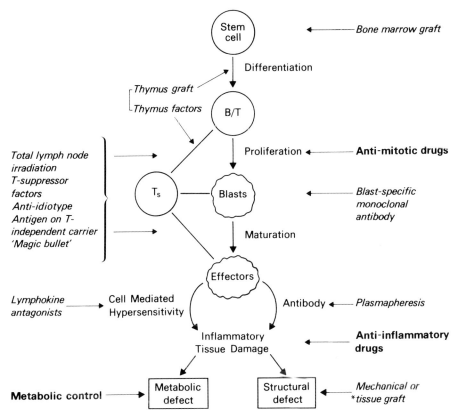

FIGURE 10.12. The treatment of autoimmune disease. Current conventional treatments are in bold type; some feasible approaches are given in italics. (*In the case of a live graft, the immunosuppressive therapy used may protect the tissue from the autoimmune damage which affected the organ being replaced.)

high doses of steroids and the same is true for serious cases of other autoimmune disorders such as SLE and immune complex nephritis where the drug helps to suppress the inflammatory lesions.

In rheumatoid arthritis, apart from steroids, anti-inflammatory drugs such as salicylates, indomethacin, phenyl-butazone and newer preparations such as fenoprofen and ibuprofen are widely used. Penicillamine, gold salts and anti-malarials such as chloroquine all find an important place in therapy but their mode of action is unknown.

Therapeutic blocking of other mediators directly concerned in immunological tissue damage will be feasible if lymphokine and complement antagonists become available. Plasma exchange to lower the rate of immune complex deposition in SLE provides only temporary benefit although it may be of value in life-threatening cases of arteritis.

While awaiting more selective therapy, conventional non-specific anti-mitotic agents such as azathioprine, cyclophosphamide and methotrexate have been used effectively in SLE, chronic active hepatitis and autoimmune haemolytic anaemia for example. It should one day be practical to correct any relevant defects in stem cells or in thymus processing by bone marrow or thymus grafting or perhaps, in the latter case, by thymic hormones.

We have already discussed the possible role of thymic factors in maintaining T-suppressor control of autoimmunity and one anticipates some interesting advances as the purified materials become available. Hybridoma technology or even gene cloning should ultimately provide the clinician with antigen-specific suppressor factors. The powerful immunosuppressive action of anti-idiotype antibodies has led to much rumination of the feasibility of controlling autoantibody production by provoking appropriate interactions.

Summary: comparison of organ-specific and non-organ-specific diseases

Organic-specific (e.g. thyroiditis, gastritis, adrenalitis)	Non-organ specific (e.g. systemic lupus erythematosus)
Differences	
1. Antigens only available to lymphoid systems in low concentration	Antigens accessible at higher concentrations
2. Antibodies and lesions organ-specific	Antibodies and lesions non-organ-specific
3. Clinical and serologic overlap—thyroiditis, gastritis and adrenalitis	Overlap SLE, rheumatoid arthritis, and other connective tissue disorders
4. Familial tendency to organ-specific autoimmunity	Familial connective tissue disease ? Abnormalities in immuno-globulin synthesis in relatives
5. Lymphoid invasion, parenchymal destruction by ?±cell mediated hypersensitivity ?±antibodies	Lesions due to deposition antigen–antibody complexes
6. Therapy aimed at controlling metabolic deficit	Therapy aimed at inhibiting inflammation and antibody synthesis
7. Tendency to cancer in organ	Tendency to lymphoreticular neoplasia

8. Antigens evoke organ-specific antibodies in normal animals with complete Freund's adjuvant.	No antibodies produced in animals with comparable stimulation
9. Experimental lesions produced with antigen in Freund adjuvant	Diseases and autoantibodies arise spontaneously in certain animals, e.g. NZB mice and hybrids and some dogs, or after injection of parental lymphoid tissue into F1 hybrids

Similarities

1. Circulating autoantibodies react with normal body constituents
2. Patients often have increased immunoglobulins in serum
3. Antibodies may appear in each of the main immunoglobulin classes
4. Greater incidence in women
5. Disease process not always progressive; exacerbations and remissions
6. Association with HLA
7. Spontaneous diseases in animals genetically programmed
8. Autoantibody tests of diagnostic value

Further reading

Allison A.C. (1971) Unresponsiveness to self antigens. *Lancet*, **ii,** 1401.

Brent L. & Holborow E.J. (eds) (1974) *Progress in Immunology.* North-Holland, Amsterdam.

Cooke A. & Lydyard P.M. (1980) The role of T cells in autoimmune diseases. In *Pathology, Research and Practice*, **1,** p. 70. Fischer Verlag, Stuttgart.

Doniach D. & Bottazzo G.F. (1977) Autoimmunity and the endocrine pancreas. *Pathobiology Annual.* Iochim H.L. (ed.). Appleton–Century–Crofts, New York.

Fudenberg H.H., Stites D.P., Caldwell J.L. & Wells J.V. (1978) *Basic and Clinical Immunology,* 2nd edn. Lange Medical Publications, Los Altos, California.

Glynn L.E. & Holborow E.J. (1964) *Autoimmunity and Disease.* Blackwell Scientific Publications, Oxford.

Johnson P.M. & Faulk W.P. (1976) Rheumatoid factor: its nature, specificity and production in rheumatoid arthritis. *Clin.Immunol.Immunopath.,* **6,** 414.

Lachmann P.J. & Peters D.K. (eds) (1982) *Clinical Aspects of Immunology,* 4th edn. Blackwell Scientific Publications, Oxford.

Maini R.N. (1977) *Immunology of the Rheumatic Diseases.* Edward Arnold, London.

Marchalonis J.J. & Cohen N. (eds) (1980) *Self/Non-self Discrimination.* Contemporary Topics in Immunobiology, vol. 9. Plenum Press, New York.

Miescher P.A. *et al.* (1978) *Menarini Symposium on Organ Specific Autoimmunity.* Schwabe & Co., Basle.

Miescher P.A. & Muller-Eberhard H.J. (eds) (1976) *Textbook of Immunopathology,* 2nd edn. Grune & Stratton, New York.

Roitt I.M. & Doniach D. (1967) Delayed hypersensitivity in autoimmune disease. *Brit. med. Bull.*, **23,** 66.

Rose N.R., Bigazzi P.E. & Warner N.L. (eds) (1978) *Genetic Control of Auto-Immune Disease.* Elsevier/North-Holland, New York.

Samter M. (ed.) (1971) *Immunological Diseases.* Little, Brown, New York.

Talal N. (ed.) (1977) *Autoimmunity.* Academic Press, New York.

Turk J.L. (1978) *Immunology in Clinical Medicine,* 3rd edn. Heinemann, London.

World Health Organization (1973) *Clinical Immunology.* Technical Report Series, no. 496.

Immunological aspects
of oral diseases

11 Oral immunity

The health of the mouth is dependent on the integrity of the mucosa which does not normally allow micro-organisms to penetrate. The mucosa is in continuity with a number of anatomical structures and these are particularly vulnerable if the oral defences are breached. It is in direct continuity with the skin of the lips at the mucocutaneous junction and with the pharynx and larynx via the oropharynx. The major and minor salivary glands open through their ducts into the mouth. The most common tissue at risk, however, is that at the junction between the gingiva and the tooth, i.e. the junctional epithelium which communicates by means of the periodontal membrane with the bone of the jaws.

The mouth is colonized by a variety of micro-organisms from the time of birth of the baby and though most of them are commensals they may become pathogenic when the host responses are altered. The factors which are responsible for maintaining oral health are the integrity of the mucosa, saliva, gingival crevicular fluid and their humoral and cellular immune components.

Mucous membrane

Surprisingly little research has been done on factors which maintain the integrity of the oral mucosa. However, a consistent finding is the lack of penetration of the intact mucous membrane by micro-organisms. Keratin might account for this only partly, as the lips, cheeks, floor of the mouth and soft palate are not keratinized (figure 11.1). In the granular layer, membrane coating granules are discharged into the intercellular space and this is associated with the formation of a barrier to the movement of substances through the epithelium. Antibodies can decrease the penetration of mucosa probably by forming immune complexes with their corresponding antigens. The basement membrane of the epithelium is another barrier to penetration of microbial and other agents. In the lamina propria adjacent to the basement membrane are a few lymphoid cells which might deal with an agent which succeeds in penetrating the overlying four barriers.

279

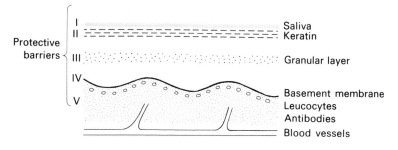

FIGURE 11.1. Protective barriers of oral mucosa.

Oral lymphoid tissues

The oral cavity is associated with extraoral lymph nodes and intraoral lymphoid aggregations. Whereas the extraoral lymph nodes are involved in the drainage of the oral mucosa, gum and teeth, the function of the intraoral lymphoid tissue is ill-understood.

EXTRAORAL LYMPH NODES

A fine network of lymph capillaries commences superficially in the mucosa of the tongue, floor of the mouth, palate, cheeks and lips, as well as from the gingiva and the pulp of the teeth. These capillaries join to form larger lymph vessels which are joined by other lymph vessels originating from a deep network in the muscle of the tongue and other structures. There is an orderly arrangement of lymph vessels which drain predominantly into the submandibular, submental, upper deep cervical and retro-pharyngeal lymph nodes, depending on the anatomical site concerned. Any microbial antigen which has gained entry through the intact epithelium into the lamina propria may enter the lymphatics directly or may be carried there by phagocytes. The antigen will then be transported to the anatomically related lymph nodes where it may induce an appropriate immune response.

INTRAORAL LYMPHOID TISSUE

Unlike the gut associated (GALT) and bronchus associated lymphoid tissue there is no well-defined oral associated lymphoid tissue. Nevertheless, there are four types of lymphoid aggregations in the mouth, each of which may play some part in the immunological surveillance of the oral tissues (figure 11.2).

(1) *Palatine tonsils* are paired lymphoid masses between the

280

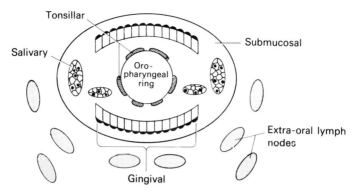

FIGURE 11.2. Organization of oral lymphoid tissue.

mouth and pharynx and are embedded between the glosso-
palatine and pharyngopalatine arches. The covering squamous
epithelium dips into the lymphoid tissue to form 10 to 20 pits.
Beneath the epithelium are found reticulum cells and lymphocytes. There are lymphoid nodules, with or without germinal
centres, and they are surrounded by lymphoid cells and a
distinctive cap of lymphocytes and plasma cells (figure 11.3).
There are no afferent but only efferent lymphatics. The crypt
epithelium, however, is specialized in allowing increased
permeability of foreign material. Antigen can penetrate the
crypt epithelium directly and it is then found in the macrophages of the germinal centre and in the perifollicular tissue.

As in lymph nodes, the lymphoid follicles contain B-cells,
whereas the perifollicular cells represent the thymus dependent
area. The B-cells proliferate in the germinal centres and
migrate into the cap as B-lymphocytes or plasma cells; hence

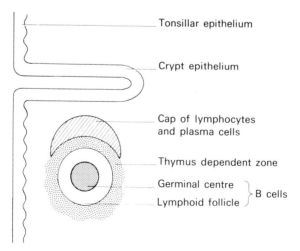

FIGURE 11.3. Organization of the palatine tonsil.

281

these cells arise locally within the tonsils. Immunofluorescence studies showed that IgG membrane staining cells are far more numerous than those with IgA, which in turn are more numerous than cells with IgM, IgD or the very rare IgE cells.

Tonsillar cells respond *in vitro* to T-cell and B-cell mitogens and antigens and give both primary and secondary antibody responses. Thus, the tonsils resemble lymph nodes in having T- and B-dependent areas, in containing both primed and un-primed cells and in that the IgG-producing cells are most numerous. They resemble GALT only in generating a signifi- cant number of IgA-forming cells and in their sub-epithelial location. However, most IgA-containing cells produce mono- mers without J chains and secretory component cannot be detected in tonsillar epithelium. The afferent pathway of antigen is directly through the covering epithelium, especially of the crypts, so that only local antigens can enter. Antibodies and sensitized cells can pass through the epithelium and there- fore may have a local protective function in guarding the entry to the digestive and respiratory tracts. Although it is likely that the immune components may spill over from the tonsils forward into the mouth, the frequent swallowing action probably carries the bulk of tonsillar antibodies and cells into the pharynx.

(2) *Lingual tonsils* are much less prominent structures on each side of the tongue, behind the circumvallate papillae. The squamous epithelium dips into the lymphoid tissue producing crypts. Ducts of mucous glands open into these crypts, flushing the cells out and this may keep the lingual tonsils free from debris and infection. As with the palatine tonsils, there are lymphoid nodules, some of which have germinal centres, and there are perifollicular diffuse lymphoid cells. However, the functional aspects of the lingual tonsils have not been studied. It is probable that they are structurally and functionally similar to the palatine tonsils.

(3) *Pharyngeal tonsils* (adenoids) are a simple mass of lym- phoid tissue, situated under the mucosa of the nasopharynx and are therefore outside the oral cavity. However, they complete the ring of lymphoid tissue separating the mouth and nose from the pharynx.

SCATTERED SUBMUCOSAL LYMPHOID CELLS

A layer of diffusely scattered lymphoid cells is found under the mucosa from the neonatal stage to old age and it is possible that occasionally some of these cells may be stimulated to proliferate into discrete lymphoid aggregations.

Lymphocytes and plasma cells are found in the major salivary glands (parotid, submandibular and sublingual), as well as in the minor salivary glands scattered under the oral mucosa. The lymphoid cells are localized in small clusters adjacent to ducts or they are scattered between acini (figure 11.6). Most of the plasma cells secrete IgA and a few IgM or IgG. It appears therefore that most of the IgA secreted in saliva is synthesized locally by the gland associated plasma cells. Furthermore, the IgA synthesized locally is dimeric, unlike the serum IgA which is monomeric.

GINGIVAL LYMPHOID TISSUE

Leucocytes are consistently found in the gingiva due to the accumulation of bacterial plaque (figure 13.2). Initially with minimal bacterial plaque the cells are predominantly lymphocytes but with the development of gingivitis there is a dramatic change to plasma cells. The ratio of T- to B cells has not been clearly defined but it appears that B-cells predominate and these form plasma cells. In subjects with clinically normal gingiva the ratio of T- to B-cells is changed from about 4:1 found in peripheral blood to about 1:3 in crevicular fluid. Seeding of lymphoid cells into an inflammatory focus has been considered to be a random process and newly stimulated blast cells have an increased non-specific affinity for inflamed tissue. Nevertheless, there appears to be some evidence that antigens can specifically select a sub-population of cells. There are two possibilities in explaining the characteristic lymphoid infiltration in the gingiva: (a) the cells originate from the regional lymph nodes, where they have been stimulated in a secondary immune response to produce blast cells and these have homed to and proliferated in the gingiva; (b) alternatively, local lymphoid cells in the gingiva are driven to proliferate by the persistent stimulation of bacterial plaque antigens and mitogens.

Clusters of plasma cells are found initially adjacent to the junctional epithelium and near the blood vessels; later the connective tissue of the gingiva may be diffusely infiltrated by these cells. IgG-producing cells predominate with a ratio of IgG to IgA varying between 4:1 and 7:1, as shown by immunofluorescent staining with specific anti-immunoglobulin conjugates. IgM cells constitute less than 1% of the plasma cells. The preponderance of IgG- over IgA-producing cells follows the pattern of a classical secondary immune response. There is evidence to suggest that a small proportion of these cells are capable of secreting specific antibodies to plaque antigens. However, most of these cells appear to produce non-reactive immunoglobulin and there are a number of inter-pretations for this. The local immune response to more than one antigen will be related to the number of stimulating antigens, so that with large numbers of antigens in bacterial plaque the chances of finding a specific antibody producing cell is rather low. Plaque contains polyclonal B-cell mitogens (e.g. lipo-polysaccharides, dextran and levan) and these may stimulate B-cells resulting in non-specific immunoglobulin formation. Furthermore, circulating blast cells or B-cells may be seeded randomly to the gingival inflammatory focus and can be stimulated by mitogenic factor released from lymphocytes to undergo further proliferation. It is therefore evident that the plasma cell infiltration of the gingiva may be the end result of a host of complex immune responses and that the immuno-globulins formed by these cells are to a great extent non-specific.

Macrophages have been detected in the gingiva with ingested bacterial plaque antigens. These macrophages may be involved in scavenging bacteria which have penetrated through the junctional epithelium. They may process the antigen and stimulate any uncommitted B-cells to produce antibodies to that antigen. Hence, antibodies passing through the gingival junctional epithelium may have two components; systemic anti-bodies and locally formed antibodies which may increase the titre of the relevant antibodies to plaque antigens.

The close relationship between protective and adverse effects is well illustrated by the gingival lymphoid tissue reactions. Spread of bacteria from the surface of the tooth may be pre-vented by coating them with antibodies, immune complex formation, phagocytosis, killing and bacteriolysis of Gram-negative bacteria by antibodies and complement. These immune responses, however, may elicit an inflammatory response through activation of the complement pathway, release of lysosomal enzymes from the phagocytes and release of endotoxin from the lysed bacteria. A local inflammation of the gum may perhaps be the price we pay for prevention of spread of the dental plaque bacteria to other parts of the body.

Summary

In addition to the extraoral lymph nodes draining the oral tissues there are four anatomically and functionally distinct intraoral lymphoid tissue aggregations.

(1) The tonsils (palatine and lingual) are the only intraoral lymphoid masses, with the classical structure of lymphoid follicles, consisting of B-cells and peri-follicular T-cells. Antigen can only penetrate directly through the covering epithelium, as there are no afferent lymphatics. Lymphoid cells from the tonsils may spill over into the mouth, but there is no evidence for a function of these cells in oral disease.

(2) Salivary gland plasma cells and lymphocytes are concerned predominantly with the synthesis of secretory IgA.

(3) Gingival aggregation of plasma cells, lymphocytes, macrophages and polymorphonuclear leucocytes is probably the most important of the four lymphoid collections in the immunological response to dental bacterial plaque.

(4) The scattered submucosal lymphoid cells have not been adequately studied.

The functional significance of the intraoral lymphoid tissue has not been clearly defined. It appears however, that an anatomical pattern of segregation has developed, with the tonsils guarding the entry into the digestive and respiratory tracts and the gingival lymphoid aggregation responding to the dental bacterial plaque accumulation. The salivary lymphoid tissue is concerned predominantly with secretory IgA synthesis and protection against infection within the salivary gland. The secretory IgA in saliva, however, may protect the oral mucosa and the tooth surface from uncontrolled bacterial colonization. The scattered submucosal lymphoid cells may act as an advanced patrol which might be stimulated into proliferation if the primary line of defence residing on the mucosal surface has failed.

Saliva

Mechanical cleansing by the muscular actions of the tongue, cheeks and lips plays an important part in maintaining hygiene of accessible sites in the mouth. This is greatly aided by saliva which in addition to lubricating the movements during speaking, chewing and swallowing makes it possible to swallow bacteria, leucocytes, tissue and food debris into the stomach where bacteria or noxious substances are inactivated. The habit of spitting, mercifully practised by few, is physiologically equally effective for the individual but has its dangers for the community in spread of infectious micro-organisms. It should be noted that there is a continuous flow of saliva which without added stimulation, that is 'the resting flow', shows an average rate of 19 ml per hour. This rate will increase with psychic stimuli, such as the thought of food, but the presence of food in the mouth acts as a powerful stimulus to salivation. There is very considerable variation in the rate of 'resting flow' of saliva between different subjects (0.5 to 111 ml per hour). At one time patients with fever and dehydration used to develop ascending infection along the ducts of the salivary glands, because of decreased salivary flow and lack of oral hygiene which resulted in stasis and infection in the ducts, often leading to a parotitis.

Lysozyme or *muramidase* is an enzyme which shows bactericidal activity by splitting the bond between N-acetyl glucosamine and N-acetyl muramic acid in the mucopeptide components of bacterial cell wall. The enzyme is a basic protein with a molecular weight of 14,000 and is found in many tissues and secretions in man, including blood leucocytes, saliva and particularly tears. The killing activity of lysozyme is most often tested with *Micrococcus lysodeikticus*.

It is somewhat surprising that although lysozyme was described by Fleming and Allison as long ago as 1922 its role as an anti-microbial factor is still rather uncertain. It may affect the development and keep down the total load of commensal organisms in the mouth, possibly by interacting with other salivary components, such as IgA. However, the oral bacterial flora appears to be resistant to lysozyme, except for *Strep. mutans*. There is nevertheless, little convincing evidence to suggest that salivary lysozyme plays an essential role in the control of caries.

Peroxidase is a heat-labile enzyme found in saliva which in the presence of thiocyanate ions and hydrogen peroxide kills *Lactobacillus acidophilus* by inhibiting the uptake of lysine, and may inactivate some streptococci by inhibiting their glycolytic enzymes. Although peroxidase can inhibit the growth of *Strep. mutans*, there is little convincing evidence that the concentration of peroxidase in saliva varies in subjects with different caries experience. Whole saliva may contain low molecular weight inhibitors of peroxidase and one of these may be hydrogen peroxide produced by some streptococci.

Lactoferrin is a heat stable protein found in saliva and milk. It has a bacteriostatic effect on a wide spectrum of micro-

organisms and may achieve its effect by depleting the environment of iron to a concentration which will fail to support
bacterial growth.

Complement. Sensitive techniques have failed to detect C3 in
parotid or submandibular saliva, but small amounts, 0.5 μg/
ml, have been found in most samples of mixed saliva. The
source of C3 in the mixed saliva is almost certainly gingival
crevicular fluid which contains high concentrations of C3. It is
evident therefore that complement dependent immune
responses and damage are unlikely to take place in saliva
because of lack of C3 and because IgA is not capable of fixing
complement.

A somewhat parodoxical finding, however, is that large
amounts of antibody to C3 (immunoconglutinin) are found in
all samples of parotid saliva, but only low titres in about one-
third of mixed salivary samples. The function of immunoconglutinins in saliva is not at all clear, but this again suggests that
complement dependent reactions are unlikely to operate in the
salivary environment.

Leucocytes. A large number of leucocytes are found in whole
saliva, and it has been estimated that leucocytes migrate at a
rate of about a milllion per minute. The leucocytes originate
from blood and migrate predominantly through the gingival
crevice into the oral cavity. Differential counts have established
that 98% to 99% of salivary leucocytes are polymorphonuclear
leucocytes, about 1% are lymphocytes and a few monocytes
and eosinophils can also be found. Cytological examination of
salivary polymorphs has shown that more than 60% of them are
poorly preserved, with rounded and fused lobes of nuclei resulting from degenerative changes. These changes have been
ascribed to saliva being hypotonic. However, few functional
studies have been carried out concerning viability, phagocytosis and release of enzymes. We have to reserve judgement
whether salivary polymorphs are effete cells which are being
disposed of, i.e. saliva represents part of the graveyard for
polymorphs. Alternatively, these cells might exert a controlling
influence on the oral microbial flora by phagocytosis, killing
and release of lysozyme, hydrolases and superoxide.

SECRETORY IgA IN SALIVA

The oral mucosa, gingiva and teeth are continuously bathed in
saliva. Assuming a resting flow of 19 ml of saliva per hour, and

TABLE 11.1. Concentration of immunoglobulins and C3 (in mg/100 ml) in four fluids

Fluid	IgG	IgA	IgM	IgG:IgA	C3
Serum	1250	220	80	5.7	150
Whole saliva*	1.4	19.4	0.2	0.07	0.05
Parotid saliva**	0.04	4.0	0.04	0.009	0
Gingival fluid	350†	110†	25†	3.2	40

*Unstimulated.
**Stimulated (from Brandtzaeg et al., 1970).
†Determined in periodontitis.

this increases with eating or decreases with sleeping, the daily secretion is about 500 ml. As saliva contains about 19 mg per 100 ml of IgA, about 100 mg of IgA is secreted daily into the mouth. In contrast, only about 1.4 mg of IgG and 0.2 mg of IgM are found per 100 ml of saliva. The relative amounts of IgG and IgM in parotid saliva are greatly reduced (table 11.1). The discrepancy between the Ig concentrations of whole saliva and parotid saliva can be accounted for only partly by the contribution of submandibular, sublingual and the minor salivary glands. The contribution made by crevicular fluid is probably

1. Major salivary glands   2. Minor salivary glands

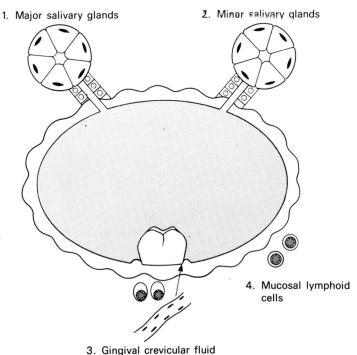

4. Mucosal lymphoid cells

3. Gingival crevicular fluid

FIGURE 11.4. Sources of immunoglobulin in whole saliva.

responsible for the increased IgG and IgM concentrations of whole saliva (figure 11.4).

Clearly IgA is quantitatively the most important immunoglobulin secreted in saliva and parotid saliva shows a ratio of IgA to IgG 400 times greater than the corresponding ratio in serum. Indeed, there is a mechanism which selectively secretes IgA and this is dependent on the presence of a secretory component (SC) (figure 11.5). Secretory IgA (mol.wt about 390,000) has three sub-components: (a) IgA molecule (mol.wt about 160,000), two of which are combined to produce a dimer of IgA by (b) J chains which are polypeptides of about 15,000 daltons, and (c) the SC, a polypeptide of about 80,000 daltons which is complexed with the IgA dimer through disulphide bonds.

There is convincing evidence to suggest that secretory IgA (sIgA) does not pass from blood to the salivary glands, to be then secreted in saliva. Immunofluorescent studies have shown that IgA is produced by plasma cells locally in the salivary glands (figure 11.6). These plasma cells produce not only heavy and light chains of IgA but also J chains which are polypeptides combining with the Fc part of IgA to produce dimeric IgA. It is significant that most of the IgA plasma cells in salivary glands produce IgA dimers and not the conventional monomeric

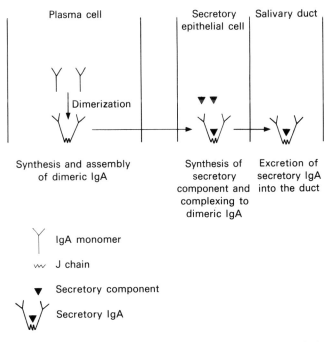

FIGURE 11.5. Synthesis, assembly and secretion of secretory IgA.

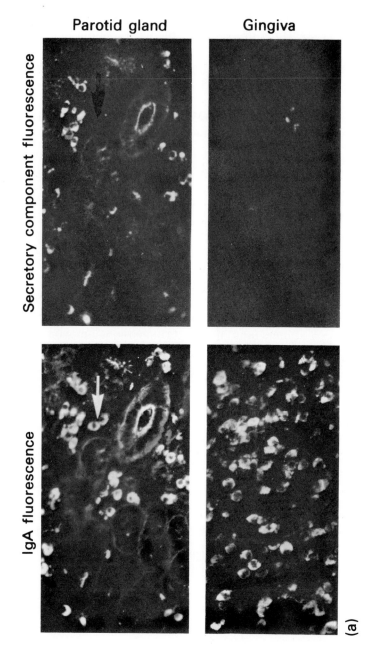

Parotid gland   **Gingiva**

Secretory component fluorescence

IgA fluorescence

(a)

FIGURE 11.6. (a) Immunofluorescent staining of sections of human parotid gland and gingiva. These sections have been treated with anti-IgA linked with a 'green' conjugate and anti-secretory component linked with a 'red' conjugate. Selective filters for 'green' and 'red' fluorescence enabled the demonstration of IgA or secretory component on the same section. Whereas most of the IgA plasma cells in the parotid gland have bound secretory component the IgA cells in the gingiva have failed to show bound secretory component. (By courtesy, from Brandtzaeg P. (1976) *J. dent. Res.*, **55**, C102–14.)

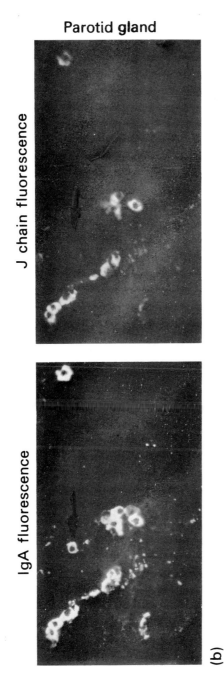

FIGURE 11.6. (b) Using similar techniques it was shown that most plasma cells in the parotid gland stained for both IgA and J chains. (Original magnification ×60.)

serum IgA. Only the dimeric IgA complexes with SC, and the affinity of SC for IgA (and indeed IgM) may be due to the dimeric (or polymeric) conformations and not necessarily the α (or μ) chains. SC appears to be synthesized by the secretory epithelial cells of salivary acini, where complexing of dimeric IgA with SC occurs. The assembled sIgA is then transported into the duct lumen and excreted into the mouth. As J chains and SC are synthesized in excess of that required to be complexed with IgA, they are found in a free state in saliva.

The origin of predominantly IgA-secreting plasma cells in the salivary gland suggests a selective mechanism for B-cells programmed to produce IgA. There are two possibilities. (a) Direct route of entry of antigenic material from the mouth to the salivary tissue may stimulate uncommitted B-lymphocytes to form IgA secreting plasma cells. This view is supported by the induction of sIgA antibodies on direct instillation of antigen into the salivary gland duct. (b) The alternative view has gained more support, that B-lymphocytes from the gut associated lymphoid tissue (GALT), that is Peyer's patches, mostly home to salivary and other secretory glands. GALT is a rich source of B-lymphocytes which can generate IgA plasma cells, whereas IgG or IgM plasma cells, with only few IgA cells, are generated from lymph nodes and blood.

The most plausible scheme illustrating antigenic sensitization, circulation and homing of IgA cells is shown in figure 11.7. Antigen from the gut lumen can be pinocytosed by the epithelial cells and reach the lymphoid follicle of Peyer's patches.

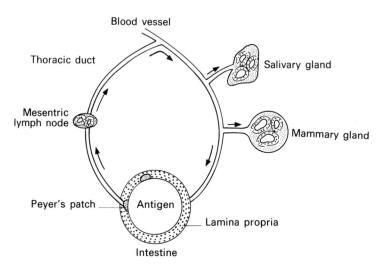

FIGURE 11.7. Antigenic sensitization in gut-associated lymphoid tissue, circulation and homing of IgA cells.

Activated lymphocytes leave Peyer's patches by the lymphatics to reach the mesenteric lymph nodes. There the cells may mature and pass into the thoracic duct where they can be recognized as blast cells with surface IgA. These cells then enter the blood stream from which they home into the lamina propria of the gut mucosa, where they differentiate into IgA plasma cells. There is also evidence that the IgA-bearing blast cells might home to other IgA-secreting glands, especially the mammary and salivary glands where they differentiate into plasma cells. Experimental work in animals and, to a lesser extent, in man have shown that oral administration of *Strep. mutans* may result in antibodies both in the saliva and in milk. As the antibody titre to the Streptococcus in serum is very low it is argued that IgA blast cells have homed from the GALT to the salivary and mammary glands. The suggestion that secretory component in these glands might bind to the blast cells which carry IgA on their surface and thereby immobilize the cells at these sites is not tenable as secretory component does not bind to these lymphocytes. Whereas antigen may well play a part in localization of large lymphocytes in the lamina propria of the intestine, there is as yet little evidence for this in the secretory glands.

Unlike systemic immune responses which have a well-established immunological memory, there is little convincing evidence for this in the local synthesis of sIgA. Thus, repeated administration of an antigen by mouth may not induce a brisk secondary response, with prolonged and high titre of antibodies. This apparent lack of memory on the part of secretory B cells might be a disadvantage in oral immunization which relies on a brisk secondary immune response, when a micro-organism is encountered, some time after immunization. It seems that a potent long-lasting response depends on immunization with live micro-organisms which may give rise to a local depot of replicating antigenic material.

Secretory IgA has at least two functional advantages: (a) it is preferentially transferred from the gland to the mucosal surface, possibly by the SC which may have special receptors on duct epithelial cells; (b) sIgA is more resistant to proteolytic degradation by bacterial and digestive hydrolases than other immunoglobulins, so that it is particularly suited to function on mucous membranes which are either colonized by a variety of micro-organisms or have potent digestive juices.

The function of sIgA has been summed up by Sir Macfarlane Burnet as an 'antiseptic paint' for mucosal surfaces. This may prevent absorption of the vast array of food and bacterial antigens from the gut and thereby prevent both overloading the immune system and development of undesirable allergic responses. A mechanism of action of sIgA which may be common to all micro-organisms is to prevent their adherence to the corresponding receptors on the mucosal surface. This mechanism would overcome the difficulty that IgA probably does not fix complement and therefore cannot induce bacterio-lysis. There is some evidence however, that sIgA combined with complement and lysozyme may cause lysis of *Escherichia coli*. sIgA antibodies to a variety of bacteria, viruses and fungi, including *Strep. mutans*, poliovirus and *Candida*, have been found in saliva. One of the functions of sIgA is neutralization of viruses.

Summary

Essential factors in the immunity of the mouth are the integrity of the oral mucosa and the functions of salivary components. Secretory IgA is the most important immunoglobulin in saliva and it may play a part in protecting the mucosa from microbial infection. The ratio of IgA to IgG is 400 times greater in parotid saliva than in serum. Indeed, there is a mechanism concerned with selective secretion of salivary IgA which is dependent on the secretory component being complexed to a dimer of IgA. IgA appears to be secreted by salivary gland plasma cells, the B-cell precursors of which may home to the salivary glands from the gut associated lymphoid tissue. Two molecules of IgA are combined by means of a J chain and the latter is also secreted by local plasma cells. Dimeric IgA is then complexed to the secre-tory component, synthesized by the epithelial cells of salivary acini, and the assembled secretory IgA is then transported into the duct lumen and excreted into the mouth. The advantage of secretory IgA is that it is more resistant to proteolytic degrada-tion than other immunoglobulins. The current view of the mechanism of action of secretory IgA is that the antibodies may combine with micro-organisms and prevent their adherence to the mucosal surface.

Gingival crevicular fluid

Components of blood can reach the dental and epithelial surfaces of the mouth by the flow of fluid through the junctional epithelium of the gingiva (figure 11.8). Some believe that the flow of fluid is secondary to the inflammation induced by microbial accumulation at the dento-gingival junction. Others

294

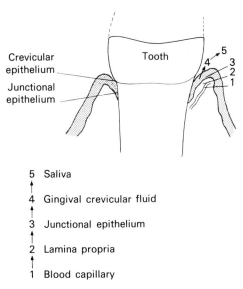

Crevicular epithelium

Tooth

Junctional epithelium

5
4
3
2
1

5 Saliva
↑
4 Gingival crevicular fluid
↑
3 Junctional epithelium
↑
2 Lamina propria
↑
1 Blood capillary

FIGURE 11.8. The origin and flow of gingival fluid.

argue that the flow is a continuous physiological process. The dispute is really academic as bacterial accumulation occurs consistently within minutes of removal of bacterial plaque, so that the induction of some inflammation at that site is unavoidable. A distinction has also been made between fluid and leucocytes; it is argued that migration of leucocytes occurs continuously but that fluid flows only as a result of inflammation. These views have been based on gross methods of collection of crevicular fluid and are unlikely to be correct. A working hypothesis, for which the evidence will be presented, is that both gingival crevicular fluid and leucocytes pass through the junctional epithelium from the gingival capillaries to the tooth surface. This flow increases greatly with inflammatory changes of gingivitis and periodontitis, as discussed in chapter 13. It is of some importance to appreciate that the total surface area of crevicular epithelium around 28 teeth is of the order of 760 mm^2 and this can increase up to 7600 mm^2 with periodontal disease.

Three principal methods have been used for the collection of gingival crevicular fluid: capillary, strip and washing methods. The capillary method uses very finely drawn out capillaries which are placed on the tooth near the gingival margin and kept there until some fluid is collected. This method works only with sufficient flow of fluid, as is found in periodontal disease. Filter strips placed on the tooth adjacent to the gingival margin will absorb crevicular fluid and the protein or other components can then be analysed. Plastic strips are similarly used to collect leucocytes by gentle pressure on the gum, squeezing the cellular content of the gingival crevice onto the strips and examining the cells microscopically. The washing method is perhaps the most suitable, as gently flushing and aspiration of saline near the gingival crevice enables both fluid and cellular components of the gingival crevice to be collected. The method has the advantages that it is simple, it can be used in normal gingiva and functional assessment of the leucocytes can be performed.

Any doubts about the physiological flow of gingival crevic- ular fluid have been recently resolved in rhesus monkeys. IgG, IgA or IgM have been separated from the serum of rhesus monkeys, labelled with ^{125}I and injected back intravenously into the monkeys. Gingival crevicular fluid was collected at short intervals of time and this showed that the labelled IgG and IgA were detected in the fluid within 30 minutes and IgM within 2 hours of injection (figure 11:9). Similarly, labelled neutrophils were detectable within 20 minutes of intravenous injection (figure 11.10). These experiments clearly establish that humoral and cellular components from blood can reach the tooth surface. Investigations of the immunological reactions of blood are therefore directly relevant to those found in crevicular fluid and they may affect the health of the tooth and gingiva. It should also be remembered that crevicular fluid passes out from the gingival crevice into the mouth, where it is mixed with saliva

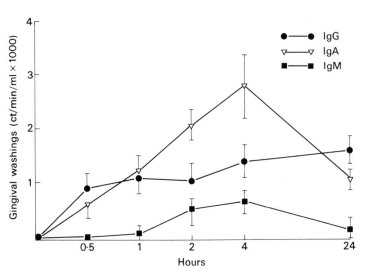

FIGURE 11.9. Sequential levels of IgG, IgA and IgM in gingival washings after intravenous injection of these immunoglobulins labelled with ^{125}I into monkeys. The means ± standard error of the mean are plotted.

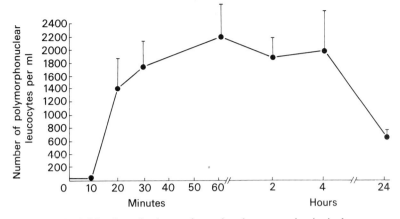

FIGURE 11.10. Number of polymorphonuclear leucocytes in gingival washings after intravenous administration of radiolabelled PMNL in rhesus monkeys. (By courtesy, from Scully C.M. & Challacombe S.J. (1979) *J. Perio. Res.* **14**, 475.)

from the major and minor glands, and imparts to 'whole saliva' a number of new characteristics.

FLUID COMPONENTS

In addition to IgG, IgA and IgM, C3, C4, C5 and C3 proactivator have been detected in gingival crevicular fluid. This suggests that both the classical and alternative complement pathways might be activated in the gingival crevice. C3 is also found in the converted form, so that complement activation may have occurred *in vivo*. Preliminary studies of crevicular fluid IgG have revealed antibodies to a number of oral microorganisms.

The presence of antigens and corresponding antibodies may lead to formation of immune complexes which will activate the classical complement pathway of $C\overline{142}$ and then C3 to release $C\overline{3a}$, $C\overline{3b}$, $C\overline{5a}$ (figure 11.11). The alternative pathway of complement can also be activated, in the absence of antibody, by plaque or some of its constituents; lipopolysaccharides from Gram-negative organisms (e.g. Veillonella), dextran from *Strep. mutans* if it becomes sulphated. These substances interact with factor D and B and properdin to generate $C\overline{3bB}$ which acts on C3 to release $C\overline{3a}$, $C\overline{3b}$ and $C\overline{5a}$. The important point to grasp here is that whilst the end results of the classical and alternative pathway appear to be identical (activation of C3) the triggering mechanism and pathways involved are very different. The relative importance of the two pathways has not been assessed,

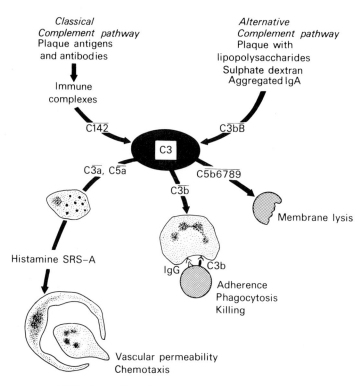

Classical
Complement pathway
Plaque antigens
and antibodies

Alternative
Complement pathway
Plaque with
lipopolysaccharides
Sulphate dextran
Aggregated IgA

Immune
complexes

C$\overline{142}$

C3

C$\overline{3bB}$

C$\overline{3a}$, C$\overline{5a}$

C$\overline{3b}$

C$\overline{5b6789}$

Membrane lysis

Histamine SRS–A

IgG

C3b

Adherence
Phagocytosis
Killing

Vascular permeability
Chemotaxis

FIGURE 11.11. Activation of complement by dental plaque.

particularly as the identification of immune complexes in the
gingiva is fraught with technical difficulties. C$\overline{3a}$ and C$\overline{5a}$
initiate vascular permeability which is an essential step in the
passage of large sized proteins (including Ig) and leucocytes
from the capillaries into the lamina propria. The same split
products C$\overline{3a}$ and C$\overline{5a}$ induce chemotactic factors for
neutrophils and monocytes, so that a chemotactic gradient is
established for directional migration of these cells from the
lamina propria to the crevicular domain. Another split product,
C3b, is concerned with binding of antigen to the C3b receptor of
neutrophils and this is the initial stage leading to ingestion of
the antigen. Whilst these biological activities of complement
have clearly defensive functions, damage to the surrounding
tissues may occur by the activated C3 generating the other
components of the complement pathway C$\overline{5b6789}$ which leads
to cell lysis. Furthermore, activation of phagocytes (neutrophils
and monocytes) leads to a release of lysosomal enzymes which
can cause a great deal of damage and potentiate the
inflammatory response.

There are a number of other components in crevicular fluid,

including albumin, transferrin, haptoglobins, glycoproteins, and lipoproteins, the functions of which have not been elucidated. Perhaps, one of the most important components are enzymes released by the cells of both the host and bacteria. Lysosomal enzymes released by phagocytic cells, proteases formed by bacteria, lysozyme, hyaluronidase and collagenase may all be intimately associated with maintenance of health or causing disease in the gingiva. The enzymes may not only affect specific tissues, such as collagen, but specific proteases have been described which selectively inactivate IgA.

CELLULAR COMPONENTS

Examination of the cells found in gingival crevicular fluid has consistently shown that neutrophils constitute by far the largest number (about 92%) of cells. The remaining cells are mononuclear, consisting of macrophages, T- and B-lymphocytes. These cells migrate continuously from blood through the junctional epithelium, where they may have ingested bacteria, into the gingival crevice. The increased proportion of neutrophils in crevicular fluid (92%) to that normally found in blood (about 70%) is consistent with the known capacity of neutrophils to migrate. This may be enhanced by the chemotactic substances formed by dental plaque, inducing neutrophils to migrate towards the tooth surface. Although about 10% of the crevicular neutrophils have seen 'active service', as they have ingested bacteria in vacuoles, over 80% are viable and functional. The cells are capable of phagocytosis of microorganisms, although the efficiency of phagocytosis is slightly impaired when compared with blood neutrophils. The phagocytic defect has been traced to the presence of C3 on the membrane of neutrophils and this may have blocked the C3b receptor responsible for opsonization. However, crevicular neutrophils show unimpaired killing capacity.

THE ROLE OF LOCAL AND SYSTEMIC IMMUNITY
IN THE IMMUNOLOGY OF THE TOOTH

A remarkable feature of the tooth surface is that it is influenced by both local salivary and systemic immune mechanisms. The line of division between the two immune mechanisms occurs near the gingival margin (figure 11.12) and this is perhaps the only site of the body where an interphase can be found between the secretory and systemic immune mechanisms. A comparison of the salivary with the gingival domain suggests that whereas

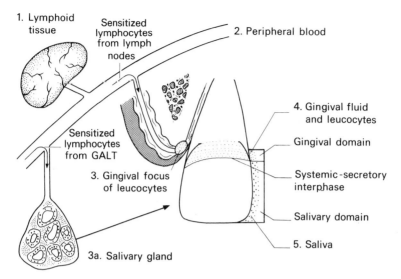

FIGURE 11.12. Gingival and salivary domains, showing the interphase between systemic and local secretory immunity; GALT, gut associated lymphoid tissue.

the salivary domain is largely dependent on the function of secretory IgA, the gingival domain is controlled by most if not all the immune components found in blood (table 11.2). It is evident that the gingival domain is influenced by more versatile and diverse immune mechanisms than the salivary domain. Of course, the pulp of the tooth is supplied by the immune components of its blood circulation and although humoral factors may influence the dentine, it is unlikely that they will reach the tooth surface.

The localization of the two domains also suggests that the gingival domain will affect both periodontal disease and approximal and cervical caries, whereas the salivary domain plays a part in fissure caries and in the protection of much of the bucco-lingual surfaces of the tooth.

ORAL FLUID

'Whole saliva' or 'mixed saliva' is a mixture of salivary gland secretions, crevicular fluid which is trapped by saliva over the gingival crevices and products of the oral mucosa. Although quantitatively oral fluid consists predominantly of salivary components, qualitatively crevicular fluid might be responsible for a number of immunologically important factors (figure 11.13). It is not clear what influence the crevicular components might have on the immune responses of oral fluid, but there is

300

TABLE 11.2. Comparison of salivary and gingival domains

	Salivary domain	Gingival domain
Localization	Bucco-lingual and occlusal surfaces, excluding the cervical zone of the tooth	Cervical and approximal sites of the tooth
Source of fluid	Salivary glands	Gingival crevicular fluid
Major Ig components	Secretory IgA	IgG, IgM, IgA
Complement	Practically absent	C3, C4, C5 demonstrated
Polymorphonuclear leucocytes	Derived from the gingival domain and over 60% are not viable	Derived from peripheral blood and over 80% are viable and capable of phagocytosis and killing
Macrophages	Not investigated	Account for about 18% of the mononuclear cells
Lymphocytes	Not investigated	T- and B-lymphocytes with a ratio of 1:3
Antigenic stimulation	Probably by antigens in the gut	Probably by some local antigens and mitogens
Chemotaxis of PMNL and macrophages	Not investigated	Both cells attracted locally by plaque-induced chemotaxis and leucocyte migration inhibition factor
Homing of lymphocytes	Circulating IgA blast cells from gut associated lymphoid tissue	Circulating IgG (and a few IgA and IgM) blast cells from lymph nodes
Type of humoral immunity	Local secretory	Systemic
Cell-mediated immunity	Not investigated but unlikely	T-cells, B-cells, blast cells and macrophages present so that cellular immunity is very likely to function
Function	Inhibition of microbial adherence	Opsonization by Ig and C3b; phagocytosis and killing; complement dependent lysis; inhibition of microbial adherence

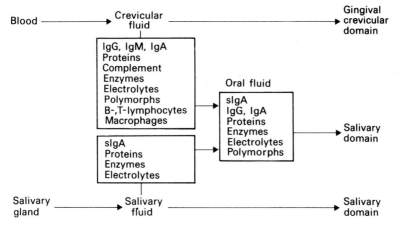

FIGURE 11.13. Humoral and cellular components in crevicular salivary and oral fluids.

little doubt that most of the polymorphs and the small amounts of IgG originate from crevicular fluid. The functional potential of oral fluid is probably enhanced by these components.

Summary

There is a continuous flow of fluid and cells from the gingival capillaries through the crevicular epithelium into the gingival crevice. The gingival crevicular fluid is probably induced by dental bacterial plaque which is usually deposited adjacent to the gingival margin. The fluid consists of IgG, IgA, IgM, complement components and a variety of enzymes. The cellular components consist mostly of neutrophils, with a few T-cells, B-cells and macrophages. It is therefore evident that gingival crevicular fluid contains most of the humoral and cellular components found in blood. The fluid and cells are capable of functioning at the tooth surface in an analogous way to that of blood in tissues. A comparison of the gingival with the salivary domain of the tooth clearly shows that in the gingival domain most immunological mechanisms may take place, whilst the salivary domain is largely dependent on secretory IgA.

Further reading

Attstrom R. & Egelberg J. (1970) Emigration of blood neutrophils and monocytes into the gingival crevices. *J. Perio. Res.*, **5**, 48.

Attstrom R., Laurell A.B., Larsson U. & Sjoholm A. (1975) Complement factors in gingival crevice material from healthy and inflamed gingiva in humans. *J. Perio. Res.*, **10**, 19.

Brandtzaeg P., Fjellanger I. & Gjeruldsen S.T. (1970) Human secretory immunoglobulins. I. Salivary secretions from individuals with normal or low levels of serum immunoglobulins. *Scand. J. Haem.*, Suppl., **12**, 58.

Brandtzaeg P. & Tolo K. (1977) Immunoglobulin systems of the gingiva. In *The Borderland between Caries and Periodontal Disease*. p. 145. Lehner T. (ed.). Academic Press, London.

Cebra J.J., Kamat R., Gearhart P., Robertson S.M. & Tzeng J. (1977) The secretory IgA system of the gut. In *Immunology of the Gut*. p. 5. Elsevier, Excerpta Medica, North-Holland, New York.

Challacombe S.J., Russell M.W., Hawkes J.E., Bergmeier L.A. & Lehner T. (1978) Passage of immunoglobulins from plasma to the oral cavity in rhesus monkeys. *Immunology*, **35**, 923.

Cimasoni G., Ishikawa I. & Jaccard F. (1977) Enzyme activity in the gingival crevice. In *The Borderland between Caries and Periodontal Disease*. p. 13. Lehner T. (ed.). Academic Press, London.

Crabbe P.A., Carbonara A.O. & Heremans J.F. (1965) The normal human intestinal mucosa as a major source of plasma cells containing gamma A-immunoglobulin. *Lab. Invest.*, **14**, 235.

Genco R.J., Mashimo P.A., Krygier G. & Ellison S.A. (1974) Antibody-mediated effects on the periodontium. *J. Periodontol.*, **45**, 330.

Genco R.J. & Taubman M.A. (1969) Secretory γ A antibodies induced by local immunisation. *Nature (Lond.)*, **221**, 679.

Husband A.J., Monie H.J. & Gowans J.L. (1977) The natural history of the cells producing IgA in the gut. In *Immunology of the Gut*. p. 29. Elsevier, Excerpta Medica, North-Holland, New York.

Jenkins G.N. (1978) *Physiology of the Mouth*. Blackwell Scientific Publications, Oxford.

Lebendiger M. & Lehner T. (1981) Characterisation of mononuclear cells in the human oral mucosa. *Archs. oral Biol.*, **26**, 1041

Mestecky J., Zikan J. & Butler W.T. (1971) Immunoglobulin M and secretory immunoglobulin A: Presence of a common polypeptide chain different from light chains. *Science*, **171**, 1163.

Ogra P.L. & Karzon D.T. (1969) Poliovirus antibody response in serum and nasal secretions following intranasal inoculation with inactivated polio-vaccine. *J. Immunol.*, **102**, 15.

Raeste A.M. (1972) The differential count of oral leukocytes. *Scand. J. dent. Res.*, **80**, 63.

Renggli H.H. (1977) Phagocytosis and killing by crevicular neutrophils. In *The Borderland between Caries and Periodontal Disease*. p. 211. Lehner T. (ed.). Academic Press, London.

Skapski H. & Lehner T. (1976) A crevicular washing method for investigating immune components of crevicular fluid in man. *J. Perio. Res.*, **11**, 19.

Sordat B., Moser R., Gerber H. & Cottier H. (1969) Differentiation pathway within germinal centers of human tonsils. *Adv. Exp. Med. Biol.*, **5**, 73.

Squier C.A., Johnson N.W. & Hopps R.M. (1976) *Human Oral Mucosa; Development, Structure and Function*. pp. 29 and 43. Blackwell Scientific Publications, Oxford.

Tomasi T.B. & Cebra J.J. (1971) Secretory immunoglobulins. In *Progress in Immunology*. p. 1481. Academic Press, London.

Waksman B.H. & Ozer H. (1977) Specialised amplification elements in the immune system. *Prog. Allergy*, **21**, 1.

Williams B.D., Challacombe S.J., Slaney J.M., Lachmann P.J. & Lehner T. (1975) Immunoconglutinins and C3 in human saliva. *Clin. exp. Immunol.*, **19**, 423.

Williams R.C. & Gibbons R.J. (1972) Inhibition of bacterial adherence by secretory immunoglobulin A: A mechanism of antigen disposal. *Science*, **177**, 697.

Wilton J.M.A. (1977) The function of complement in crevicular fluid. In *The Borderland between Caries and Periodontal Disease*. p. 223. Lehner T. (ed.). Academic Press, London.

12 Immune responses to dental bacterial plaque

The nature of dental plaque

MICROBIAL COLONIZATION OF THE MOUTH OF THE INFANT

The mouth of the newborn is sterile, but microbial colonization begins within hours of birth of the baby (figure 12.1). *Strep. salivarius* constitutes the bulk of cultivable bacteria on the first day. *Veillonella alcalescens*, lactobacilli and *Candida albicans* may

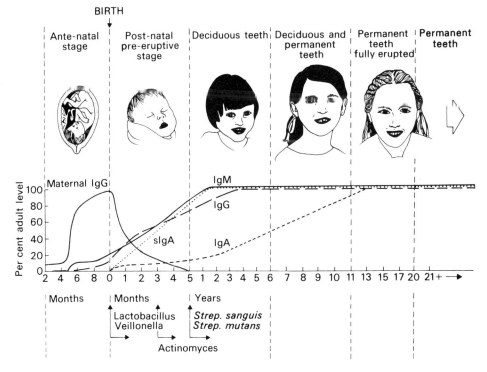

FIGURE 12.1. Fetal and post-natal development of the immune components and their relationship to oral bacterial colonization and eruption of teeth in the infant. T-lymphocytes and C3 appear at about 4 months *in utero*; T-lymphocytes reach 100% of the adult value at birth and C3 reaches adult level by 6 months of age.

also appear on the first day. Actinomyces and other anaerobes may appear months later, but *Strep. sanguis* and *Strep. mutans* follow the eruption of deciduous teeth. These micro-organisms are normally found in the oral cavity. The ecological balance between the oral micro-organisms is dependent on the nutritional requirements, as well as the effect of various metabolites and bacteriocins on certain micro-organisms. This balance can be upset by nutritional factors; for instance increased intake of sugar may increase the population of *Candida* and *Strep. mutans* to give rise to candidiasis and caries. It is not clear to what extent immunological factors may affect colonization by micro-organisms, but it is probable that they may influence both qualitatively and quantitatively the balance between different micro-organisms.

THE DEVELOPMENT OF DENTAL BACTERIAL PLAQUE

Dental plaque is an aggregation of a large number and variety of micro-organisms on the tooth surface (figure 12.2). The ecology of dental plaque is extremely complex, with bacterial commensalism, competition and antagonism playing important parts in the nature and properties of plaque. Initially, aerobic organisms attach to a surface pellicle consisting probably of a glycoprotein. Gram-positive cocci and rods appear first and *Strep. sanguis* is perhaps the most prevalent organism. The bacteria form microcolonies which often develop in columns perpendicular to the tooth surface. There is then a shift to anaerobic organisms, such as veillonellae, actinomyces and fusobacteria. A complex microbial flora develops due to a variety of interacting factors. The development of anaerobic conditions with increased bacterial accumulation, nutritional interaction between plaque bacteria and the formation of extracellular polysaccharides mediating interbacterial adhesion may determine the properties of plaque. Thus, formation of lactic acid by *Strep. mutans* can be utilized in the metabolism by *Veillonella alcalescens,* so that the latter increases in number. Dextran formed from sucrose may mediate interbacterial aggregation between *Strep. mutans* or *Strep. sanguis* and *Actinomyces viscosus.* Salivary agglutinins may also play a part in aggregating certain bacteria.

Fully formed plaque contains about 2.5×10^7 aerobic and 4.6×10^7 anaerobic organisms per mg of plaque. If oral hygiene is deliberately not practised, up to 50 mg of removable bacterial plaque may accumulate on the teeth.

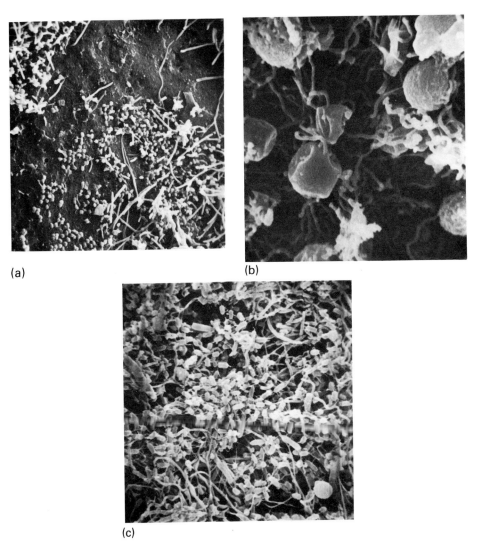

(a)

(b)

(c)

FIGURE 12.2. Scanning electron micrograph of dental microbial plaque showing: (a) cocci and filamentous organisms, × 1540; (b) spirochaetes attached to erythrocytes, × 2750; (c) mixed microbial flora, × 2750. (By courtesy of H.N. Newman (1977) In *The Borderland between Caries and Periodontal Disease*. p. 79. Lehner T. (ed.). Academic Press, London.

THE COMPONENTS OF DENTAL PLAQUE

Dental bacterial plaque may be considered to have three functional components (figure 12.3): (a) Cariogenic organisms of which *Strep. mutans, Lactobacillus acidophilus* and *Actinomyces viscosus* are most important; (b) periodontal disease inducing organisms of which *Bacteroides asaccharolyticus (gingivalis)* and *Actinobacillus (actinomycetemcomitans)* appear to be particularly significant, but other organisms, such as *Actino-*

307

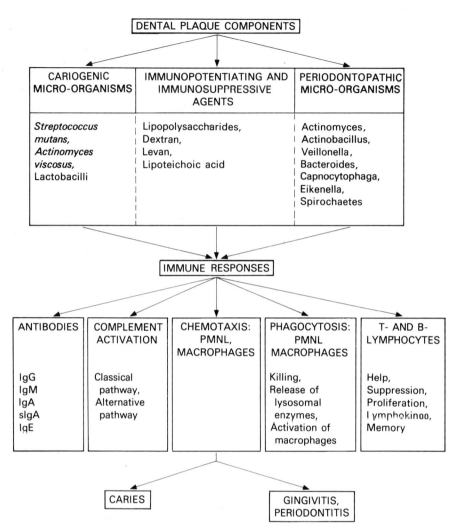

FIGURE 12.3. The effect of the three principal plaque components on the immune response in the development of caries and periodontal disease.

myçes viscosus, *Bacteroides melaninogenicus*, *Veillonella alcalescens*, Fusobacteria and Spirochaetes are also involved; (c) adjuvant and suppressive agents, the most potent of which are lipopolysaccharides (LPS), dextrans, levans and lipoteichoic acids (LTA). The aetiological roles of cariogenic and periodontal disease inducing bacteria will be discussed in the corresponding sections. The effects of adjuvant and suppressive agents on the immune responses to plaque bacteria will be discussed here. Dental plaque contains 0.01% LPS, about 8.5% soluble dextrans (with predominantly α1−6 linkages), about 1.4% of insoluble dextrans (with mostly α1−3 linkages), 1% levan and an undetermined quantity of LTA.

In order that dental plaque should be able to induce an immune response or cause direct toxic effects it must penetrate through the epithelial barrier of the gingival crevice. Indeed, the junctional epithelium is a highly permeable tissue which allows substances, probably up to a molecular weight of 700,000, to pass from the gingival sulcus to the connective tissue and vice versa. The substances pass through the intercellular spaces of the junctional epithelium and among the large variety of substances tested, tritium-labelled collagenase, albumin and endotoxin are particularly significant.

Dental plaque and the immune response

SPECIFIC CELLULAR IMMUNE RESPONSES TO DENTAL PLAQUE

Dental plaque broken up by ultra-sonication can induce increased DNA synthesis of lymphocytes which have been previously sensitized to some of the plaque antigens. Both T- and B-lymphocytes respond to plaque antigens, as indeed they respond to different components of single bacteria; T-lymphocytes respond to the protein fraction, whereas B-lymphocytes respond to the lipoprotein of veillonella. There is a significant correlation between the proliferative response of lymphocytes stimulated by dental plaque, as compared with single organisms, such as *Veillonella alcalescens*, or *Actinomyces viscosus*. However, the effect of plaque on lymphocytes is not additive, in that it does not reflect the summated effect of the individual antigens, of which there might be a very large number.

Sensitized lymphocytes also respond to dental plaque by the release of soluble mediators or lymphokines. These are released by both T- and B-cells, though some lymphokines, such as mitogenic and chemotactic factors are released predominantly by T-cells and others, such as osteoclast activating factor (OAF), by B-cells. A release of macrophage migration inhibitory factor might localize macrophages to the site of lymphocyte activation. Another mediator, lymphotoxin, is cytotoxic for human gingival fibroblasts which are concerned in laying down collagen in the periodontal membrane. OAF is also released by activated lymphocytes and causes bone resorption, as measured by the release of ^{45}Ca from fetal rat bone, so that it may cause destruction of the supporting alveolar bone. The release of mitogenic factor may recruit unsensitized lymphocytes to proliferate, so that the cellular reactions are boosted.

309

It is assumed that there must be a suppressor mechanism to halt the damaging reactions, though such a mechanism has not been demonstrated formally. Probably both specific and non-specific suppressor cells and factors may be released in controlling the cellular reactions.

MATERNAL-FETAL IMMUNE RESPONSES TO PLAQUE ANTIGENS

At birth the newborn infant has a normal concentration of IgG which crosses the placenta from the mother to the infant (figure 12.1). It is therefore not surprising that the infant will have maternal IgG antibodies to plaque bacteria, such as *Strep. mutans*, *Veillonella alcalescens* or *Actinomyces viscosus* (figure 12.4). However, IgM and IgA do not cross the placental barrier and at birth the infant can synthesize only about a fifth of the normal amount of IgM. As no IgM antibodies to plaque bacteria are found in the infant at birth, though they are present in the mother, this is reasonable evidence that the infant does not produce any antibodies to the mother's dental plaque; antigenic stimulation *in utero* would have induced IgM antibodies.

The cellular responses to maternal plaque antigens in the infant appear to reflect the maternal pattern of sensitization. Sensitized lymphocytes to dental plaque, *Strep. mutans* (figure 12.5), *Veillonella alcalescens* and *Actinomyces viscosus* are detected only in those infants whose mothers have sensitized lymphocytes to these antigens, associated with the presence of dental plaque and gingival inflammation.

Whilst it is clear that accumulation of dental plaque in the pregnant woman will be associated with sensitized lympho-

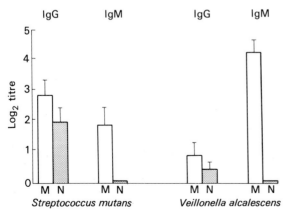

FIGURE 12.4. Antibodies in maternal (M) and neonatal (N) serum; mean and standard error of the mean given.

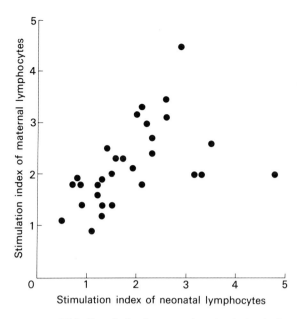

FIGURE 12.5. Correlation between the stimulation indices of maternal and neonatal lymphocytes to *Strep. mutans*. Stimulation index refers to the ratio of DNA synthesis in the antigen stimulated to that of the unstimulated lymphocytes.

cytes, there is little understanding of the mechanism involved in sensitization of the fetal lymphocytes. It is reasonably certain that maternal lymphocytes normally do not cross the placental barrier. One view is that bacterial plaque from the mother passes through the placenta to the fetus and sensitizes the fetal lymphocytes directly. An alternative view is that fetal lymphocytes may become sensitized by means of a transfer factor-like substance from the mother.

A full complement of surface immunoglobulin-bearing B-lymphocytes are found in neonatal blood and these cells respond to B-cell mitogens, such as LPS and dextran. Surface Ig-bearing B-lymphocytes are detectable from about 9 weeks of gestation and by 15 weeks the proportion of cells bearing each Ig class reaches adult values. However, the capacity of B-lymphocytes to synthesize Ig lags behind the appearance of surface immunoglobulin bearing cells. This has been demonstrated by using pokeweed mitogen which has the property of transforming B-lymphocytes to plasma cells which contain cytoplasmic Ig. These were detectable at about 15 weeks of gestation and at birth IgM-containing cells reach 12%, IgG 2% and IgA 0.5% of adult values. The full adult values are only reached at about 4 months after birth. Hence the functional capacity of B-lymphocytes to synthesize cytoplasmic Ig appears later than surface Ig-bearing B-lymphocytes. The ontogeny of cytoplasmic Ig-synthesizing cells parallels more closely the development of serum Ig than that of the surface Ig-bearing cells. The sequence of development of the Ig-synthesizing cells is in the order of IgM, IgG and IgA and this is the same sequence as that found with the serum immuno-globulins. The latter, however, reach adult values only by the age of 1 year for IgM, 6 to 7 years for IgG and about 12 years for IgA. Although there is some doubt about the stage of maturation of T-lymphocytes at birth, these cells respond well to at least two T-cell stimulants; to HLA antigens in the mixed leucocyte reaction and to phytohaemagglutinin. T-lymphocyte responses are detectable from about 15 weeks of gestation.

Complement is synthesized by the fetus at about 15 weeks and the total complement, C1, C3, C4, and C5, at birth reaches about half the adult level. By 6 months, however, the full adult level is found.

Since oral colonization by veillonella or lactobacilli occurs within days of birth, it is taking place in the presence of maternal IgG antibodies and the infant's lymphocytes are sensitized to these bacteria. There is, however, no certainty that the humoral or cellular agents reach the bacteria at the mucosal surface of the mouth. With the eruption of the deciduous teeth from the age of about 6 months, the systemic immune compo-nents may enter the gingival crevicular domain and then pass into the oral cavity. It might be significant that just before the eruption of deciduous teeth, that is at 3–5 months after birth, the maternal IgG antibodies disappear from the infant because of catabolism of IgG. There is no information available as to the persistence of neonatal lymphocyte sensitization but inspired guesswork would suggest that it may well last about 6 months. It is also uncertain whether by 6 months the infant has produced any IgM or IgG antibodies to oral micro-organisms. It seems, however, that there may exist a critical timing between the physiological hypogammaglobulinaemia resulting from the clearance of maternal IgG, formation of antibodies by the infant, the presence of sensitized lymphocytes and bacterial colonization of the erupting deciduous teeth. The role of anti-bodies and sensitized lymphocytes in oral and dental coloniza-tion might have an effect on the balance of microbial population in the mouth.

The effects of plaque accumulation *in vivo* on the immune response have been tested in dental students. They were asked to abstain from oral hygiene for 28 days and the plaque accumulation, gingival inflammation and cellular and humoral immune responses were tested sequentially (figure 12.6). Accumulation of dental bacterial plaque and the associated gingival inflammation were correlated with an increase in lymphocyte transformation and release of macrophage migra-

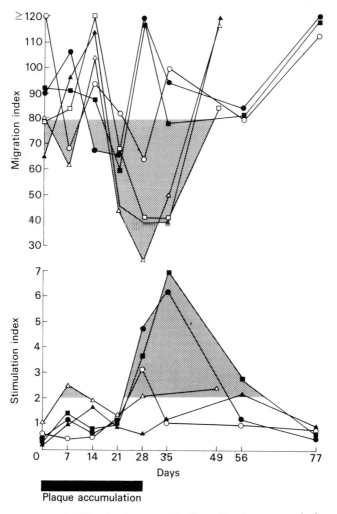

FIGURE 12.6 The development of cell-mediated responses during experimental gingivitis in six subjects. Profiles of the sequential lympho-proliferative responses and macrophage migration inhibition to *Veillonella alcalescens* are shown. The shaded areas indicate the significant change.

313

tion inhibition factor (MIF). Lymphocytes were activated by sonicates of autologous bacterial plaque, streptococci, veillonella, actinomyces and some unrelated antigens. Both cellular responses were of limited duration and had returned to base-line values 28 days after plaque was removed. In contrast, serum haemagglutinating and complement fixing antibodies to these antigens were not increased.

These results clearly show that accumulation of dental bacterial plaque adjacent to the gingiva can stimulate the cell-mediated immune response by presumably some of the plaque antigens penetrating the junctional epithelium. As the response is often biphasic it is possible that suppressor cells might also be stimulated to turn off the cellular reactions. Furthermore, memory cells to some plaque antigens may also be stimulated, as has been observed by repeating the plaque accumulation experiment in the same subjects (figure 12.7). Significant lymphocyte transformation was found earlier, it was greater in magnitude and lasted longer in the second as compared with the first plaque accumulation experiment. These immunological features are usually ascribed to secondary immune responses, or to enhancement of an existing immune state. It suggests that bacterial plaque *in vivo* can induce a recall of immunological memory for plaque antigens at the cellular level. It is not clear at present whether this is a measure of T- or B-lymphocyte memory, but both might be involved, since pooled dental plaque and veillonella specifically can stimulate T- and B-lymphocytes to undergo blast cell transformation.

ADJUVANT EFFECT OF DENTAL PLAQUE

Dental plaque may act as an endogenous adjuvant potentiating the responses of both T- and B-lymphocytes. It can augment the *in vitro* antibody-forming cell response to sheep erythrocytes and this effect appears to be dependent on the capacity to activate T-helper cells which affect the response of the B-antibody-forming cells. Indeed, dental plaque can replace partially the requirement for T-helper cells. It is probable that the immunopotentiating effects of plaque are due to its content of polyclonal B-cell mitogens. LPS from Gram-negative bacteria, dextran synthesized by *Strep. mutans* and *sanguis* and probably levan synthesized by *Actinomyces viscosus* are the most likely candidates as they potentiate the responses to mitogens and antigens.

The immunopotentiating effect of plaque has been first observed in man. A group of dental students abstained from

314

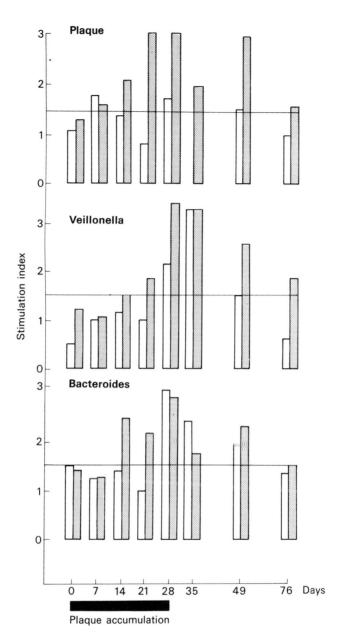

FIGURE 12.7. Evidence for a secondary immune response to dental plaque organisms after a second episode of experimental gingivitis. Mean sequential lymphoproliferative responses with first (blank columns) and second (shaded columns) episodes of gingivitis.

oral hygiene for 28 days and this was associated with plaque accumulation and a significant increase in the gingival index of inflammation (figure 12.8). Lymphocyte cultures were prepared from the peripheral blood of these students and the

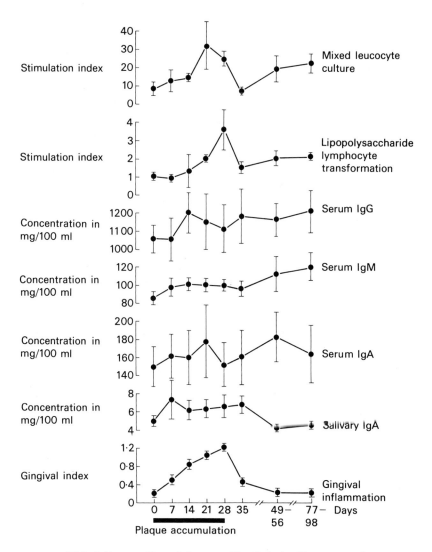

FIGURE 12.8. Adjuvant effect of plaque on T-cells (mixed leucocyte culture response) and B-cells (lipopolysaccharide response). The serum and salivary immunoglobulin concentrations are also given; mean and standard error of the mean are given.

T-lymphocyte function was tested by the mixed leucocyte culture reaction and the B-lymphocyte function by stimulation with LPS. A significant increase in DNA synthesis (figure 12.8), as well as macrophage migration inhibition factor, was correlated with maximal plaque accumulation and gingival inflammation. There was also a slight increase in the serum immunoglobulin concentrations. The immunopotentiating effect of dental plaque accumulation on human lymphocytes *in vivo* has been confirmed with the responses to at least two of the plaque components, namely LPS and levan *in vitro*.

The mechanism of adjuvants is complex but four points need to be emphasized in relation to dental plaque. (a) The persistence of dental plaque along the gingival margin enables LPS, dextran and levan to be released continuously over an extensive epithelial surface. (b) Dental plaque or LPS are potent agents causing release of lysosomal hydrolases from macrophages and these cells may be involved in the action of adjuvants. (c) In order for dextran to potentiate immune responses and to activate the alternate pathway of complement it must be negatively charged. Indeed, sulphated macromolecules are found in dental plaque, some of which are sulphated glycoproteins. Negatively charged polysaccharides can be formed by *Strep. mutans* and *sanguis* which incorporate labelled phosphate into soluble and insoluble high molecular weight polysaccharides. In addition to the negative charge of dextrans which may be necessary for adjuvanticity, the $\alpha1-3$, $\alpha1-6$ and $\alpha1-4$ linkages may influence their adjuvanticity, especially as the $\alpha1-3$ linked dextran is resistant to degradation and is slowly metabolized. (d) Recruitment and proliferation of immuno-competent cells both in the gingival mononuclear cell infiltration and the draining lymph nodes may follow exposure to high local concentrations of antigens.

POLYCLONAL B-CELL MITOGENS

A variety of bacteria and their products are capable of non-specific stimulation of B-lymphocytes to produce immunoglobulins and these substances are termed polyclonal B-cell mitogens. Among the most important are LPS from Gram-negative bacteria, dextrans, levans and antigens from *Actinomyces viscosus*. However, a number of other Gram-negative organisms associated with periodontal disease have potent polyclonal B-cell activating properties. B-cell hyper-reactivity has been demonstrated in some patients with severe periodontitis, with staphylococcal A protein which is also a potent B-cell activator. Polyclonal B-cell activation might account for the increase in the concentration of immunoglobulins in experimental gingivitis and in periodontitis, but its biological role in the development of periodontal disease is unknown. It is possible that the non-specific activation of B-cells to produce antibodies and lymphokines might be involved in the development of periodontal disease.

Serum IgG, IgM and IgA antibodies to most oral micro-organisms have been found in control subjects and an increase in antibody titre was not detected in patients with periodontal disease. The evidence suggests that dental plaque organisms elicit a serum antibody response as part of the host response to any microbial antigen. However, recent antibody studies with *Bacteroides gingivalis (asaccharolyticus)*, using the sensitive ELISA technique have shown a significant increase in serum IgG antibodies in patients with periodontitis as compared with controls. The possibility has therefore been raised that this might be the causative organism of periodontal disease.

IMMUNOSUPPRESSION INDUCED BY DENTAL PLAQUE COMPONENTS

Although dental plaque has not been formally shown to have immunosuppressive properties, this has been demonstrated with LPS, dextran, levan and LTA. It may be confusing that the same B-cell mitogens may have adjuvant and suppressive properties, but this is dependent among other factors on the sequence of administration. LPS or levan administered before an antigen causes suppression, but when given after the antigen they enhance the immune response. Both high zone and low zone tolerance can be induced in mice by polysaccharides so that the dose is also important. This applies to the branched native levans and the predominantly $\alpha1-6$ linked, near-linear dextran. LTA present in a variety of Gram-positive bacteria (e.g. streptococci and lactobacilli) can also depress the immune response if administered before the antigen.

It is worth noting that soluble levans are synthesized by *Strep. mutans* and *Actinomyces viscosus*. *Strep. mutans* can also synthesize a continuous series of dextrans with a variable proportion of $\alpha1-6$ and $\alpha1-3$ linkages. Furthermore, LPS is released from Gram-negative and LTA from Gram-positive bacteria. The net result of all these agents may be complex and whether enhancement or suppression will result may depend on the proportion of $\alpha1-3$ to $\alpha1-6$ linked dextrans, branching, negative charge and sequence of adding mitogen and antigen.

Specific suppressor T-cells to oral microbial antigens have now been described, so that active suppression also plays a role in the development of both periodontal disease and dental caries.

IMMUNO-GENETIC CONTROL OF T-CELL
HELPER AND SUPPRESSOR FUNCTION

T-cell helper and suppressor functions to a protein antigen prepared from *Strep. mutans* have now been investigated in mice, monkeys and man. A reciprocal relationship has been established between helper and suppressor cells in man. This relationship is antigen dose-dependent and appears to be related to the HLA-DR antigens. Thus, with DRw6 lymphocytes help is elicited with 1 ng and suppression with 10–1000 ng of streptococcal antigen. Conversely, DR4 lymphocytes release helper activity with 1000 ng and suppressor activity with 1 to 100 ng of the antigen. These observations suggest that immune responses to the cariogenic microorganism *Strep. mutans* might be under genetic control of the DR (Ia) antigens or in linkage disequilibrium with these antigens.

THE EFFECT OF DENTAL PLAQUE ON THE
COMPLEMENT PATHWAY

The possibility has been discussed (see p. 297) that plaque antigens, in the presence of antibodies, may form immune complexes which may activate the classical complement pathway (figure 11.11). However, plaque and some of its components, especially lipopolysaccharides, can activate the alternative complement pathway. Some Gram-positive plaque bacteria (e.g. *Strep. mutans*, *Strep. sanguis* and *Actinomyces viscosus*) can activate both the classical and alternative complement pathways. The activation of either of the two complement pathways might be the mechanism which triggers off the complex inflammatory responses by releasing C3a and C5a which initiate vascular permeability (figure 2.3). C3a and C5a induce the release of histamine from mast cells and platelets and this may account for the increased vascular permeability. A kinin-like substance is also released following the action of C1s on C2 and this increases vascular permeability directly. It is worth reminding ourselves that the essential step in the inflammatory process is increased vascular permeability which allows exit of proteins and cells from the capillaries to the surrounding connective tissue.

C3a and C5a also cause platelet aggregation which may result in intravascular clotting; this may minimize the spread of bacteria but may also increase local damage by depleting the blood supply. The cleavage product C3a has other properties, in that it is cytotoxic to various cells, including fibroblasts. As

319

normal fibroblast function is important in maintaining the collagen fibres of the periodontal membrane, it can be seen that generating C3a may affect the integrity of periodontal membrane by killing fibroblasts.

The effects of C3a and C5a on chemotaxis and C3b on phagocytosis will be discussed below. However, among the later components of complement activation C5b6789 is cytotoxic to membranes of cells and micro-organisms. The cytotoxic mechanism functions most effectively when the complement components are assembled on the surface of the cell. C8 appears to be the essential lytic component, with its action being significantly enhanced by C9. The terminal components of complement also give rise to the synthesis of prostaglandin E1 which can cause bone resorption. Thus, radiolabelled calcium is released from cultured rat fetal bones in the presence of fresh serum, but not when it is incubated in heated or C6-deficient serum. Bone resorption was correlated with prostaglandin synthesis and was inhibited by indomethacin which blocks prostaglandin synthesis. Activation of both the classical and alternative pathways can be involved in bone resorption and the significance of this is evident in periodontal disease in which perhaps the most important factor is loss of bone supporting the teeth.

THE EFFECT OF DENTAL PLAQUE ON PHAGOCYTES

The transport of phagocytes from blood vessels to extra-vascular sites is an active process mediated by chemotactic factors induced by the C3a and C5a products of complement activation. Chemotaxis has been studied particularly with LPS and as little as 0.05 μg of LPS from *Veillonella alcalescens* will elicit chemotactic activity. Both PMNL and monocytes are attracted by the chemotactic factors and particularly PMNL appear in large number. This has been demonstrated *in vitro*, using Boyden chambers with two compartments, separated by a micro-filter which allows migration of PMNL from one chamber towards the chemotactic factor in the other. Chemotaxis has also been shown *in vivo* by assessing the migration of PMNL before and after solubilized dental plaque has been applied to the gingival crevices of beagle dogs. There is another mechanism which may be involved in the localization of macrophages and PMNL, that is macrophage or leucocyte migration inhibition factor released by stimulating lymphocytes with plaque extracts.

320

The accumulated phagocytes are then involved in phago-cytosis which can be non-specific but is greatly enhanced by opsonization. This is achieved by IgG antibodies combining with the antigens and then binding to the Fc receptor on the phagocyte (figure 11.11). Another means of opsonization is by an antigen combining with IgG or IgM antibodies which will generate C3b and this will bind to the C3b receptor on the phagocyte. Phagocytosis of plaque components may have a dual function: (a) bacteria and their products are ingested and the bacteria may be killed by a variety of enzyme reactions; (b) antigens may be processed and then passed on to immunocompetent cells to induce an immune response.

Dental plaque and LPS are very potent agents which induce phagocytes to release hydrolytic enzymes. Gram-positive bacteria derived from dental plaque were capable of inducing the release of lysosomal hydrolases from PMNL, if the bacteria synthesized extracellular polysaccharides. Dental plaque stimulates macrophages to release lysosomal hydrolases and in addition the cells appear to be activated, as shown by an increase in size and the content of certain non-lysosomal enzymes. Collagenase is also secreted by macrophages activated by LPS and can degrade native collagen. The lyso-somal enzymes are potent agents which can cause tissue damage.

Summary

The effects of dental plaque on the immune response are varied and complex and this is not surprising if the nature of plaque is considered. The large number of Gram-positive and negative bacteria and their products, such as LPS, LTA, dextrans and levans enable most of the immunological mechanisms so far examined to be activated. Both complement pathways are activated, lymphocytes are stimulated, lymphokines are released and macrophages are activated. The large number of polyclonal B-cell mitogens may play an important part in lymphocyte stimulation: An immuno-genetic control of T cell helper and suppressor functions has been suggested with at least one dental plaque antigen and is associated with the HLA-DR or related antigens. These potent reactions might be modulated by the potentiating and suppressive effects of some of the plaque components and may result in a localized chronic inflammatory response. The direct toxic effects of plaque components on the gingival tissues may contribute further to the inflammatory reaction.

Passive transfer of IgG antibodies and cellular sensitization to plaque antigens from the mother to the infant is of great interest. It may influence oral bacterial colonization of the newborn and the development of active immunity to some of the bacterial antigens by the infant. Although serum antibodies to plaque microbial antigens are found in practically all normal subjects, there might be significant increase in titres in patients with periodontal disease to some organisms which play an important part in the development of the disease (e.g. *Bacteroides gingivalis*).

Further reading

Adinolfi M. (1974) The development of lymphoid tissues and immunity. In *Scientific Foundations of Paediatrics*. p. 333. Heinemann, London.

Alford C.A., Frank Wu L.Y., Blanco A. & Lawton A.R. (1975) *The Immune System and Infectious Diseases*. Fourth International Congress of Immunology.

Carlsson J. (1967) Presence of various types of non-haemolytic streptococci in dental plaque and in other sites of the oral cavity in man. *Ondont. Revy*, **18**, 55.

Gibbons R.J. (1980) Adhesion of bacteria to the surfaces of the mouth. In *Microbial Adhesion to Surfaces*. p. 35. Berkeley R.C.W., Lynch J.M., Melling J., Rutter P.R. & Vincent B. (eds). Ellis Horwood, Chichester.

Gibbons R.J. & van Houte J. (1975) Dental caries. *Ann. Rev. Med.*, **26**, 121.

Horton J.E., Oppenheim J.J., Chan S.P. & Baker J.J. (1976) Relationship of transformation of newborn human lymphocytes by dental plaque antigen to the degree of maternal periodontal disease. *Cell. Immunol.*, **21**, 153.

Horton J.E., Oppenheim J.J. & Mergenhagen S.E. (1974) A role for cell-mediated immunity in the pathogenesis of periodontal disease. *J. Periodont.*, **45**, 351.

Horton J.E., Raisz L.G., Simmons H.A., Oppenheim J.J. & Mergenhagen S.E. (1972) Bone resorbing activity in supernatant fluid from cultured human peripheral blood leukocytes. *Science*, **177**, 793.

Ivanyi L. & Lehner T. (1970) Stimulation of lymphocyte transformation by bacterial antigens in patients with periodontal disease. *Archs. oral Biol.*, **15**, 1089.

Ivanyi L. & Lehner T. (1971) Lymphocyte transformation by sonicates of dental plaque in human periodontal disease. *Archs. oral Biol.*, **16**, 1117.

Ivanyi L. & Lehner T. (1974) Stimulation of human lymphocytes by B-cell mitogens. *Clin. exp. Immunol.*, **18**, 347.

Ivanyi L. & Lehner T. (1977) Interdependence of *in vitro* responsiveness of cord and maternal blood lymphocytes to antigens from oral bacteria. *Clin. exp. Immunol.*, **30**, 252.

Ivanyi L., Topic B. & Lydiard P.M. (1981) The role of Ty lymphocytes in cell mediated immunity in patients with periodontal disease. *Clin. exp. Imm.*, **46**, 633.

Kahnberg K.E., Lindhe J. & Hellden L. (1976) Initial gingivitis induced by topical application of plaque extract. *J. Perio. Res.*, **11**, 218.

Krasse B. (1977) Microbiology of the gingival plaque. In *The Borderland between Caries and Periodontal Disease.* p. 5. Lehner T. (ed.). Academic Press, London.

Lehner T. (1980) Future possibilities for the prevention of caries and periodontal disease. *Brit. dent. J.*, **149**, 318.

Lehner T. (1982) Cellular immunity in periodontal disease: an overview. In: *Host-Parasite Interactions in Periodontal Diseases.* p. 202. Genco R.J. & Mergenhagen S.E. (eds). American Society for Microbiology, Washington, D.C.

Lehner T., Lamb J.R., Welsh K.I & Batchelor J.R. (1981) Association between HLA−DR antigens and helper cell activity in the control of dental caries. *Nature*, **292**, 770.

Lehner T., Wilton J.M.A., Challacombe S.J. & Ivanyi L. (1974) Sequential cell-mediated immune responses in experimental gingivitis in man. *Clin. exp. Immunol.*, **16**, 481.

Lindhe J. & Hellden L. (1972) Neutrophil chemotactic activity elaborated by human dental plaque. *J. Perio. Res.*, **7**, 297.

Loesche W.J. (1976) Chemotherapy of dental plaque infections. *Oral Science Rev.*, **9**, 65.

Mouton C., Hammond P.G., Slots J. & Genco R.J. (1981) Serum antibodies to oral *Bacteroides asaccharolyticus (Bacteroides gingivalis)*: relationship to age and periodontal disease. *Infect. Immun.*, **31**, 182.

Newman M.G., Socransky S.S., Savitt E.D., Propas D.A. & Crawford A. (1976) Studies of the microbiology of periodontosis. *J. Periodont.*, **47**, 373.

Schroeder H.E. (1977) Histopathology of the gingival sulcus. In *The Borderland between Caries and Periodontal Disease.* p. 43. Lehner T. (ed.). Academic Press, London.

Smith S., Bick P.H., Miller G.A., Ranney R.R., Rice P.L., Lalor J.H. & Tew J.G. (1980) Polyclonal B-cell activation: severe periodontal disease in young adults. *Clin. Immunol. Immunopath.*, **16**, 354.

Socransky S.J. (1977) Microbiology of periodontal disease−present status and future considerations. *J. Periodont.*, **48**, 497.

Taichman N.S. & McArthur W.P. (1976) Interaction of inflammatory cells and oral bacteria: release of lysosomal hydrolases from rabbit polymorphonuclear leukocytes exposed to Gram-positive plaque bacteria. *Archs. oral Biol.*, **21**, 257.

Tempel T.R., Snyderman R., Jordan H.V. & Mergenhagen S.E. (1970) Factors from saliva and oral bacteria, chemotactic for polymorphonuclear leukocytes: Their possible role in gingival inflammation. *J. Periodont.*, **41**, 71.

Wilton J.M.A. (1982) Polymorphonuclear leukocytes of the human gingival crevice: clinical and experimental studies of cellular function in humans and animals. In *Host−Parasite Interactions in Periodontal Diseases.* p. 246. Genco R.J. & Mergenhagen S.E. (eds). American Society for Microbiology, Washington D.C.

323

13

Immunology of periodontal disease

Dental plaque in the development of gingival and periodontal diseases

Dental bacterial plaque initiates gingival inflammation and since plaque is found in almost all subjects it follows that gingivitis affects most people. The transition from chronic gingivitis to destructive periodontitis in most instances appears to be related to age. Whereas bacteria trigger off the inflammatory reaction, it now appears that the host immune responses may be involved in both the chronic gingival inflammation and the progression to a detructive periodontitis. This may take many years or decades, with breakdown of the periodontal ligament and loss of supporting bone, leading to pocket formation, loosening and eventually loss of the teeth.

The causative factors responsible for periodontal disease are not known but deposits of bacterial plaque are thought to be involved in the pathogenesis of this disease. There are two views concerning the microbial aetiology: (a) that the non-specific pathogenic potential of the mixed organisms in dental plaque, (b) that specific organisms are responsible for the development of periodontal disease. The specific microbial aetiology hypothesis has recently received support from the observations that *Bacteroides gingivalis (asaccharolyticus)* is the predominant organism isolated from both human and monkey periodontal disease. Furthermore, a specific type of juvenile periodontitis is associated with another organism *(Actinobacillus actinomycetemcomitans)*.

A close relationship has been found between accumulation of bacterial plaque and gingivitis and during this process a change occurs from a predominantly Gram-positive coccal form to a complex population of filamentous organisms, spirochaetes, vibrios and Gram-negative cocci. Of the Gram-positive organisms, *Actinomyces viscosus* appears to be especially involved in the development of gingivitis. Gram-negative organisms are thought to be essential in the development of periodontal disease. *Veillonellae, bacteroides, actinobacilli, capnocytophaga* and *spirochaetes* have been implicated in this disease. The cell walls of the Gram-negative organisms contain lipopolysaccharides and those of the Gram-positive organisms have lipoteichoic acids, dextrans or levans which may be responsible for a variety of immunological functions (see pp. 313–21).

Local immunopathology of the gingiva and periodontium and systemic immune responses

Quantitative analysis of the histopathological and ultra-structural changes in experimental gingivitis and periodontal disease have suggested four stages of development: initial, early, established and ·advanced lesions. Parallel studies between the immunopathological changes in the gingiva and the systemic immune responses have not been carried out during plaque-induced experimental gingivitis. Nevertheless, sequential studies make it possible to relate the local immunopathological changes with the systemic immune responses (figure 13.1).

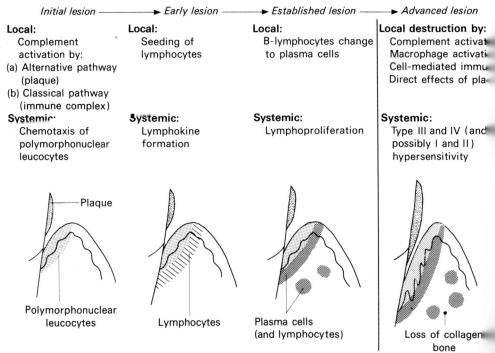

FIGURE 13.1. Diagrammatic representation of the local immunopathological and systemic immune responses during the four stages of development of periodontal disease.

Initial lesion

As bacteria and their products are normally found on teeth it is difficult to distinguish between the normal and pathological tissue reactions. In the relatively plaque-free subjects or animals, small numbers of leucocytes migrate through the junctional epithelium towards the gingival crevice (figure 13.2).

Local immunopathology. The initial lesion is an acute inflammatory response which develops within 2 to 4 days of plaque accumulation. The lesion is localized to the gingival sulcus and the adjacent junctional epithelium and connective tissue. The gingival blood vessels dilate and there is exudation of fluid, with immunoglobulin (especially IgG) complement, fibrin and PMNL being found in the extravascular space. A few lymphocytes and macrophages are also found in the junctional epithelium and the adjacent connective tissue. The initial lesion may be a response to the generation of chemotactic substances by the bacterial plaque antigens.

Systemic immunity. Serum antibodies to a variety of plaque bacteria are present at this stage, so that immune complexes might well be formed with some of the plaque antigens. The immune complexes will activate the classical complement pathway and LPS and other plaque substances may activate the alternative pathway. The biological effects of complement activation seem to be adequate to account for the initial lesion; C3a and C5a induce increased vascular permeability and are chemotactic for polymorphonuclear leucocytes (PMNL) which may account for the inflammatory changes.

Early lesion

A dense lymphoid cell infiltration develops within 4 to 7 days of plaque accumulation at the site of the initial lesion. The early lesion is often found in the normal gingiva, when plaque control is not practised efficiently.

Local immunopathology. Lymphocytes constitute 75% of the leucocyte infiltration and there are only a few plasma cells (figure 13.3). Most of the lymphocytes are of the T-cell series with a small number of B-cells. There are some macrophages and blast cells. Fibroblasts adjacent to lymphocytes show degenerative changes and there is a localized loss of collagen fibres. The exudation of serum immunoglobulins, complement,

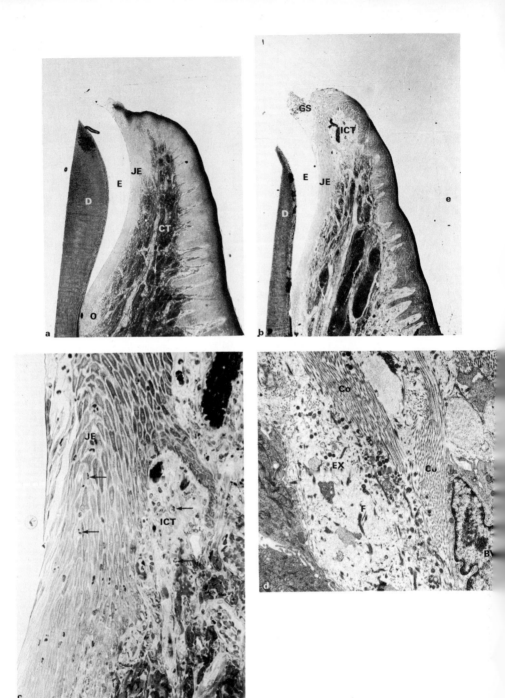

fibrinogen and leucocytes is increased. The gingival crevicular fluid and leucocytes reach a maximum level 6 to 12 days after the onset of clinical gingivitis.

Systemic immunity. Lymphoid cells, especially newly stimulated blast cells in the circulation have a heightened, non-specific affinity for inflamed tissue and may therefore be seeded into the gingival focus of inflammation developed in the initial lesion. Lymphocytes at this stage are capable of releasing at least some mediators, such as leucocyte migration inhibition and mitogenic factor and these may augment the localization of leucocytes and proliferation of lymphocytes (figure 13.6).

Established lesion

This develops within 2 to 3 weeks of plaque accumulation and its distinguishing feature is the prominent plasma cell infiltration, as compared with the lymphoid infiltration in the early lesion (figure 13.4). It is probable that some of the B-lymphocytes found in the early lesion have been stimulated by some plaque antigens to differentiate into plasma cells.

Local immunopathology. The lesion is still confined to a small site adjacent to the gingival sulcus but consists of numerous plasma cells (figure 13.4). However, clusters of plasma cells are also

---

FIGURE 13.2. Pathological features of the initial lesion.

(a) A bucco-lingual section of normal marginal gingiva from a beagle dog kept completely free of microbial plaque. Dense collagen bundles and the subgingival plexus of blood vessels comprise the connective tissue (CT). The junctional epithelium (JE) does not have rete ridges and covers the cervical enamel (E). The dentine of the crown is indicated (D). Note the absence of a gingival sulcus (compare to (b)).

(b) A bucco-lingual section from a dog with experimentally induced initial gingivitis. Lateral to the gingival sulcus (GS) is an acutely inflamed and infiltrated connective tissue (ICT). The junctional epithelium (JE), enamel (E), and the dentine (D) are indicated.

(c) A higher magnification of an inflamed region from (b). Note the relative absence of collagen fibres and the presence of numerous polymorphonuclear leucocytes (arrows) in the infiltrated connective tissue (ICT) and junctional epithelium (JE).

(d) An electron-microscope view of an area of connective tissue adjacent to the junctional epithelium, showing exudate (EX), deposits of fibrin (F), remnants of collagen fibres (Co), lysosomal bodies free in the tissues, and part of a blood vessel (BV).

(a) ×35; (b) ×35; (c) ×216; (d) ×5400.

(Figures 13.2–5 by courtesy of R.C. Page & H.E. Shroeder; from *Lab. Invest.* (1976) **33**, 235.)

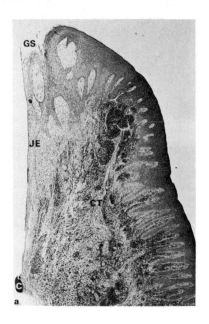

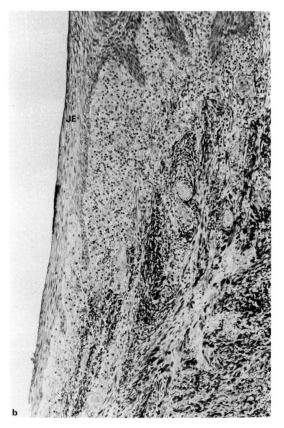

FIGURE 13.3. Pathological features of the early lesion.

(a) Bucco-lingual section from the gingiva of a human premolar. A gingival sulcus (GS) is present; the junctional epithelium (JE) has proliferated as shown by the rete ridges and there is a dense round cell infiltrate in the connective tissue (CT). C, cementum.

(b) A higher magnification of the junctional epithelium (JE) and infiltrated connective tissue shown in (a). Note the virtual absence of collagen fibres and the presence of a dense round cell infiltrate.

(c) (See p. 327). An electron microscopic view of a portion of the junctional epithelium and infiltrated connective tissue from (b). The fibroblasts (FI) show pathological changes consisting of vacuolated cytoplasm and paucity of nuclear chromatin. The fibroblasts are surrounded by a dense population of lymphocytes (L) and only remnants of collagen fibres (Co) are present.

(d) (See p. 327.) An electron microscope view of a medium-sized lymphocyte (ML) closely apposed to a damaged altered fibrosis (FI). Note the swollen rough endoplasmic (rer) cisternae and the large amount of smooth, cytoplasmic membranes in the fibroblast.

(a) ×35; (b) ×96: (c) ×405; (d) ×15,900.

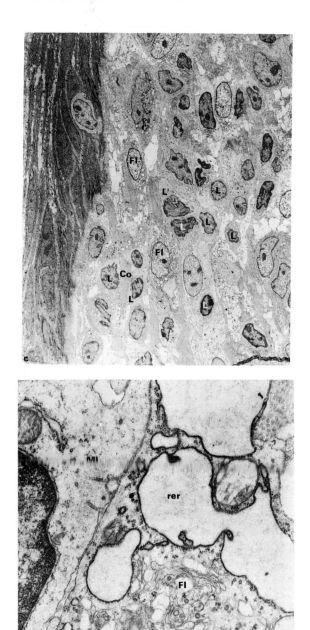

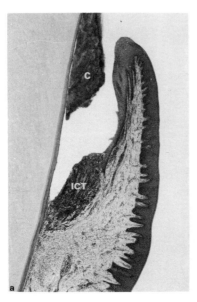

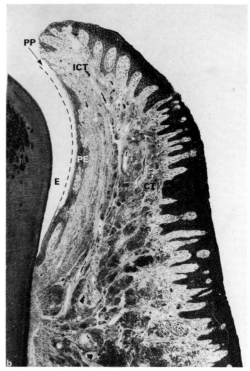

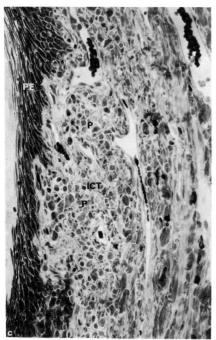

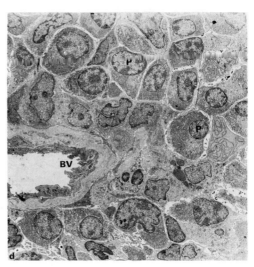

found among blood vessels and collagen fibres. Most of the plasma cells produce IgG, some IgA and a few IgM. There are also some T-lymphocytes. Extra-vascular connective tissue and the junctional epithelium contain immunoglobulin, complement and probably immune complexes. The junctional and oral epithelium may proliferate apically into the connective tissue and there is loss of collagen. The gingival sulcus may deepen and the junctional epithelium may be converted into a pocket. A significant recent finding is that lymphocytes isolated from gingival tissue responded by *in vitro* proliferation to oral bacteria and this correlated well with the response of peripheral blood lymphocytes (see pp. 336–7).

Systemic immunity. The proliferative response of lymphocytes to plaque antigen becomes evident at 14 to 21 days of plaque accumulation. Specific plaque antigens may be involved in this process, but the polyclonal B-cell mitogens found in plaque (LPS, dextran and levan) might also act as potent activators. As both T- and B-lymphocytes are stimulated by plaque antigens and newly stimulated blast cells are preferentially seeded to inflammatory foci, there is a continuous supply of these cells in the established lesion. Plasma cells are secretory end cells, so that for the established lesion to be maintained for years or decades (as it often is) a continuous influx of lymphocytes is required.

Another significant feature of the established lesion is the development of the adjuvant effect after 14 days of plaque accumulation (figure 12.8). The adjuvant effect may boost the local immune response and non-specific stimulation of peripheral blood T- and B-lymphocytes. This may exacerbate the local reaction and may be responsible for the persistence of the

FIGURE 13.4. Pathological features of the established lesion.

(a) A bucco-lingual aspect of a human tooth with a gingival pocket filled with calculus (C). There is a small area of infiltrated connective tissue (ICT) covered by pocket epithelium near the base of the pocket.

(b) A bucco-lingual section of a dog tooth with a periodontal pocket (PP). Note the pocket epithelium (PE) and an adjacent narrow band of infiltrated connective tissue (ICT) extending from the gingival margin apically. The dotted line indicates the location of the enamel surface (E) before demineralization.

(c) A higher magnification of the pocket epithelium (PE) and infiltrated connective tissue (ICT) shown in (b). Plasma cells (P) predominate in the infiltrate.

(d) An electron microscopic view of the dense plasma cell (P) infiltration around a blood vessel (BV) in the connective tissue.
(a) × 35; (b) × 35; (c) × 348; (d) × 2880.

established lesion. Any influence of the adjuvant property of dental plaque on systemic immunity needs to be further explored, especially as it may affect the overall immunological load of the host.

A slight increase in salivary IgA concentration was found in experimental gingivitis but a corresponding increase in antibody titres to oral micro-organisms was not detected.

Advanced lesion

The established lesion can persist for many years and the change into the advanced lesion marks the transition from a chronic and successful defence reaction to a destructive immunopathological mechanism. It is not certain what factors are responsible for the progression from an established to an advanced lesion. There is little doubt that this transition is crucial in the health of the periodontium and there are two principal schools of thought: (a) that the host immune responses may be involved; (b) that some specific micro-organism in dental plaque may be responsible for the development of the advanced lesion. *Bacteroides gingivalis* (asaccharolyticus) has been recently singled out as a potentially significant organism and increased serum antibody titres support this view.

Local immunopathology. This stage is recognized clinically as periodontitis, with pocket formation, ulceration of the pocket epithelium, destruction of the collagenous periodontal ligament and bone resorption. These changes lead to mobility and eventually loss of the tooth. The features of acute vasculitis are maintained, with the further development of chronic inflammation and reparative fibrosis. The pathological changes now extend apically and laterally, with a dense infiltration of plasma cells, lymphocytes and macrophages (figure 13.5). There is a

---

FIGURE 13.5. Pathological features of the advanced lesion.

(a) Mesio-distal section through the interdental tissue of lower front teeth of an adult. The marginal gingiva and the alveolar bone (AB) have receded to the apical one-third of the roots. The root surfaces are covered with calculus, and long fingers of pocket epithelium extend into the infiltrated connective tissue (ICT).

(b) A bucco-lingual section of a dog tooth. A deep periodontal pocket (PP) filled with plaque (P) is present (arrow). The lateral wall of the pocket consists of pocket epithelium (PE) and a band of infiltrated connective tissue (ICT).

(c) A higher magnification of the infiltrated tissue (ICT) adjacent to the pocket epithelium (PE). The infiltrate contains many plasma cells (P).
(a) ×9; (b) ×35; (c) ×192.

breakdown of the epithelial barrier between plaque and periodontal tissue and this might be associated with a significant change in the immune responses and permit direct access of plaque antigens and metabolites. The essential feature of this stage of periodontal disease is that there is irreversible loss of periodontal ligament and bone, with a progressive increase in

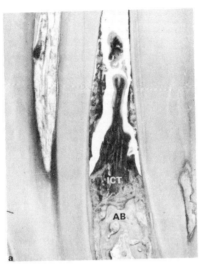

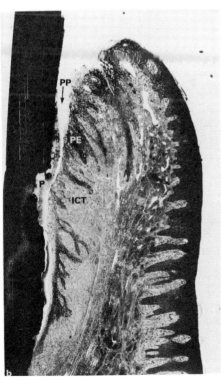

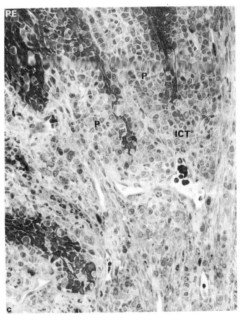

pocket formation. Gingival fluid collected at this stage contains high concentrations of IgG, IgA, IgM and complement, as well as a predominantly PMNL infiltration.

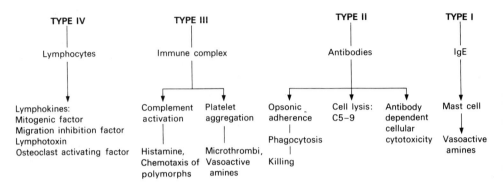

FIGURE 13.6. The complex nature of immune responses postulated in the immunopathogenesis of periodontal disease.

Systemic immunity. It is now becoming clear that the chronic destructive process may involve all the mechanisms known to contribute to the immunopathology of chronic lesions. The complexity of the development of the advanced lesion of periodontal disease will become evident when it is appreciated that type IV, type III, type II and type I immune reactions have been implicated (in this order of importance; figure 13.6). Whilst all these reactions may contribute to the complex mechanism of bacterial elimination and the inevitable tissue destruction and tissue repair, the biological significance of any one mechanism is not known. The diverse mechanisms will be briefly described though some aspects have been dealt with in the section on the immune responses to dental plaque (chapter 12).

Immunological mechanisms

CELL-MEDIATED HYPERSENSITIVITY (TYPE IV)

The activation of cell-mediated immunity (CMI) by plaque antigens stimulates T- and B-lymphocytes to proliferate. A sub-population of T-lymphocytes may be cytotoxic to periodontal tissue. Lymphocytes maintain a supply of soluble mediators; leucocytes migration inhibition factor may immobilize further macrophages and PMNL, chemotactic factor may attract further leucocytes, lymphotoxin may damage fibroblasts and osteoclast activating factor may cause further bone resorption.

Tissue destruction enables more plaque antigen to enter the periodontal tissue, thereby activating further immune reactions which leads to a vicious cycle. An intriguing possibility might be the activation of suppressor cells and factors which might check some of the cellular or humoral immune responses. Lymphocyte activity can be modulated *in vitro* by serum factors, by stimulating or inhibitory antibodies, or their immune complexes. Activation of lymphocytes by one of the plaque bacteria such as Veillonella seems to depend not only on the presence of sensitized lymphocytes but also on stimulating factors present in sera from patients with gingivitis or mild and moderate periodontitis. A depression of lymphocyte transformation, in the presence of autologous serum from patients with severe periodontitis, has been ascribed to a serum inhibitory factor, but suppressor T cells with Fc-y receptors are also involved. This has now been demonstrated not only with peripheral blood lymphocytes but also lymphocytes isolated from gingival tissue.

Attempts to correlate quantitatively the stimulation index of lymphocytes with the periodontal index of disease have not been successful. There are considerable individual variations in the CMI immune responses, and the pattern of cellular responses might be an indication of the patient's sensitization to plaque antigens. The hypothesis that needs to be examined is whether the pattern of cellular responses is related to the susceptibility to develop periodontal disease. Identifying subjects especially prone to periodontal disease would aid greatly in prognosis and in the preventive measures that need to be applied to different individuals.

The existence of an immunological memory for plaque antigens has been clearly established (see p. 314). It is therefore of interest to note that cellular immune response to some plaque antigens may persist for some time after the teeth are extracted. However, this might also be associated with the persistence of some micro-organisms, such as Actinomyces or Veillonella in the edentulous mouth. Further evidence of an immunological memory and the presence of a suppressive agent is that in those patients with severe periodontitis whose lymphocytes are not stimulated by plaque antigens, significant lymphocyte stimulation results within 2 weeks of extraction of the diseased teeth.

TYPE III OR IMMUNE-COMPLEX-MEDIATED HYPERSENSITIVITY

Due to technical difficulties immune complexes have not as yet been satisfactorily demonstrated in periodontal disease. Nevertheless, the presence of plaque antigens and antibodies suggests that immune complexes (IC) might be formed. This has been demonstrated by direct immunofluorescent staining for Ig and C3. Furthermore gingival crevicular fluid PMNL have membrane bound IgG, IgM and C3 (figure 13.7) and the C3b but not Fc receptors are blocked. These findings are consistent with the presence of IC in the gingival domain. The IC may activate the classical complement pathway to produce a number of biologically active mediators (see pp. 297–8). These will induce an increased vascular permeability, platelet aggregation, chemotaxis of phagocytes, opsonization and phagocytosis of micro-organisms and antigens, and killing of micro-organisms. This is associated with the release of lysosomal enzymes, both by PMNL and macrophages, and will cause local damage. The macrophage is a particularly versatile cell, capable of secreting collagenase which can degrade collagen of the periodontal ligament. The generation of C567 complexes may bind to the surface of normal adjacent cells and bind C8 and C9, resulting in cell lysis.

Complement activation can also cause bone resorption and both the classical and alternative pathways are involved. This type of bone resorption is mediated by prostaglandins which can be inhibited by indomethacin, a prostaglandin inhibitor.

The cellular immune responses are also influenced by

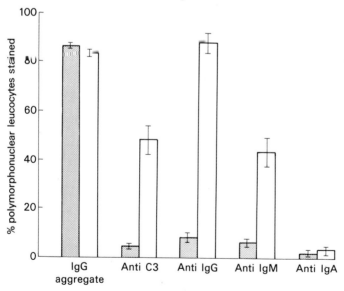

FIGURE 13.7. Binding of aggregated IgG and staining for surface immunoglobulin and complement of peripheral blood (shaded columns) and crevicular (blank columns) polymorphonuclear leucocytes. Vertical bars are ± standard deviation of the mean.

products of complement activation; C3b can interact with receptors on lymphocytes stimulating these cells to produce lymphokines. This mechanism illustrates a link up between the type III and type IV hypersensitivity reactions.

Activation of the alternative complement pathway should be considered here as this may result in a similar reaction to that induced by IC in the classical pathway. Plaque, LPS and peptidoglycans from plaque bacteria can activate the alternative complement pathway, thereby augmenting activation of the classical pathway. The macrophage may again play an important role, because it secretes factor B, C3 and cathepsin G which participate in the alternative complement pathway.

TYPE II OR ANTIBODY-DEPENDENT HYPERSENSITIVITY

Antibodies to periodontal tissue have not been detected, though during the early days of discovery of autoimmunity the latter has been invoked as a cause of periodontitis, without any evidence. The three components of type II hypersensitivity, that is (a) antibody binding to cell surface antigens and causing phagocytosis, (b) antibody-dependent killer cell activity and (c) the lytic function of the later components of complement might, however, be involved in attempts to eliminate plaque bacteria. Antibody and complement-mediated phagocytosis and killing are the most important mechanisms dealing with Gram-positive organisms. Complement-dependent lysis, without the aid of phagocytes, is effective with Gram-negative organisms. Both these mechanisms are working overtime in an effort to keep clear the periodontal tissue from the mass of organisms in dental plaque. However, it should be noted that these mechanisms have not, as yet, been demonstrated directly against the cells of periodontal tissue and therefore type II hypersensitivity should not be considered for the time being as playing an essential part in periodontal disease.

TYPE I OR ANAPHYLACTIC HYPERSENSITIVITY

The evidence in favour of type I hypersensitivity has been the observation that mast cells are found in the normal gingiva but they decrease in number with inflammation. IgE has been found in normal gingiva and it coats some plaque bacteria. Antigen might induce degranulation of the mast cells associated with IgE and release histamine and other vasoactive substances. It is of interest that increased levels of prostaglandins E1 and E2 were found in gingivitis and these may also cause increased vascular permeability.

Consideration of the wealth of immune protective-destructive mechanisms in periodontal disease makes one wonder how the tissue avoids total destruction for so many years. The first point to make is that the biological significance of any of the experimental findings needs to be explored before their function *in vivo* can be fully assessed. However, nature has introduced a complex network of checking or inhibitory mechanisms to prevent the immune-inflammatory reactions from getting out of control. Some of these have already been noted.

Cell-mediated immunity can be suppressed by inducing suppressor cells and factors, and their potential importance in the control of the various stages of periodontal disease needs to be explored. Indeed, T-suppressor cells with Fc-y receptors have been identified in advanced periodontal disease and these may inhibit the normal immune responses. Serum inhibitory factors have been reported in severe periodontitis. Macrophages secrete prostaglandins which may also inhibit the cellular reactions. The complement pathway can be inhibited by a number of agents, especially C3 inactivator which breaks down C3b, as well as by proteinase inhibitors.

Dental plaque itself contains a number of immunosuppressive agents of which the best known are lipopolysaccharide, lipoteichoic acid, dextran and levan. Lipopolysaccharides can depress cellular immune responses, whereas lipoteichoic acid suppresses the antibody responses. High-zone and low-zone B-cell tolerance can be induced by high and low doses of branched native levan and predominantly α1–6 linked dextran. Finally, some of the plaque bacteria are capable of producing specific proteinases which inhibit certain classes of immunoglobulins. Thus, *Strep. sanguis* produces a proteinase which specifically cleaves IgA. Modulation of the immune mechanism by microbial products and by the host immune responses may therefore play an important part in regulation of the host-microbial relationship.

IMMUNOSUPPRESSION AND IMMUNOSTIMULATION IN PERIODONTAL DISEASE

The influence of immunodeficiency on periodontal disease will be further discussed in relation to immunodeficiency diseases (pp. 338–92). However, particularly relevant here are the studies with immunosuppressive and immunostimulating agents. In an interesting experiment in beagle dogs, administration of antithymocyte serum had little effect on gingival inflammation. On the other hand, administration of anti-neutrophil serum, or treatment with cobra venom factor which renders the dogs complement deficient, induced severe inflammatory and necrotic gingival changes. These findings can be interpreted to suggest that the complement-neutrophil axis is more important in the development of gingivitis than cell-mediated immunity. The effect, however, of anti-thymocyte serum treatment varies greatly and B-lymphocyte functions are not affected, so that further work is required before any conclusions are drawn.

Patients treated with immunosuppressive drugs used in renal transplantation have significantly decreased gingival and periodontal disease in an age and sex matched population. This could be due to the anti-inflammatory effect of corticosteroids used, but a plausible interpretation is that suppression of cell-mediated immunity by the immuno-suppressive effects of the corticosteroid and anti-metabolite drugs is responsible for the decreased periodontal disease. The reverse effect, that is increased gingival inflammation, was observed by using the immunopotentiating drug levamisole which stimulates cell-mediated immunity. Hence, the use of immunosuppressive and immunostimulating drugs in man decreases or increases gingival inflammation and these changes are best interpreted by their effects on cell-mediated immunity.

JUVENILE PERIODONTITIS (PERIODONTOSIS)

This is a rare but important disease which affects one or several teeth in young people under the age of 21 years. There is rapid destruction of the periodontal ligament and the supporting bone leading to loosening and then loss of the teeth. Three immunological defects have been found in this condition. (a) There is little or no activation of the patients' lymphocytes to increased DNA synthesis, though production of macrophage migration inhibition factor is intact when stimulated with bacteria concerned with periodontal disease. (b) An increase in the concentrations of serum IgG, IgA and IgM suggests polyclonal B-cell activation. (c) There is a defect in chemotaxis of PMNL and this may be due to inhibitors directed against both the cells and the chemotactic factor.

It is therefore possible that patients with juvenile periodontitis develop a rapidly advancing disease early in life, because of defects in the immunological responses to some micro-organisms. Recent evidence suggests that *Actinobacillus*

341

actinomycetemcomitans (a name that evokes instant empathy) may cause this type of periodontitis. Raised serum IgG antibodies to this organism have been found in juvenile periodontitis but not in controls or patients with the adult type of periodontal disease. This organism appears to have a cytotoxic effect on neutrophils in the periodontium which may in turn decrease phagocytic removal of the organism.

Summary

Gingival and periodontal disease is induced by dental bacterial plaque. There are four immunopathological stages which have systemic immune counterparts. (a) The initial lesion is found in the normal state with a localized inflammatory response of polymorphonuclear leucocytes; complement activation and chemotaxis generated by plaque antigens and possibly immune complexes may account for this stage. (b) The early lesion shows a localized infiltration of predominantly T- with a few B-lymphocytes. In the circulation lymphocytes are sensitized at this stage to plaque antigens, as shown by their ability to release lymphokines. (c) The established lesion is characterized by a localized plasma cell infiltration and peripheral blood lymphocytes can be stimulated to proliferate with plaque antigens. This stage can persist for years, with early pocket formation. (d) The advanced lesion marks the transition to a destructive immunopathological mechanism, with ulceration of the pocket epithelium and localized destruction of collagen and bone. This is a progressively destructive process leading to loss of teeth. The immunological processes are complex and may involve type IV, III, II and I reactions, with the protective-destructive mechanisms of lymphocyte and macrophage functions, antibodies and complement activation. These reactions are modulated by immunopotentiating and immunosuppressive agents and a number of inhibitory responses have developed to prevent the immune reaction from getting out of control.

Further reading

Allison A.C., Schorlemmer H.U. & Bitter-Suermann D. (1976) Activation of complement by the alternative pathway as a factor in the pathogenesis of periodontal disease. *Lancet*, **ii**, 1001.

Attstrom R. (1975) The roles of gingival epithelium and phagocytosing leukocytes in gingival defence. *J. Clin. Perio.*, **2**, 25.

Baehni P., Tsai C.C., McArthur W.P., Hammond B.F. & Taichman N.S. (1979) Interaction of inflammatory cells and oral microorganisms: VIII,

Detection of leukotoxic activity of a plaque-derived Gram negative micro-organism. *Infect. Immun.*, **24**, 233.

Clagett J.A. & Page R.C. (1978) Insoluble immune complexes and chronic periodontal diseases in man and the dog. *Archs. oral Biol.*, **23**, 153.

Cianciola L.J., Genco R.J., Patters M.R., McKenna J. & Van Oss C.J. (1977) Defective polymorphonuclear leukocyte function in a human periodontal disease. *Nature*, **265**, 445.

Genco R.J., Mashimo P.A., Krygier G. & Ellison S.A. (1974) Antibody-mediated effects on the periodontium. *J. Periodontol.*, **45**, 330.

Goodson J.M., Dewhirst F.E. & Brunetti A. (1974) Prostaglandin E2 levels and human periodontal disease. *Prostaglandins*, **6**, 81.

Horton J.E., Leiken S. & Oppenheim J.J. (1972) Human lymphoproliferative reaction to saliva and dental plaque deposits. An *in vitro* correlation with periodontal disease. *J. Periodont.*, **43**, 522.

Horton J.E., Oppenheim J.J., Mergenhagen S.E. & Raisz L.G. (1974) Macrophage—lymphocyte synergy in the production of osteoclast activating factor. *J. Immunol.*, **113**, 1278.

Horton J.E., Raisz L.G., Simmons H.A., Oppenheim J.J. & Mergenhagen S.E. (1972) Bone resorbing activity in supernatant fluid from cultured human peripheral blood leukocytes. *Science*, **177**, 793.

Ivanyi L. (1980) Stimulation of gingival lymphocytes by antigens from oral bacteria. In *The Borderland between Caries and Periodontal Disease*, II. pp. 125–134. Lehner T. & Cimasoni G. (eds). Academic Press, London.

Ivanyi L. & Lehner T. (1970) Stimulation of lymphocyte transformation by bacterial antigens in patients with periodontal disease. *Archs. oral Biol.*, **15**, 1089.

Ivanyi L. & Lehner T. (1977) The effect of Levamisole on gingival inflammation in man. *Scand. J. Immunol.*, **6**, 219.

Ivanyi L., Topic B. & Lydiard P.M. (1981) The role of Tγ lymphocytes in cell mediated immunity in patients with periodontal disease. *Clin. Exp. Immun.*, **46**, 633.

Lehner T. (1982) Cellular immunity in periodontal disease: an overview. In *Host-Parasite Interactions in Periodontal Diseases*. pp. 202–216. Genco R.J. & Mergenhagen S.E. (eds). American Society for Microbiology, Washington, D.C.

Lehner T., Wilton J.M.A., Challacombe S.J. & Ivanyi L. (1974) Sequential cell-mediated immune responses in experimental gingivitis in man. *Clin. exp. Immunol.*, **16**, 481.

Lehner T., Wilton J.M.A., Ivanyi L. & Manson J.D. (1974) Immunological aspects of juvenile periodonitis (periodontosis) *J. Periodontol.*, **45**, 261.

Mackler B.F., Altman L.C., Wahl S., Rosenstreich D.L., Oppenheim J.J. & Mergenhagen S.E. (1974) Blastogenesis and lymphokine synthesis by T and B lymphocytes from patients with periodontal disease. *Infect. Immun.*, **10**, 844.

Mackler B.F., Faner R.M., Schur P., Wright T.E. & Levy B.M. (1978) IgG subclasses in human periodontal disease. *J. Periodontal Res.*, **13**, 433.

Mouton C., Hammond P.G., Slots J. & Genco R.J. (1981) Serum antibodies to oral Bacteroides asaccharolyticus (*Bacteroides gingivalis*): relationship to age and periodontal disease. *Infect. Immun.*, **31**, 182.

Nisengard R.J., Beutner H.E. & Hazen S.P. (1968) Immunologic studies of periodontal disease. IV. Bacterial hypersensitivity and periodontal disease. *J. Periodontol.*, **39**, 329.

Nobreus N., Attstrom R. & Egelberg J. (1974) Effect of anti-thymocyte serum on development of gingivitis in dogs. *J. Perio. Res.*, **9**, 227.

Page R.C. & Schroeder H.E. (1976) Pathogenesis of inflammatory perio-dontal disease: A summary of current work. *Lab. Invest.*, **33**, 235.

Sandberg A.L., Raisz L.G., Goodson J.M., Simmons H.A. & Mergenhagen S.E. (1977) Initiation of bone resorption by the classical and alternative complement pathways and its mediation by prostaglandins. *J. Immunol.*, **119**, 1378.

Schenkein H.A. & Genco R.J. (1977) Gingival fluid and serum in periodontal diseases. I. Quantitative study of immunoglobulins, complement com-ponents, and other plasma proteins. *J. Periodontol.*, **48**, 772.

Schenkein H.A. & Genco R.J. (1977) Gingival fluid and serum in periodontal diseases. II. Evidence for cleavage of complement components C3, C3 proactivator (factor B) and C4 in gingival fluid. *J. Periodontol.*, **48**, 778.

Schroeder H.E. (1977) Histopathology of the gingival sulcus. In *The Borderland between Caries and Periodontal Disease*. p. 43. Lehner T. (ed.). Academic Press, London.

Schuller P.D., Freedman H.L. & Levins D.W. (1973) Periodontal status of renal transplant patients receiving immunosuppressive therapy. *J. Periodontol.*, **44**, 167.

Schwartz J. & Dibblee M. (1975) The role of IgE in the release of histamine from gingival mast cells. *J. Periodontol.*, **46**, 171.

Smith S., Bick P.H., Miller G.A., Ranney R.R., Rice P.L., Lalor J.H. & Tew J.G. (1980) Polyclonal B-cell activation: severe periodontal disease in young adults. *Clin. Immunol. Immunopath.*, **16**, 354.

Tanner A.C., Haffer C., Bratthall G.T., Visconti R.A. & Socransky S.S. (1979) A study of the bacteria associated with advancing periodontitis in man. *J. Clin. Periodontol.* **6**, 278.

Taichman N.S., McArthur W.P., Tsai C.C., Baehni P.C., Shenker B.J., Berthold P., Evian C. & Stevens R. (1982) Leukocidal mechanisms of *Actinobacillus actinomycetemcomitans*. In *Host–Parastie Interactions in Periodontal Diseases*. p. 261. Genco R.J. & Mergenhagen S.E. (eds). American Society for Microbiology, Washington, D.C.

Taubman M.A., Ebersole J.L. & Smith D.J. (1982) Association between systemic and local antibody and periodontal diseases. In *Host–Parasite Interactions in Periodontal Diseases*. p. 283. Genco R.J. & Mergenhagen S.E. (eds). American Society for Microbiology, Washington, D.C.

Tolo K. & Brandtzaeg P. (1982) Relation between periodontal disease activity and serum antibody titres to oral bacteria. In *Host–Parasite Interactions in Periodontal Diseases*. p. 270. Genco R.J. & Mergenhagen S.E. (eds). American Society for Microbiology, Washington, D.C.

Van Dyke T.E., Levine M.J. & Genco R.J. (1982) Periodontal diseases and neutrophil abnormalities. In *Host–Parasite Interactions in Periodontal Diseases*. p. 235. Genco R.J. & Mergenhagen S.E. (eds). American Society for Microbiology, Washington, D.C.

Wilton J.M.A. (1977) The function of complement in crevicular fluid. In *The Borderland between Caries and Periodontal Disease*. p. 223. Lehner T. (ed.). Academic Press, London.

Wilton J.M.A. (1982) Polymorphonuclear leukocytes of the human gingival crevice: clinical and experimental studies of cellular function in humans and animals. In *Host–Parasite Interactions in Periodontal Diseases*. p. 246. Genco R.J. & Mergenhagen S.E. (eds). American Society for Micro-biology, Washington, D.C.

14 Immunology of dental caries

Dental decay (caries) is the most common disease of mankind. It has reached epidemic proportions in modern times, since a fine consistency diet, rich in refined sugars has been consumed The prevalence of caries in developed countries is greater than 97% and has been increasing in developing countries, with the increase in popularity of highly refined sugar. The development of dental caries requires: (a) the presence of cariogenic bacteria that are capable of rapidly producing acid below the critical pH required for dissolving enamel, and (b) a sugar in the diet that favours colonization of these bacteria and that can be metabolized by the bacteria to form acid. This process can be interfered with by the presence of an effective immune response (figure 14.1).

There are a number of cariogenic organisms which can be defined by their ability to colonize teeth, to reduce the pH to about 4·1 in the presence of a suitable sugar substrate and to induce caries in germ-free animals. *Strep. mutans, Strep. sanguis, Lactobacillus acidophilus* and *Actinomyces viscosus* fulfil most of these

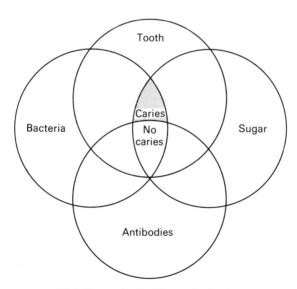

FIGURE 14.1. Four principal factors in the development of caries.

criteria. However, *Strep. mutans* appears to be the most efficient cariogenic organism as it induces caries rapidly in germ-free rodents.

Strep. mutans and caries

As most of the immunological studies in caries have been concerned with *Strep. mutans* these will be described in some detail. It should, nevertheless, be remembered that the other organisms may also contribute to the disease. *Strep. mutans* is a

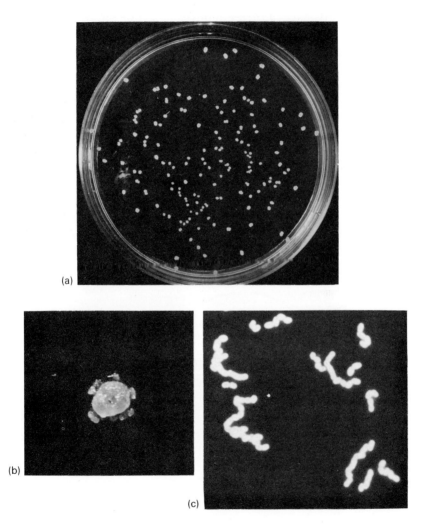

FIGURE 14.2. (a) Colonies of *Streptococcus mutans* grown on mitis salivarius agar. (b) Single colony surrounded by globules of dextran (×10). (c) Chains of streptococci stained by fluorescent antibody (×1100).

facultative anaerobic, non-haemolytic acidogenic organism, producing extracellular and intracellular polysaccharides (figure 14.2). The organism fulfils Koch's postulates as a cause of dental caries.

(1) *Strep. mutans* is found in the plaque of carious teeth and cannot usually be isolated in the absence of caries.

(2) The organism can be grown in pure culture.

(3) Infection of germ-free rats or normal hamsters with *Strep. mutans* has induced caries.

(4) The organism can then be recovered from the carious lesion and grown in pure culture.

(5) Antibodies to this organism are increased in patients with caries.

Strep. mutans has been separated into seven serotypes (a to g) by means of precipitating and immunofluorescence techniques. The serotype antigen appears to be a polysaccharide residing in the cell wall of the coccus and over 70% of *Strep. mutans* isolated from man appear to belong to serotype c; the next most common is serotype d.

The structure and antigenic composition of *Strep. mutans* are of considerable importance in our understanding of the immune responses to this organism. As any other Gram-positive coccus it consists of a cell wall and protoplast membrane which enclose the protoplast of the organism (figure 14.3) The matrix of the cell wall consists of a cross-linked

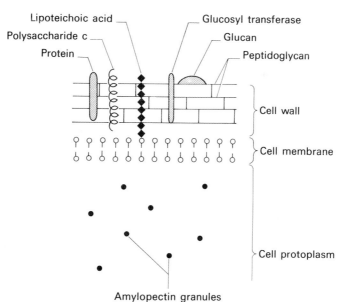

FIGURE 14.3. Cell wall constituents of *Strep. mutans*.

peptidoglycan which is composed of N-acetyl amino sugars, N-acetylmuramic acid and numerous peptides. The surface antigens of the cell wall are involved in the immunogenicity of the organism. A large number of antigens have been identified, of which the most important are proteins, including the enzyme glucosyl transferase which converts sucrose into dextran (polymer of glucose). Hence, in the presence of sucrose *Strep. mutans* is surrounded by a large bulk of dextran (figure 14.2). The other major protein antigens have been termed strepto-coccal antigens I, II, I/II and III (see below). The group specificity resides in the group carbohydrate (a to g) and these are polymers of glucose, rhamnose, galactose or galactosamine. Serotype c (e and f) contains only polymers of glucose and rhamnose, whereas serotype d has in addition galactose. Lipo-teichoic acid (LTA) is derived from the protoplast membrane but penetrates the cell wall to function as a surface component. LTA has a carbohydrate substituent which may endow LTA with some specificity. The other component of LTA is glycerol phosphate which produces a backbone common to Gram-positive bacteria and is probably responsible for most of the cross-reactions between LTA.

Proteins

The constitutive enzyme glucosyltransferase (GTF) converts sucrose into glucan (dextran), which may be responsible for adhesion of *Strep. mutans* to the tooth surface. Three protein antigens (I, II, III) have been identified on examination of culture supernatant and cell extracts of *Strep. mutans* (serotype c). Streptococcal antigens (SA) I and II appear to be two determinants present in a single molecule termed antigen I/II. Antigen I/II has a molecular weight of 185,000 and this is consistent with the sum of the molecular weights of antigens I (150,000) and antigen II (48,000), as determined by poly-acrylamide gel electrophoresis. Antigen III has a molecular weight of about 40,000. Immunization with GTF and the protein antigens I, II and I/II but not III protect against caries. It is of considerable interest that antigen I/II appears to have similar cross-reactivities between the different serotypes of *Strep. mutans* as those established for the group carbohydrates.

Polysaccharides

(1) *Extracellular dextran (glucan)* is synthesized in large amounts by the action of glucosyltransferase (dextransucrase).

348

Strep. mutans synthesizes predominantly an $\alpha(1-3)$ linked water insoluble dextran, termed mutan. Glucosyltransferase from *Strep. sanguis*, however, synthesizes predominantly the $\alpha(1-6)$ linked water soluble dextran. The differences in solubility of these two polysaccharides may reflect the greater efficiency of *Strep. mutans* in the formation of plaque and caries.

(2) *An extracellular levan (fructan)* is synthesized to a limited extent by *Strep. mutans* but larger quantities are produced by *Strep. salivarius* and *A. viscosus*. Although levan is found in plaque, it can be rapidly hydrolysed by plaque bacteria so that unlike dextran it is not efficient in plaque formation.

(3) *An intracellular amylopectin* is an iodine staining polysaccharide found in *Strep. mutans* and dental plaque. Amylopectin is synthesized when exogenous carbohydrate is available and forms an intracellular storage material. The intracellular amylopectin is metabolized to lactic acid when environmental carbohydrate becomes depleted and this may be responsible for the prolonged acid formation inside the plaque.

The most important source of acid is glucose which may enter plaque from a diet, but quantitatively the most important source of glucose is sucrose. Plaque bacteria and *Strep. mutans* contain invertase which hydrolyses sucrose to glucose and fructose. Glucose metabolism will depend on a cytochrome system and the supply of oxygen to the plaque streptococci. Since streptococci do not possess a cytochrome system but contain the Embden-Meyerhof glycolytic enzymes, glucose will be converted to lactic and other organic acids. The pH inside the plaque may fall within 2–3 minutes of rinsing the mouth with glucose or sucrose from a level of about 6.5 to 5; the critical pH below which decalcification of enamel occurs is thought to be about 5.5. Caries is the end result of a complex sequence of microbial and biochemical processes terminating in acid formation, which attacks the tooth enamel to cause caries.

Immunology of caries in man

SALIVARY ANTIBODIES

The role of non-specific salivary factors, such as the buffering capacity, lysozyme, lactoferrin and peroxidases, have been discussed earlier (p. 286). Although there may be some differences in these salivary components between subjects with high and low caries experience, a consistent and meaningful pattern has not been found. However, the concentration of secretory IgA in whole saliva is significantly less in subjects with high caries as compared with those having low caries experience. This evaluation may be dependent on the rate of secretion of saliva which is notoriously difficult to standardize and a greater proportion of the IgA may be contributed by submaxillary than parotid saliva.

Specific secretory IgA antibodies to *Strep. mutans* have been detected in saliva by the haemagglutination and agglutination assays. However, contrary to expectations from the IgA concentrations, a significant increase in salivary IgA antibodies to *Strep. mutans* was not found in subjects with low caries experience (figure 14.4). It appears that the salivary IgA antibodies increase with the number of past carious lesions, so that they may reflect the cumulative caries experience. Salivary IgA antibodies to *Strep. mutans* have been induced in man by swallowing daily capsules filled with 10^{10} organisms, but the duration of the antibody titre was limited, even on secondary immunization. This is consistent with the view that the secretory, unlike systemic immunity lacks an effective memory for antigens.

As salivary IgA antibodies may function by preventing bacterial adherence to enamel, it is possible that this mechanism is highly efficient in most subjects, as the exposed smooth surfaces of teeth seldom develop caries. However, the

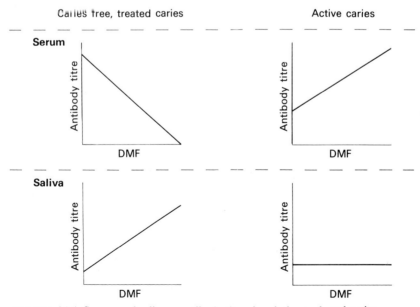

FIGURE 14.4. Serum and salivary antibody titres in relation to dental caries.

development of caries at the susceptible sites (fissures, approximal and cervical sites) may not be accessible to the salivary components and a protective relationship has not been found between the antibody titre and caries index.

MILK IgA

A further source of antibodies and cells in the mouth of the baby is breast milk. This contains secretory IgA, complement, PMN and macrophages which are capable of opsonization, phagocytosis and killing of micro-organisms. Indeed, epidemiological studies have shown that breast fed babies are less susceptible to infection than artificially fed babies. It might be significant that human milk contains antibodies to *Strep. mutans*, so that breast fed babies receive an additional supply of IgA antibodies, as well as phagocytic cells which may alter the pattern of microbial colonization of the mouth.

SERUM ANTIBODIES

Serum antibodies to cell, cell wall and the culture supernatant rich in glucosyltransferase (GTF) of *Strep. mutans* have been studied in adults and children. Using the haemagglutination test which assays predominantly IgM antibodies and complement fixation test which assays IgG antibodies, both classes of antibodies have been found in man. A significant negative correlation has been found (figure 14.4) between the titre and caries index in adults free of caries but some with treated caries (i.e. fillings). A reverse, namely positive correlation was found (figure 14.4) in subjects with the disease (caries) at the time of blood test, between the antibody titre and caries index. Sequential studies showed that the development of caries is associated with a modest but significant increase in serum IgG and IgM antibodies to *Strep. mutans*, as is the case with any infection. The somewhat small change in the antibody level may reflect the chronic nature of caries which may take many months to develop. It is therefore particularly significant that if the carious lesion is treated by removing it and filling the cavity, the serum antibody titre falls and salivary antibodies increase (figure 14.5). No relationship was found with *Strep. sanguis, Actinomyces viscosus* or *Lactobacillus casei*.

In children 2 to 5 years of age, in whom only the deciduous dentition has erupted, the concentration of IgA and IgG may not have reached adult values. The fluorescent antibody test was used with the cells of *Strep. mutans* to assay the IgG, IgM and IgA antibodies. Unlike the adult population, a significant

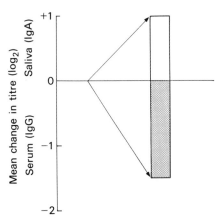

FIGURE 14.5. Fall in serum IgG antibody titre and rise in salivary IgA antibodies within 8 months of removing caries.

relationship between caries and the IgG or IgM antibodies to *Strep. mutans* was not found. However, the ratio of IgG to IgA showed a significant negative correlation so that the child with an immature immunological system and a shorter exposure to dental plaque and *Strep. mutans* than the adult, responds in a way comparable to that found in the rhesus monkey (p. 365). IgG antibodies may be protective, whereas IgA antibodies may interfere with the function of IgG antibodies, so that it is the proportion of the two classes of antibodies which seems to be a measure of protection against caries.

It is of interest to note that IgG antibodies to *Strep. mutans* are transferred from the mother to the infant, but due to the limited half-life of these passively transferred antibodies they are cleared from the infant 3 to 6 months after birth (figure 12.1). There is no information available, as to the antibody titre to *Strep. mutans* in the 6 to 24 months period which is probably a crucial period, not only in the development of the dentition, but also in the qualitative and quantitative development of dental bacterial plaque.

OPSONIZATION, PHAGOCYTOSIS AND KILLING

Serum antibodies are capable of opsonizing *Strep. mutans* and this appears to be particularly a function of the IgG class of antibodies. Polymorphonuclear leucocytes have specific receptors for the Fc part of IgG to enable the antibody bound *Strep. mutans* to adhere to the polymorphonuclear membrane. The complex is then internalized in vacuoles called phagosomes which may combine with the lysosomes of the leucocyte to form phago-lysosomes. The organism will then be killed by the action of the lysosomal enzymes. Complement is another opsonizing agent but it lacks immunological specificity. Both IgG and IgM antibodies may activate complement when combined with the antigen and generate C3b for which there are receptors on polymorphonuclear leucocytes. Opsonization, phagocytosis and killing by polymorphonuclear leucocytes or macrophages might be one of the essential protective functions against colonization by *Strep. mutans*.

CELLULAR IMMUNE RESPONSES

Strep. mutans can induce human lymphocytes both to proliferate and to release macrophage migration inhibition factor. These functions are good evidence for the presence of cell-mediated immunity to the most important cariogenic organism in man. Although the response of lymphocytes is rather modest, this can be boosted by the immunopotentiating effect of plaque accumulation (figure 14.6). Under these conditions a negative correlation was established between the caries index and stimulation index of lymphocytes (figure 14.7) and this is consistent with the findings between serum antibody and the caries index. Hence, the lower the caries index the higher are the lymphoproliferative responses and antibody titres. As the stimulated cells are T-lymphocytes, it is probable that they represent the T-cell helper population which is involved in helping B-cells to produce antibodies.

A minimum of four sets of cells and their products cooperate in the outcome of antigenic stimulation (figure 14.8). These are the antigen presenting cell (macrophage), T-helper, T-suppressor and B-cells, and the helper or suppressor activity appears to be associated with the HLA-DR locus.

Specific helper activity in boosting the number of antibody forming cells is induced by about 1 ng of streptococcal antigen from DRw6 lymphocytes, whereas higher doses induce suppressor activity (figure 14.9). The converse is found with DR4-typed lymphocytes, in that 1000 ng is required to induce helper function whereas 1 ng induces suppression. Under biological conditions 1 ng but not 1000 ng of antigen is a likely dose to reach the immune system. Hence, DRw6 subjects would be likely to respond with a helper and DR4 subjects with a suppressor function to a low dose of antigen.

A surprising feature in the studies of the maternal-fetal relationship was to find that if the mother's lymphocytes are sensitized to *Strep. mutans*, so are the lymphocytes of the newborn (figure 12.5). It is not clear as yet, how long these

353

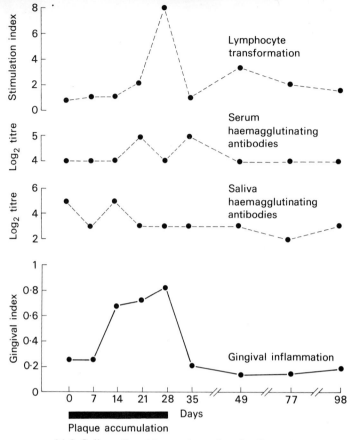

FIGURE 14.6. Cell-mediated immunity and antibodies to *Strep. mutans* during and after plaque accumulation.

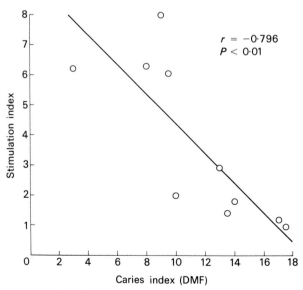

FIGURE 14.7. A negative correlation between the proliferative response of lymphocytes to *Strep. mutans* and the DMF index of caries.

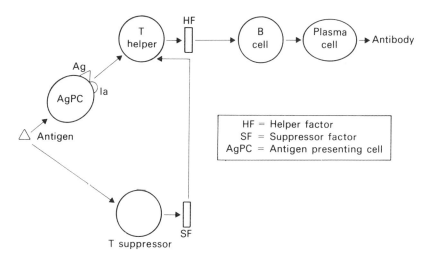

FIGURE 14.8. Regulation of the immune response to *Strept. mutans* antigen.

lymphocytes remain sensitized. If, as it might be assumed, sensitization has been acquired passively *in utero* by a soluble lymphocyte factor from the mother, then sensitization may be of short duration. Nevertheless, the effect of IgG antibodies and lymphocytes sensitized to *Strep. mutans* in the first months of life on the development of an active immune response in the child and colonization by *Strep. mutans* should be an exciting field for investigation.

APPARENT FAILURE OF NATURAL IMMUNITY IN
PROTECTION AGAINST DENTAL CARIES

As more than 99.9% of the populations of Western countries develop caries, any natural immunity seems to be hopelessly ineffective. Yet the data concerning humoral and cellular immunity to *Strep. mutans* would suggest that these may have a protective function. This apparent contradiction can be interpreted on the basis that *Strep. mutans* is a poor immunogen, particularly as it preferentially colonizes enamel surfaces. Sensitization to the organism might depend on the entry of a sufficient dose of antigenic material through the junctional epithelium of the gingiva to immunologically competent cells and the efficiency of this route of immunization is questionable. Indeed, natural immunization induces a low antibody titre which is relatively higher in IgM than IgG antibodies and these may not be directed against an essential antigen of *Strep. mutans*. The T-cell response to *Strep. mutans* also appears to be of a low order of magnitude and may need boosting for the sensitization to be detected.

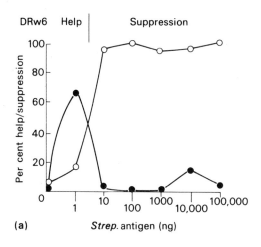

(a) *Strep.* antigen (ng)

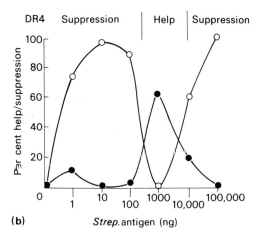

(b) *Strep.* antigen (ng)

FIGURE 14.9. Helper and suppressor activities of (a) HLA-DRw6, and (b) HLA-DR4, lymphocytes to streptococcal antigen.

It can be assumed that *Strep. mutans* in saliva is swallowed and although the organism does not colonize the gut mucosa, it may nevertheless, induce an immune response in the gut associated lymphoid tissue. Sensitized cells may then home to salivary gland to produce the IgA antibodies found in saliva. We have seen that the antibody titre in saliva increases with the caries index, so that salivary antibodies lack a protective relationship to caries but may be an indirect index of the frequency and possibly magnitude of colonization by *Strep. mutans*.

The ability of man to produce an effective immune response to *Strep. mutans* may depend on the Ia (immune associated)

356

gene. This might have developed only in the few individuals who are caries free. It appears, however, that man has the potential to mount the cellular and humoral immune responses to Strep. mutans but that under conditions of natural immunization these are usually inadequate.

Prevention of dental caries by immunization

As dental decay fulfils the criteria of an infectious disease, the possibility of preventing it by vaccination has been pursued recently. The rationale is that immunization with Strep. mutans should induce an immune response which might prevent the organism from colonizing the tooth surface and thereby prevent decay. The attractions of this approach are numerous. As a vaccine would be administered before the deciduous dentition has erupted—at about 6 months of age—it would prevent the disease in children who show the greatest incidence of caries. In spite of some recent distractions, the public is well disposed to vaccination and as individual parents would make the decision whether to have their child vaccinated, the principle of individual freedom would not be violated. The vaccine could be given at the same time as that against diphtheria and tetanus. Immunity could be boosted at intervals thereafter to provide life-long protection. The existing delivery system of immunization could be used, without any additional financial burden being incurred.

Rats and monkeys have been largely used in the immunization studies. The principal design in most of the experiments has been first to immunize the animals with cells of Strep. mutans and an adjuvant, as frequently as is necessary to attain high antibody levels, and to follow this by implanting the same organism in the mouth and placing the animals on a high sucrose diet. The corresponding control animals are maintained under identical conditions of diet and bacterial implantation, but they are sham-immunized, that is they are injected with saline instead of the vaccine. The teeth are then examined for the number of Strep. mutans colonized and for the number of carious lesions produced. Blood and saliva are assayed for antibody titres to Strep. mutans. Some of the experiments have been so designed as to aim for salivary immunity and others for systemic immunity.

357

These experiments were performed mostly in rats and monkeys.

(1) *Periglandular salivary immunization* was used in one experimental design in which repeated subcutaneous injections of killed *Strep. mutans* in Freund's complete adjuvant were administered adjacent to the salivary glands. This was followed by implantation of the same organism by swabbing the teeth with the live *Strep. mutans* and maintaining the rats on rat cakes containing about 54% of sucrose. The results of these experiments showed that the immunized rats had a lower mean caries score than the sham-immunized rats and that this was associated with salivary IgA class of antibodies. These antibodies, directed to a cell surface antigen, might interfere with adherence of *Strep. mutans* to the tooth. Alternatively, salivary antibodies may be directed against glucosyltransferase and by inhibiting the enzyme function less dextran is formed and therefore fewer bacteria adhere to the tooth surface. Whilst both these mechanisms may operate, the rats also developed serum antibodies, mostly of the IgG class, the titre of which was probably about five times greater than that in saliva. Serum antibodies may therefore have also been concerned in the protection against caries. Indeed, a similar immunization regime in monkeys elicited only serum antibodies

The possibility that antibodies to glucosyltransferase may interfere with adherence of *Strep. mutans*. has been further tested by immunization with preparations of glucosyltransferase, instead of whole cells of *Strep. mutans*. These experiments have confirmed that salivary antibodies are induced which inhibit glucosyltransferase enzyme activity and result in a lower mean caries score and sometimes a reduction in the number of *Strep. mutans* on the teeth of immunized animals. However, again the serum glucosyltransferase inhibiting antibodies were consistently higher than salivary antibodies.

(2) *Salivary gland immunization by combined periglandular injection and instillation of Strep. mutans into the parotid duct.* Combined immunization of irus monkeys by multiple periglandular injections, followed by retrograde ductal installation of *Strep. mutans* resulted in both salivary IgA and serum IgG and IgA antibodies. There was a reduction in the number of *Strep. mutans* on the teeth and although this could be ascribed to salivary antibodies, the serum antibody titres were much higher than those

in saliva. This regime also led to some functional impairment of the salivary gland.

(3) *Parenteral immunization.* Killed *Strep. mutans* was administered to germ-free rats in the drinking water for 45 days, before implantation of live *Strep. mutans*, and then throughout the experimental period. A significant reduction in caries was related to an increased level of salivary IgA antibodies to *Strep. mutans*, as the serum antibody titre was minimal. That IgA can be involved in the protection against caries has been established by passive transfer of secretory IgA antibodies in the milk of lactating rats to their litter. However, unlike IgG antibodies which are absorbed by the gastrointestinal tract of the offspring to enter the blood and are found in both serum and saliva, this has not been demonstrated for IgA antibodies. It must remain therefore an unresolved question whether passive transfer of IgA in the milk has a protective value by directly preventing

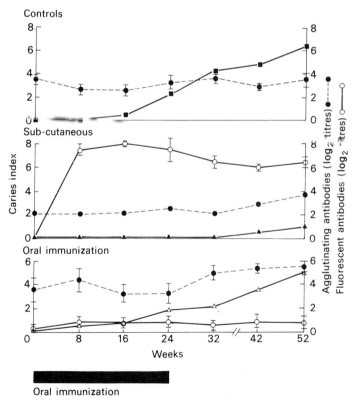

FIGURE 14.10. The effect of oral or subcutaneous immunization on the development of caries and on salivary IgA and serum IgG antibodies in rhesus monkeys.

adherence of *Strep. mutans* to the tooth or indirectly by being absorbed into the blood circulation and then affecting the tooth via crevicular fluid or saliva.

Oral immunization with *S. mutans* did not induce secretory IgA in monkeys. Daily addition of 10^{11} cells of *Strep. mutans* in capsules filled with 10^{11} organisms produced small increases in secretory IgA. Oral immunization failed to reduce caries significantly (figure 14.10), as compared with subcutaneous immunization. The rise in secretory antibodies produced was small and of short duration, even after secondary immunization. This was similar to an experiment in man in whom ingestion of *Strep. mutans* in gelatin capsules resulted in an increase in secretory IgA antibodies in saliva, although for a limited time only. Immunological memory in secretory IgA responses is rather limited and this may curtail the value of oral immunization.

(4) *Oral submucous immunization* has been introduced both in the irus and rhesus monkeys in order to induce a local immune response. Cells or cell walls were mixed with an adjuvant and injected under the mucosa into the buccal sulci of the four quadrants of the mouth. Although the serum antibody response was comparable to that elicited by subcutaneous immunization, the salivary antibody titres were only marginally higher. This method of immunization resulted in a significant reduction in caries which was similar to that found with subcutaneous immunization. As the immunological advantages of oral submucous immunization are questionable and this is an untried route which might lead to some discomfort and possibly complications it has not been pursued energetically.

EXPERIMENTAL DESIGN AIMED FOR
SYSTEMIC IMMUNE RESPONSES

Although some experiments in rats were designed to elicit systemic immunity, this approach has been pursued mostly in irus and rhesus monkeys. Initially intravenous injections of live *Strep. mutans* were used in irus monkeys, and later oral submucous injections of cell wall preparations. Recently the purified streptococcal protein antigens I/II, I and II have been administered subcutaneously.

The rhesus monkey model has been developed to induce caries and to immunize the monkeys in a way that would be acceptable in man. The significance and advantages of using this sub-human primate will be mentioned briefly. The teeth are similar to human teeth—in their number, morphology and eruption of deciduous and permanent teeth. The sequence of cusp formation and calcification in the first permanent molars is comparable to that in man. The pattern of approximal, cervical and fissure caries and the rate at which caries develops in the deciduous dentition is consistent with that found in man. The monkeys acquire *Strep. mutans* (serotype c) naturally, without resorting to artificial implantation of large numbers of the organism which might alter the bacteriological balance and act as a further route of immunization. The monkeys are fed entirely on a human type of diet. It contains about 15% of sucrose, and its consistency and content are similar to those used by man. Effective immunization can be induced by one subcutaneous injection. of killed *Strep. mutans* (plus an adjuvant), boosted, if necessary, 6 months later. So the site and frequency of injections are similar to those used in man. The immune responses also parallel those found in man, in the major serum antibody classes and in the T- and B-lymphocyte responses.

The experimental model was so designed as to assess the effect of immunization on caries development of the deciduous

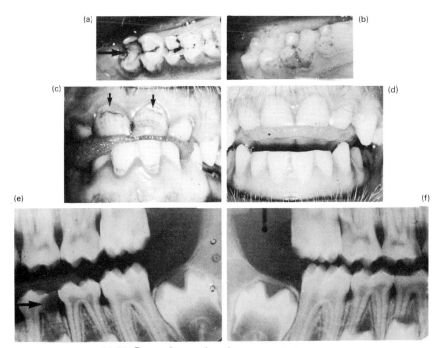

FIGURE 14.11. Protection against fissure, cervical and approximal caries in immunized (b, d, f), as compared with control (a, c, e), monkeys; arrows indicate caries.

dentition and first permanent molars within 6 to 12 months (figure 14.11). Immunization reduced approximal, cervical and fissure caries by 60% to 80%. The reduction in caries is associated with a reduction in the number of *Strep. mutans* in the plaque of the immunized monkeys.

The development of antibodies

A subcutaneous injection of killed cells of *Strep. mutans* in Freund's incomplete adjuvant elicits IgG, IgM and IgA classes of antibodies (figure 14.12). Sequential studies of these isotypes to *Strep. mutans* over a period of 3 years have shown that the IgG antibodies are well maintained at a high titre, IgM antibodies progressively fall and IgA antibodies increase slowly in titre. The antibody sequence of IgG–IgM–IgA is consistent with that found in secondary immunization and suggests that rhesus monkeys must have been exposed to *Strep. mutans* or some cross-reacting organism before active immunization started.

The development of serum IgG antibodies takes place within 2 months of immunization, reaching a titre of up to 1:1280,

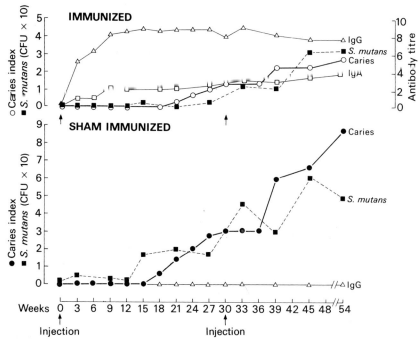

FIGURE 14.12. Sequential IgG and IgA antibody titres to *Strep. mutans* after a subcutaneous injection of killed *Strep. mutans* in Freund's incomplete adjuvant and boosted at about 6 months, without the adjuvant; sham-immunized monkeys were injected with saline. (CFU, colony forming units.)

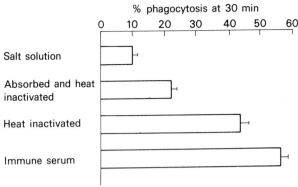

% phagocytosis at 30 min

FIGURE 14.13. Phagocytosis of *Strep. mutans* by polymorphonuclear leucocytes (PMNL). The effects of absorption of antibodies by *Strep. mutans* and of removal of complement by heat inactivation are shown. Control of Hank's balanced salt solution was used. Mean and standard error of the mean are given.

with no change in antibodies being found in the corresponding sham-immunized monkeys. The increase in salivary IgA antibodies is very modest and not significantly different between the immunized and sham-immunized monkeys. Most of the antibody assays utilized the classical complement fixation, haemagglutination, agglutination, precipitation and fluorescent tests. A functional opsonizing antibody assay for phagocytosis and killing of *Strep. mutans* by blood polymorphonuclear

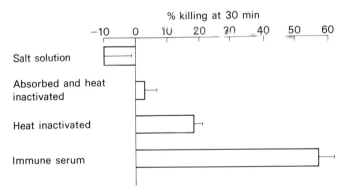

% killing at 30 min

FIGURE 14.14. Killing of *Strep. mutans* by PMNL. The effects of absorption of antibodies by *Strep. mutans* and of removal of complement by heat inactivation are shown. Control of Hank's balanced salt solution was used. Mean and standard error of the mean are given.

leucocytes has been used. A very sensitive radioimmunoassay has also been used to estimate *antibodies to the streptococcal antigen I/II*, not only in *serum* but also in *crevicular fluid*. These studies have established *in vitro* that *Strep. mutans* is opsonized by high dilution of antibodies and by complement which leads to ingestion and killing of the organisms (figures 14.13, 14.14).

Protection against caries was associated predominantly with increased serum IgG antibodies. This is consistent with the findings that IgG unlike IgA antibodies are involved in opsonization of *Strep. mutans*. Indeed, there is convincing evidence to suggest that IgA can interfere with the function of IgG by inhibiting IgG mediated bacterolysis, phagocytosis and chemotaxis of polymorphonuclear leucocytes. It must be therefore evident that under certain conditions, induction of IgG antibodies and high titres of IgA antibodies can be counterproductive as the IgA antibodies may interfere with the protective function of IgG and thus cancel any protective effect of immunization.

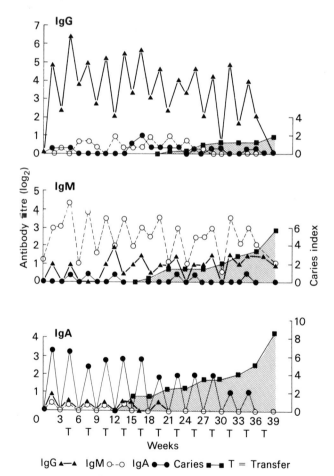

FIGURE 14.15. Prevention of the development of caries (shaded area) by passive transfer of IgG but not IgA or IgM fractions separated from serum of monkeys immunized with *Strep. mutans*.

364

The classical approach to demonstrate the protective effect of immunization is by passive transfer of antibodies from immunized donors to non-immune recipients. Indeed, this has been carried out in rhesus monkeys. Passive transfer of immune serum at 3-weekly intervals with IgG, IgM and IgA antibodies to *Strep. mutans* failed to induce protection against dental caries. However, when separated IgG, IgM and IgA sera were given, IgG induced significant protection but IgA or IgM antibodies to *Strep. mutans* did not (figure 14.15). It appears therefore that in active and passive immunization in monkeys, and in natural immunity in man, IgG antibodies are essential in immunity against dental caries.

Cell-mediated immunity

Skin delayed hypersensitivity *in vivo* and the lymphoproliferative and leucocyte migration inhibition reactions *in vitro* are induced by immunization with *Strep. mutans* (figures 14.16, 14.17). The skin induration is maximal at 24 to 48 hours after intradermal injection of the streptococcal antigen. Histological examination of the injected site is consistent with delayed hypersensitivity by the appearance of lymphocytes and macrophages, although there is an admixture of polymorphonuclear

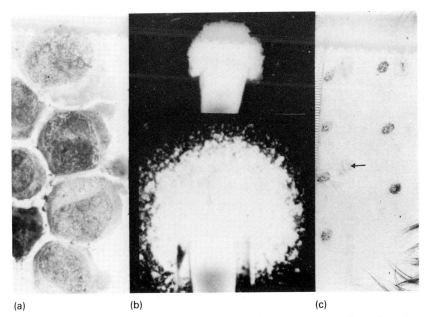

(a)   (b)   (c)

FIGURE 14.16. Cell-mediated immunity to *Strep. mutans*. Transformation of lymphocytes to blast cells (a), macrophage migration inhibition (b) and skin delayed hypersensitivity (c); arrowed reaction induced by *Strep. mutans*.

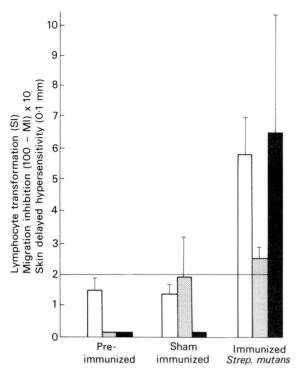

FIGURE 14.17. Skin delayed hypersensitivity (solid black columns), blast cell transformation of lymphocytes (blank columns) and leucocyte migration inhibition (shaded columns) induced by *Strep. mutans* in pre-immunized, sham-immunized (controls) and immunized monkeys. Mean and standard error of the mean, are given.

leucocytes. The increased DNA synthesis of lymphocytes from immunized monkeys stimulated with *Strep. mutans* is a T-cell dependent reaction, as shown by separating the cells on a nylon wool column. The type of cell involved in the leucocyte migration inhibition reaction has not been determined. Although it is probably T-cell dependent, B-cells are also capable of releasing lymphokines. Skin delayed hypersensitivity reaction and the lymphoproliferative response to *Strep. mutans* have been significantly correlated with IgG and IgA but not IgM antibody titres. This finding is consistent with the observation that IgG and IgA antibodies are T-cell dependent to a greater extent than IgM antibodies. The role of cell-mediated immunity has been further explored by the use of transfer factor. This showed that protection against dental caries can be elicited by passive transfer of whole immune serum and cellular immunity, but not by cellular immunity or immune serum alone. The results of active and passive immunization suggest that immuno-regula-

366

tion of T- and B-cell interactions plays an important part in the mechanism of protection against dental caries.

Direct assays of *T-cell helper* and *suppressor factors* after immunization of rhesus monkeys with cells or the streptococcal antigen I/II revealed that both factors are produced within 5 days of immunization. However, a significantly greater amount of *helper factor* was found in immunized than in control monkeys, so that T-cell helper activity is one of the essential objects of immunization, in order to elicit a prompt and effective antibody response from B cells. It is also of interest that the antigenic specificities of the T-cell helper factor and B-cell derived antibodies are similar and this argues in favour of *antigen receptors* on T- and B-cells sharing antigen specificities.

The results of systemic immunization (figure 14.18) suggest that a significant reduction in caries is associated with a reduction in the number of *Strep. mutans* and an increase in the IgG, IgM and IgA antibody titres, skin delayed hypersensitivity and DNA synthesis of lymphocytes. However, a significant change in the salivary IgA antibodies to *Strep. mutans* was not detected.

The passage of immunoglobulins from serum to crevicular fluid. Antibodies to streptococcal antigen I/II have now been detected directly in *gingival crevicular fluid*, and a significant correlation has been established between *serum* and *crevicular fluid antibodies* to antigen I/II. *IgG antibodies to antigen I/II* were found

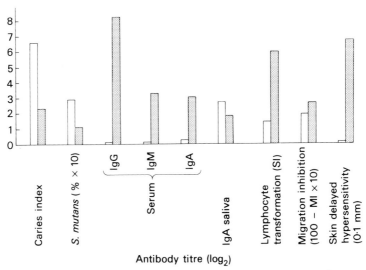

FIGURE 14.18. Antibodies and cell-mediated immune responses to *Strep. mutans* and the number of *Strep. mutans* in immunized (shaded columns) and control (blank columns) monkeys.

in both serum and crevicular fluid and were associated with protection against dental caries. These findings are consistent with the hypothesis that serum IgG antibodies pass from the circulation into gingival crevicular fluid, from where they enter the oral fluid, so that they may function in both the crevicular and salivary domains of the tooth.

Local gingival immune response. The possibility that the local gingival focus of plasma cells may contribute to the systemic antibodies passing into the gingival domain has to be considered. Although preliminary examination for antibody forming plasma cells to *Strep. mutans* in the gingiva has failed, this additional local source of antibodies cannot be excluded. It has been calculated that up to 20% of the IgG in gingival fluid of man and monkeys might be derived from local synthesis. Cell-mediated immune responses might also be generated locally; as macrophages, T- and B-lymphocytes and blast cells have been found in crevicular fluid.

IMMUNE MECHANISMS IN THE
PREVENTION OF CARIES

The experiments in rats and monkeys suggest two principal immune mechanisms of protection against caries. One involves saliva and acts on the salivary domain and the other involves gingival crevicular fluid which affects the gingival domain (figure 14.19). The salivary glands produce secretory IgA antibodies either by direct immunization of the salivary glands or more likely by immunization of the gut associated lymphoid tissue, from where sensitized B-cells may home to the salivary glands (figure 14.19). The salivary IgA antibodies have, of course, direct access to the tooth surface. They may prevent *Strep. mutans* from adhering to the enamel surface or they may prevent formation of dextran by inhibiting the activity of glucosyltransferase.

The gingival crevicular mechanism involves all the humoral and cellular components of the systemic immune system which may exert its functions at the tooth surface. There is now sufficient evidence to postulate what may happen after subcutaneous immunization with *Strep. mutans*. The organism is phagocytosed and probably undergoes antigenic processing by macrophages. In the central lymphoid tissue T- and B-lymphocytes are sensitized with formation of T-helper and suppressor cells and factors. These may play an essential part in modulating the formation of IgG, IgA and IgM classes of

368

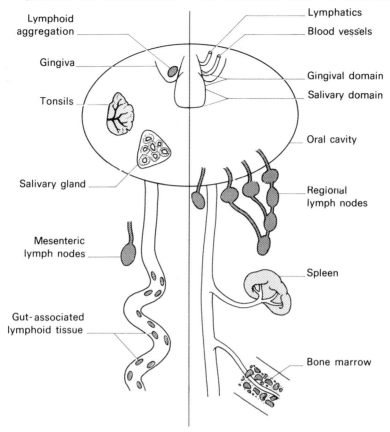

ORAL AND GUT IMMUNIZATION   LYMPHATIC AND VASCULAR IMMUNIZATION

Lymphoid aggregation

Gingiva

Tonsils

Salivary gland

Mesenteric lymph nodes

Gut-associated lymphoid tissue

Lymphatics

Blood vessels

Gingival domain

Salivary domain

Oral cavity

Regional lymph nodes

Spleen

Bone marrow

FIGURE 14.19. The mechanisms involved in oral as compared with systemic (subcutaneous) immunization.

antibodies by B-lymphocytes. Soluble mediators may be induced by antigenic stimulation of sensitized lymphocytes and these may be functioning particularly at the periphery. Transport of antibodies, complement, sensitized lymphocytes, PMNL and macrophages occurs via the blood supply to the gingiva and then through the junctional epithelium into crevicular fluid. Chemotactic factors for PMNL and monocytes can be generated by plaque antigens, lipopolysaccharides, and immune complexes and these will activate the classical or alternative complement pathways to generate C3a and C5a which are chemotactic for phagocytes. PMNL and macrophages may be immobilized at this site by antigenic stimulation of sensitized lymphocytes which may release macrophage and leucocyte inhibitory factors. IgG antibodies and complement play an essential part in opsonization; IgA is not effective and may indeed interfere with opsonization by IgG antibodies. Opsonization leads to binding, phagocytosis and killing by phagocytes and this could be the principal immune mechanism against *Strep. mutans*. Inhibition of adherence by IgA or IgG antibodies in the gingival domain needs to be examined. Local T- and B-lymphocyte responses to antigen may supplement the immune responses elicited centrally and increase the effective antibody titre and the number of phagocytes adjacent to the site of bacterial colonization.

It should not be particularly surprising that two different immune mechanisms may be involved in protection against caries. We know this to be true of other vaccines. The most recent example is poliomyelitis, in which both subcutaneous and local immunization by mouth are effective, yet different immune mechanisms seem to operate. It is, of course, possible that both systemic and local immunity might be necessary in the protection against caries and we have now the immunological and bacteriological knowledge to test these concepts.

SAFETY ASPECTS

There is some evidence that hyperimmunized rabbits with whole cells of *Strep. mutans*, injected intra-venously or subcutaneously in Freund's incomplete adjuvant may induce *antibodies to heart muscle*. A comprehensive series of safety tests will therefore have to be carried out before immunization trials can be started in man. However, experience with rhesus monkeys for over 10 years has not revealed any systemic side-effects or lesions at the site of injection if Aluminium hydroxide or Freund's incomplete adjuvant was used as adjuvant. Haematological indices were unchanged and no abnormalities were found in the heart, lungs, kidneys, liver or brain on post-mortem examination. Examination of serum for *cross-reactive antibodies to heart muscle* by immunofluorescence and radio-immunoassay were negative. Anti-IgG antibodies were also not detected. It seems then that the findings in hyperimmunized rabbits may not be applicable to conventional immunization in the sub-human primate or indeed in man.

Summary

Dental caries is a disease caused by bacteria utilizing sugar in the diet for the production of acid. *Strep. mutans* is by far the most efficient cariogenic organism in germ-free rats and it is correlated with the presence of caries in man. Hence, most of our immunological knowledge about caries concerns *Strep. mutans*. In man, serum IgG, IgA and IgM antibodies, as well as cell-mediated immunity to *Strep. mutans* can be correlated with the DMF index of caries. Salivary IgA antibodies are also found. Although man has the potential to mount humoral and cellular immune responses to *Strep. mutans* under natural conditions, the immunity achieved is largely ineffective. This might be associated with the HLA-DR locus as some DRw6 lymphocytes generate helper factor with 1 ng of streptococcal antigen and these subjects are caries resistant. Most other subjects require 1000 ng of the antigen to release a corresponding amount of helper factor and since it is unlikely that such a large dose will reach the immune system, most of these subjects are caries prone.

In the last decade immunization experiments with *Strep. mutans* have been successfully carried out in rats and monkeys, with a significant reduction in caries. There are two principal immunological mechanisms of protection against caries. One involves salivary IgA antibodies which are probably induced by immunization of the gut associated lymphoid tissue, from where sensitized B-cells may home to salivary glands. Salivary antibodies may prevent *Strep. mutans* from adhering to the tooth surface and thereby prevent caries. The alternative mechanism involves all the humoral and cellular components elicited

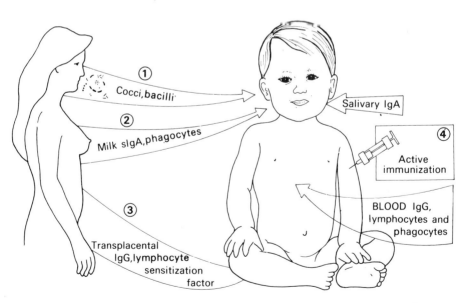

FIGURE 14.20. Four preventive immuno-microbiological measures from gestation to childhood.

371

by systemic immunization. Antibodies, complement, poly-morphonuclear leucocytes, lymphocytes and macrophages pass from the gingival blood vessels to the gingival domain of the tooth. Bacterial colonization of the tooth can therefore be influenced by systemic immunity and an important mechanism is probably that of IgG-induced opsonization, binding, phago-cytosis and killing of *Strep. mutans* by phagocytes.

From these basic principles we can see that there are at least four possible immuno-microbiological means of changing the pattern of oral colonization during the pre- and post-natal period (figure 14.20).

(1)   Passive transfer of maternal immune responses through the appropriate control of the mother's dental condition during pregnancy.

(2)   Encouragement of breast feeding to determine if natural oral immunization during pregnancy might affect the immune responses in the milk.

(3)   Environmental control of potential dental pathogens, especially in the mouth of the mother and nursing staff.

(4)   Active immunization with *Strept. mutans* may prevent colonization of the teeth by this organism.

Further reading

Arnold R.R., Mestecky J. & McGhee J.R. (1976) Naturally occurring secretory immunoglobulin A antibodies to *Streptococcus mutans* in human colostrum and saliva. *Infect, Immunol.*, **14**, 355.

Dowen W.H., Cohen B., Cole M.F. & Colman G. (1975) Immunisation against dental caries. *Brit. dent. J.*, **139**, 45.

Bratthall D. (1970) Demonstration of five serological groups of streptococcal strains resembling *Streptococcus mutans*. *Odont. Revy*, **21**, 143.

Challacombe S.J. & Lehner T. (1980) Salivary antibody responses in rhesus monkeys immunized with *Streptococcus mutans* by the oral, submucosal or subcutaneous routes. *Archs. Oral. Biol.*, **24**, 917.

Challacombe S.J. & Lehner T. (1976) Serum and salivary antibodies to cariogenic bacteria in man. *J. Dent. Res.*, **55**, C139.

Fitzgerald R.L. & Keyes P.H. (1960) Demonstration of the etiological role of Streptococci in experimental caries in the hamster. *J. Am. dent. Ass.*, **61**, 9.

Evans R.T., Emmings F.G. & Genco R.J. (1975) Prevention of *Streptococcus mutans* infection of tooth surfaces by salivary antibody in irus monkeys (*Macaca fascicularis*). *Infect. Immun.*, **12**, 302.

Gibbons R.J. & van Houte J. (1975) Dental caries. *Ann. rev. Med.*, **26**, 121.

Guggenheim B. & Newbrun E. (1969) Extracellular glucosyltransferase activity of an HS strain of *Streptococcus mutans*. *Helv. odont. Acta*, **13**, 84.

Hamada S. & Slade H.D. (1980) Biology, immunology, and cariogenicity of *Streptococcus mutans*. *Microbiological Reviews*, **11**, 331.

Ivanyi L. & Lehner T. (1978) The relationship between caries index and stimulation of lymphocytes by *Streptococcus mutans* in mothers and their neonates. *Archs. oral Biol.*, **23**, 851.

Krasse B. (1977) Microbiology of the gingival plaque. In *The Borderland between Caries and Periodontal Disease*. p. 5. Lehner T. (ed.). Academic Press, London.

Lamb J.R., Kontiainen S. & Lehner T. (1980) A comparative investigation of the generation of specific T cell helper function induced by *Streptococcus mutans* in monkeys and mice. *J. Immunol.*, **124**, 2384.

Lamb J.R., Kontiainen S. & Lehner T. (1979) The generation of specific T cell suppressor function induced by *Streptococcus mutans* in monkeys and mice. *Infect. Immunol.*, **26**, 903.

Lehner T. (1980) Future possibilities for the prevention of caries and periodontal disease. *Brit. dent. J.*, **149**, 318.

Lehner T., Challacombe S.J. & Caldwell J. (1975) Immunological and bacteriological basis for vaccination against dental caries in rhesus monkeys. *Nature*, **254**, 517.

Lehner T., Challacombe S.J., Wilton J.M.A. & Caldwell J. (1976) Cellular and humoral immune responses in vaccination against dental caries. *Nature*, **264**, 69.

Lehner T., Lamb J.R., Welsh K.I. & Batchelor J.R. (1982) Association between HLA–DR antigens and helper cell activity in the control of dental caries. *Nature*, **292**, 770.

Lehner T., Russell M.W. & Caldwell J. (1980) Immunisation with a purified protein from *Streptococcus mutans* against dental caries in rhesus monkeys. *Lancet*, **i**, 995.

Lehner T., Russell M.W., Challacombe S.J., Scully C.M. & Hawkes J.E. (1978) Passive immunisation with serum and immunoglobulins against dental caries in rhesus monkeys. *Lancet*, **i,** 693.

Mestecky J., McGhee J.R., Arnold R.R., Michalek S.M., Prince S.J. & Babb J.L. (1978) Selective induction of an immune response in human external secretions by ingestion of bacterial antigen. *J. Clin. Invest.*, **61**, 731.

Michalek S.M. & McGhee J.R. (1977) Effective immunity to dental caries: Passive transfer to rats of antibodies to *Streptococcus mutans* elicits protection. *Infect. Immun.*, **17**, 644.

Michalek S.M., McGhee J.R.., Mestecky J., Arnold R.R. & Bozzo L. (1976) Ingestion of *Streptococcus mutans* induces secretory immunoglobulin A and caries immunity. *Science*, **192**, 1238.

Orland F.J., Blayney J.R., Harrison R.W., Reiymers J.A., Trister P.C., Ervin R.F., Gordon H.A. & Wagner M. (1955) Experimental caries in germ free rats incubated with enterococci. *J. Am. Dent. Ass.*, **50**, 259.

Russell M.W., Bergmeier L.A., Zanders E.D. & Lehner T. (1980) Protein antigens of *Streptococcus mutans* purification and properties of a double antigen and its protease-resistant component. *Infect. Immunol.*, **28**, 486.

Russell M.W. & Lehner T. (1978) Characterisation of antigens extracted from cells and culture fluids of *Streptococcus mutans* serotype c. *Arch. Oral Biol.*, **23**, 7.

Scully C.M. & Lehner T. (1979) Bacterial and strain specificities in opsonisation, phagocytosis and killing of *Streptococcus mutans*. *Clin. exp. Immunol.*, **35**, 128.

Smith D.J., Taubman M.A. & Ebersole J.C. (1980) Local and systemic antibody response to oral administration of glucosyltransferase antigen complex. *Infect. Immunol.*, **28**, 441.

Taubman M.A. & Smith D.J. (1974) Effects of local immunisation with *Streptococcus mutans* on induction of salivary immunoglobulin A antibody and experimental dental caries in rats. *Infect. Immun.*, **9**, 1079.

Taubman M.A. & Smith D J. (1977) Effects of local immunization with glucosyltransferase fractions from *Streptococcus mutans* on dental caries in rats and hamsters. *J. Immunol.*, **118**, 710.

Williams R.C. & Gibbons R.J. (1972) Inhibition of bacterial adherence by secretory immunoglobulin A: A mechanism of antigen disposal. *Science*, **177**, 697.

Wilton J.M.A., Renggli H.H. & Lehner T. (1977) A functional comparison of blood and gingival inflammatory polymorphonuclear leucocytes in man. *Clin. exp. Immunol.*, **27**, 152.

15

Immunology of oral infections

There are two common oral infections caused by known organisms: (a) *Herpes simplex* virus infection and (b) Candidiasis caused by the fungus *Candida*.

Herpes virus infections

Clinical or subclinical primary infection by *Herpes simplex* virus type I is commonly acquired in early childhood, in the second and third years of life. Primary herpetic infection in the first year is very rare, possibly because most mothers have neutralizing antibodies to the virus which are transferred through the placenta to the fetus. Placental transfer of cellular immunity may also take place in a small proportion of fetuses. Serum virus complement fixing and neutralizing antibodies are found in about 50% of children at 5 years of age.

PRIMARY HERPETIC GINGIVO-STOMATITIS

Primary herpetic infection is usually seen in the mouths of young children and less frequently in adults. The disease is recognized by an acute onset of sore mouth and often throat, fever, diffuse inflammation of the gum, followed by formation of vesicles and ulcers of the oral mucosa, and regional lymphadenitis. Infants display considerable fretfulness, sleeplessness and refusal to eat. Initially there are crops of small ulcers but these coalesce to produce large, shallow, irregular ulcers with surrounding inflammation. The natural course of this infection is 7 to 14 days and healing of ulcers occurs spontaneously.

Herpetic keratitis is not often associated with herpetic stomatitis, and encephalitis is extremely rare but may occasionally complicate the stomatitis. Herpetic infection of the nail-bed is sometimes seen in dentists who have treated patients with herpes labialis. Recurrences of herpetic lesions in the mouth are very rare. Extraoral recurrent herpetic infection, however, commonly affects the lips.

Herpes simplex virus (HSV) is a DNA virus which first gains entrance into epithelial cells of the oral mucosa. Virus replication takes place inside the nucleus and this is associated with formation of intranuclear inclusion bodies and giant cells. As more epithelial cells become infected, degenerative and oedematous changes give rise to vesicular formation, and these rupture early resulting in ulcers. The incubation period for primary herpetic infection is between 2 and 7 days.

Within the first week of onset of clinical manifestations (therefore within 2 weeks of viral infection) sensitized lymphocytes to HSV can be detected in the peripheral blood (figure 15.1); at this time significant antibodies or macrophage migration inhibition factor (MIF) is not found. However, after 2 weeks significant antibody titres and MIF appear, whilst the stimulation index of lymphocytes falls. Recovery from infection coincides therefore with the appearance of antibody and of MIF. Infection with HSV in animals is also associated with an early development of delayed skin hypersensitivity or the lymphoproliferative response, to be followed by that of antibody and MIF formation. In animals antibody alone was not protective against dissemination of HSV and macrophages

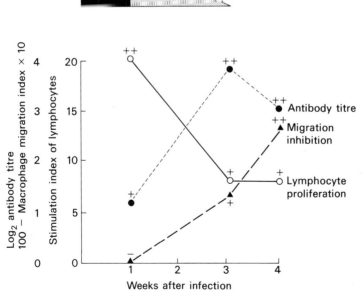

FIGURE 15.1. Immune responses in primary *Herpes simplex* virus infection.

were required. MIF may immobilize macrophages to the site of the infection and it may also enhance their viricidal activity.

Seropositive subjects give delayed hypersensitivity reactions to HSV and *in vitro* sensitized lymphocytes from these subjects will undergo blast cell transformation (figure 15.2) and produce the following lymphokines: macrophage migration inhibition factor, lymphotoxin, chemotactic factor and interferon. In addition the lymphocytes are cytotoxic for HSV infected target cells. There are a number of cytotoxic mechanisms and their action may depend upon the surface markers of both effector and target cells (figure 15.3). It is a remarkable feature of HSV that within less than 6 hours of infection the infected cell surface acquires two surface markers; a virus-specific glycoprotein antigen and Fc receptor for IgG. Antibodies may combine with the surface antigen and cell lysis is caused by complement activation. Antibody dependent cellular cytotoxicity is a particularly sensitive killing mechanism and both the virus-specific surface antigen and the Fc receptor of the infected cell might be involved. The Fc receptor of the killer cell may combine with the Fc portion of IgG antibody and the Fab portion with the HSV antigen on the cell surface. Alternatively

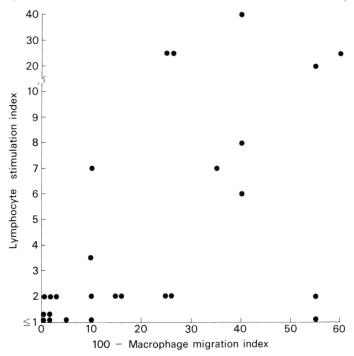

FIGURE 15.2. Correlation between lymphocyte transformation and macrophage migration inhibition with *Herpes simplex* virus type I in normal adults.

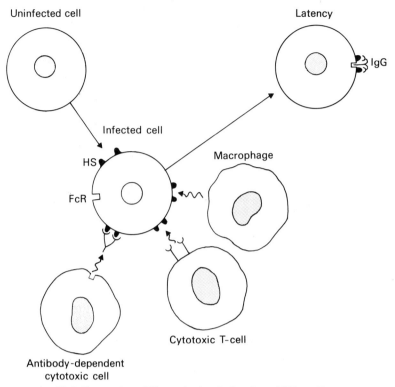

Uninfected cell

Latency

IgG

Infected cell

HS

FcR

Macrophage

Cytotoxic T-cell

Antibody-dependent
cytotoxic cell

FIGURE 15.3. Expression of *Herpes simplex* viral antigen (HS) and Fc receptors (FcR) on the surface of an infected cell and their possible role in killing and latency. The macrophage effect is non-specific.

immune complexes of HSV and IgG antibodies could bind to the Fc receptors of both the target and effector cells and result in killing of the target cell.

LATENCY OF HSV

It is now clearly recognized in man that HSV often remains latent after the primary infection, for years and probably throughout life. The propensity of HSV to gain entrance into the nucleus of a cell where it may remain dormant in a non-replicating phase has been the subject of great interest. Although oral epithelial cells and salivary glands have been considered as the reservoirs for latency of HSV, there is now convincing evidence both in man and in animals that the trigeminal ganglion is the principal reservoir for HSV. The virus can be grown from trigeminal ganglia in man. HSV can also be recovered from the trigeminal ganglia in 65% of mice which had the virus inoculated into the lips or cornea. Both clinical and subclinical infection in animals can result in latency.

The mode of entry of HSV to the trigeminal ganglion is not clear, but it appears that during primary infection of the oral mucosa the virus may be sequestrated to the neurons as a result of neurotropism of the virus, or the inaccessibility of mononuclear killer cells to the nerves. HSV may enter the demyelinated nerve endings and undergo centripetal axonal migration to the nerve cells in the trigeminal ganglion (figure 15.4). The mechanism of latency is unknown and it has been suggested that as the neuron is a non-replicating cell it may lack the specific transcriptase capable of producing the virus, so that both the virus and host cell are maintained. Considerable progress has been made recently by the elegant demonstration that IgG antibodies to HSV are necessary for latency. The hypothesis has been suggested that the Fab sites of antibody will bind to the HSV surface antigens and the Fc site to the Fc receptor, as a result of conformational changes in the antibody molecule (figure 15.3). Double binding of Fc receptor and HSV antigen by the antibody may suppress the viral genome, but the cell is not damaged because the Fc site is not available for complement or 'K cell' binding. This hypothesis accounts for the necessity of IgG antibodies for the manifestation of latency and confers a biological significance on the induction of Fc receptor to the infected cell. Recently this hypothesis has been supported by the finding that when HSV-induced Fc receptor on the cell surface is engaged with IgG or its Fc fragment, viral replication is significantly inhibited.

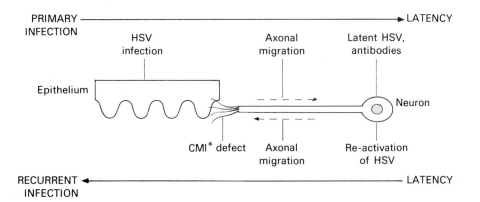

* Cell-mediated immunity

FIGURE 15.4. Primary infection, latency and recurrent infection by *Herpes simplex* virus (HSV).

This very common condition is limited to the vermillion border of the lips and adjacent skin, and it is often referred to as a 'cold sore'. A single vesicle or a crop of vesicles may develop a day after the prodromal phase of a tingling or burning sensation. The duration of the lesion varies usually between 3 and 10 days and the lesion recurs at various intervals for many years. A number of activating factors will precipitate recurrent HSV infection and among the most common are sunlight, cold, fever, stress, trauma, menstruation and section of the sensory root of the trigeminal ganglion. It is not clear whether there is a common mechanism for the various activating factors, but one possibility is that some alteration in the surface charge of neurons may induce weakening of the IgG bond to the Fc and/or Fab binding sites, or may cause shedding of the Fc receptors and/or membrane antigens. Removal of the double binding may induce derepression of HSV which may then undergo replication. The virus will then migrate centrifugally along the axon and will be shed at the nerve endings (figure 15.4). There is now ample evidence for axonal transport of proteins and organelles; there is a slow and a fast axonal flow rate and the latter, which may be greater than 40 mm per day, might account for recurrent HSV infection 2 days after section of the sensory root of the trigeminal ganglion. Once the virus is shed at the nerve endings a lesion may not appear if the cellular immunity is intact and the virus will be shed into the mouth, as is found in 2% of the normal population. However, in the presence of a selected cell-mediated immunodeficiency the virus will replicate at the epithelial site of shedding and produce a recurrent lesion. The constant site for recurrences might be due to the involvement only of some neurones which innervate a restricted peripheral epithelial area.

A number of cellular defects have been recorded in patients with recurrent *Herpes labialis*. A deficiency of MIF production and decreased cytotoxicity by sensitized lymphocytes (probably T-lymphocytes) to unrelated target cells may play a part in recurrent infection. T-lymphocytes produce interferon and decreased interferon production has been correlated with an increased frequency of recurrent HSV infections. Recently, careful sequential studies of recurrent HSV infection have shown a cyclical pattern of proliferation of lymphocytes and the release of MIF (figure 15.5). Recurrent HSV infection appears to coincide with a minimal lymphoproliferative response and MIF formation. Although lymphocyte stimulation is low it is

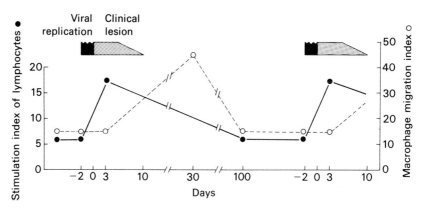

FIGURE 15.5. Cellular immune responses in recurrent *Herpes simplex* virus infections.

still moderately positive and increases rapidly within about 7 days. In contrast the MIF reaction is weak or negative and takes more than 14 days to be converted into a functional response. Recurrent HSV infection appears therefore to be related to a defect in lymphocyte function which consists of sluggish formation of MIF. A rapid influx of macrophages and killer cells might be necessary to prevent the HSV to replicate and produce a recurrent lesion. These responses are functions of T-lymphocytes and antibodies are intact, with perhaps slight variation in titre during recurrent infections. Recurrent HSV infection is envisaged to occur in two stages: (a) HSV in the trigeminal ganglion is released from its latent stage, permitting virus replication, axonal migration and shedding from the nerve endings near the epithelium, and (b) a selective deficiency in cell-mediated immunity will permit the virus to proliferate and cause a local lesion. The significance of cellular immunity is highlighted by the intractable HSV infections found in cell-mediated immunodeficiency states and in patients receiving immunosuppressive therapy.

Laboratory diagnosis

The clinical diagnosis of primary herpes virus infection can be confirmed in the laboratory by showing a rise in *complement fixing* or *neutralizing antibody* titres of at least three dilution steps. This requires two or more specimens of blood collected at or near the onset of the clinical manifestations and during the convalescent period. *Intra-nuclear inclusion bodies* can often be demonstrated on direct cytological examination of the epithelial cells. However, *virological culture* is the definitive method in confirming the diagnosis.

The diagnosis of recurrent *Herpes labialis* is usually clinically straightforward, though the above laboratory aids can also be used. However, a rise in the level of antibodies is variable and sometimes not observed.

Candidiasis

Candida is a commensal organism of the gastrointestinal tract in man. The oral carrier rate in a normal population varies between 20% and 40%. The genus *Candida* contains a number of species which are associated with disease in man. *Candida albicans* is the principal organism associated with infection but other species such as *C.parapsilosis* and *C.kruseii* are also pathogenic for man. *C.albicans* is a dimorphic fungus with two growth phases, the yeast form and the hyphal form (figure 15.6).

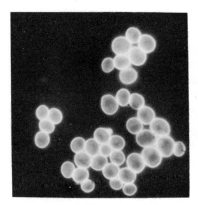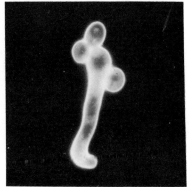

FIGURE 15.6. Yeast cells (left) and a hypha of *Candida albicans* (right) shown by the fluorescent antibody test.

ORAL CANDIDIASIS

There are four varieties of oral candidiasis and these are superficial infections, usually caused by *C.albicans*.

Acute pseudomembraneous candidiasis

This disease, commonly referred to as 'thrush' is seen in infants as well as in debilitated adults, particularly in diabetes and malignant diseases, especially leukaemia and lymphoma. Iatrogenic agents are also important predisposing factors; antibiotics, corticosteroids and immunosuppressive drugs seem to enhance candida infection. Local antibiotic and corticosteroid treatment can enhance oral candidiasis. Clinical

382

manifestations of thrush are usually symptomless white papules or cotton-wool like exudates which can be rubbed off leaving an erythematous mucosa.

Acute atrophic candidiasis

This may follow acute pseudomembraneous candidiasis and is usually associated with broad spectrum antibiotic therapy; hence, referred to as 'antibiotic-sore tongue'. It is the only type of oral candidiasis that is consistently painful, showing a smooth erythematous tongue, with angular cheilitis and, less often, inflamed lips and cheeks.

Chronic atrophic candidiasis

This type of *Candida* infection is better known as 'denture stomatitis' for it presents as a diffuse erythema of the palate, limited to the denture-bearing mucosa. The denture covering the palatal mucosa predisposes to proliferation of *Candida*. The lesion is usually symptomless but is often associated with angular cheilitis.

Chronic oral hyperplastic candidiasis

This is a less common type of candidiasis which presents as a firm white patch which cannot be rubbed off and commonly affects the tongue, cheeks and lips. The lesion may persist for years, it is resistant to antimycotic treatment and has been referred to as 'candidal leukoplakia'.

CHRONIC MUCO-CUTANEOUS CANDIDIASIS

Although this disease is much less common, it has attracted a great deal of attention because of its intractable nature and the association with a variety of immunodeficiencies. The disease is characterized by persistent, superficial candida infection of the mouth, nails and skin, sometimes producing granulomatous masses over the face and scalp. It can be associated with endocrine disorders, especially Addison's disease and hypo-parathyroidism.

DISSEMINATED CANDIDIASIS

In contrast to superficial candidiasis affecting the mucous membranes and skin. *Candida* can occasionally spread to internal organs (kidney, heart, liver, brain). This occurs usually under the influence of iatrogenic agents, in patients suffering from other debilitating diseases.

Laboratory diagnosis

A culture from the lesion usually yields *C.albicans,* and direct examination of scrapings shows *Gram-positive hyphae* and *yeast cells* of *Candida.* Biopsy of the lesion in chronic oral hyperplastic candidiasis and chronic muco-cutaneous candidiasis is helpful, as in addition to the superficial invasion of epithelium by *Candida* hyphae, there is parakeratosis and usually extensive epithelial hyperplasia. The lamina propria and dermis show an intense mononuclear cell infiltration with a large proportion of plasma cells. Serological tests can also be helpful when there is a rise in antibody titre.

IMMUNOLOGICAL FEATURES OF CANDIDIASIS

Serum antibodies

Agglutinating, precipitating, complement fixing and fluorescent antibodies have been used in investigating candidiasis. It should, however, be appreciated that most, if not all, normal subjects have been exposed to *Candida.* Indeed, about 60% of a clinically uninfected population shows agglutinating antibodies to *Candida* Precipitating antibodies are found less commonly in normal subjects and are therefore of greater diagnostic value in disease.

A differential serum fluorescent antibody titre is found between patients with candidiasis and controls; an IgG antibody titre greater than 1 : 16 appears to be significant. A parallel study of fluorescent, agglutinating and precipitating antibodies to *C. albicans* revealed that precipitating antibodies belong to the IgG class, whereas agglutinating antibodies reside in the IgG, IgM and IgA classes. The three antibody tests and the three classes of antibodies were found in muco-cutaneous candidiasis, as well as in candida endocarditis. Immuno-absorption studies suggest that the three serological tests estimate antibodies to mannan and not to the protein determinants of *C.albicans.*

Secretory IgA antibodies

These are found in saliva in increased titres in patients with oral

384

candidiasis, but not in some patients with chronic muco-cutaneous candidiasis. The relationship between salivary IgA and serum IgG, IgM and IgA antibodies to *C.albicans* runs in parallel in the control, carrier and oral candidiasis group of subjects and this suggests that antigenic stimulation initiated in the mouth and probably in the alimentary canal induced both local secretory and systemic antibody response. This relationship, however, breaks down in patients with chronic muco-cutaneous candidiasis.

Opsonization, phagocytosis and killing of Candida

Antibody and complement are necessary for optimal phagocytosis of *Candida* by polymorphonuclear leucocytes (PMNL) or macrophages. Both opsonizing agents are found in normal serum which can induce phagocytosis and killing of live *Candida* blastospores. The hyphal forms, however, can escape phagocytosis, particularly if they are large in size.

Immune complexes of *Candida* and antibodies activate the classical complement pathway, but whole *C.albicans* or soluble extracts of the blastospores activate the alternative pathway of complement. Indeed, depressed levels of serum complement have been recorded and C3 and properdin have been found in biopsies of some patients with chronic muco-cutaneous candidiasis. Phagocytic defects have been reported in patients prone to develop candidiasis, but these patients have usually been treated with antibiotics, steroids or cytotoxic drugs. The agents are associated with depressed phagocytosis and antibiotics such as tetracycline and gentamycin inhibit C3 consumption.

Poor resistance to *Candida* infection can be found in patients with high titres of *Candida* antibodies and normal complement levels, so that other factors may be more important in the defence against *Candida*. Indeed, a *Candida* clumping factor has been found in practically all normal sera and this factor seems to be absent in muco-cutaneous and systemic candidiasis and is reduced in diabetes, leukaemia and carcinoma. Furthermore, a candidacidal factor has also been found in normal human serum and inhibiting antibodies to this factor have been detected in some patients with muco-cutaneous candidiasis. The biological role of these factors is not clear, but they are not antibodies.

Normal PMNL and monocytes can kill *C.albicans in vitro* and the principal mechanisms of killing is mediated by myeloperoxidase and hydrogen peroxide. Some patients with leukaemia show a depression of killing of *C. albicans* by PMNL.

Systemic candidiasis can also be associated with the absence of myeloperoxidase in phagocytes. The defect, however, might reside in migration of the phagocytes to the inflammatory site. Such a chemotactic defect has been found in PMNL of patients susceptible to *Candida* infections (e.g. diabetes) and in PMNL and monocytes of patients with chronic muco-cutaneous candidiasis. It is of interest that cell wall mannan and complement are chemotactic for PMNL.

Cell-mediated immunity

Cutaneous delayed hypersensitivity reactions and *in vitro* tests to *C.albicans* in a normal population are usually positive, though the actual incidence varies with the protein/mannan ratio of the antigen and the population tested. Positive skin induration 24 to 48 hours after intradermal administration of *C.albicans* antigen varies between 46% and 94%. The lymphocyte transformation and macrophage migration inhibition tests show similar variations and these can be attributed to a lack of standardization of these tests. However, there is a positive correlation between the lymphoproliferative response, macrophage migration inhibition and antibody titre in control subjects.

It is generally thought that cell-mediated immunity (CMI) plays a more important part than humoral immunity in the protection from *Candida* infection, because often the antibody titre is not impaired. The best evidence for the significance of CMI in the protection from chronic candidiasis is derived from the study of patients with genetic defects of T-lymphocyte function, secondary to thymic defects. These patients suffer from intractable chronic muco-cutaneous candidiasis from birth and are unable to eliminate *C.albicans* from the mucosal surfaces, although systemic candidiasis is surprisingly rare. Thus, candidiasis is found in patients with defective generation or differentiation of lymphoid stem cells, as can be seen in the Swiss type of agammaglobulinaemia and in thymic aplasia or dysplasia. Patients with B-lymphocyte defects alone are not susceptible to candidiasis, unless they also have a concurrent T-cell deficiency as in the severe combined immunodeficiency syndromes.

However, it should be appreciated that most patients with chronic muco-cutaneous candidiasis do not suffer from any one of the very serious deficiencies of CMI. Most patients have a variable defect in one or more components of CMI. A spectrum of increasing cell-mediated immunodeficiencies is found in chronic muco-cutaneous candidiasis. Chronic oral hyperplastic candidiasis has a cellular immune defect involving lymphocyte cytotoxicity, macrophage migration inhibition and skin delayed hypersensitivity to *C.albicans*. However, in the more extensive muco-cutaneous candidiasis the cellular defects may also be directed against unrelated antigens and to mitogens. There is frequently a dissociation between the various defects, so that in some patients the skin delayed hypersensitivity may be intact but MIF production by lymphocytes is impaired. In others there may be a dissociation between MIF production and the lymphoproliferative response. Serum IgG, IgM and IgA antibodies also fail to show a consistent relationship and they are increased in some but decreased in others. These inconsistencies might be associated with the function of T-helper and suppressor cells. Indeed, there is now evidence that T-suppressor cells might be responsible for some of the cellular defects in chronic muco-cutaneous candidiasis.

Further evidence in favour of CMI playing a significant part in protection against *Candida* is the beneficial effect from therapeutic procedures which restore CMI. Transplantation of bone marrow, thymus or immunocompetent lymphocytes, as well as injections of transfer factor resulted in clinical improvement and restoration of some of the CMI markers.

The complexities of the cellular, humoral and phagocytic immune mechanisms of protection against *Candida* suggest that nature has provided a number of inter-related and possibly compensatory mechanisms. A defect in some of the components of the defence reaction may result in disease. The biological significance of any one of the mechanisms described is unknown and the probability cannot be excluded that some of these might be *in vitro* phenomena, without necessarily any *in vivo* significance.

Summary

It is a surprising feature that bacterial infections of the oral mucosa are rather uncommon but that a viral (*Herpes simplex*) and a fungal (*Candida*) infection are commonly found. Most if not all people have been exposed to *Herpes simplex* and *Candida* in the form of clinical or subclinical infection and the carrier rate of the latter is about 30%. Latency of *Herpes simplex* is the viral counterpart of bacterial carrier mechanism and must be rather common, though the prevalence has not been determined. Hence, most subjects in a normal control population will be sensitized to both organisms and yield antibodies and cell-mediated immune reactions.

Herpes simplex virus infection is characterized by early primary clinical or subclinical infection, followed by latency and, commonly, recurrence of the viral infection. Cellular immunity and antibodies to *Herpes simplex* are induced during primary infection. The virus becomes latent in the trigeminal ganglion and there is some evidence that latency might be dependent on antibodies. Recurrent herpetic infection seems to occur in patients with a selective deficiency in T-cells which are concerned with the formation of some lymphokines.

Candidiasis can manifest itself in an acute or chronic form and a number of predisposing factors have been recorded. Immunodeficiencies of cellular, humoral or phagocytic components play an important part, especially in chronic muco-cutaneous candidiasis. The diversities of the immune defects makes this a particularly interesting disease to study.

Oral manifestations of immunodeficiencies

Both primary and secondary immunodeficiencies may have oral manifestations. Recurrent throat infections, recurrent oral ulceration, herpes virus infections, candidiasis and severe gingivitis are the most common features. Although the oral features may not be of great importance in relation to the systemic manifestations of the disease, nevertheless oral lesions may be the presenting features and therefore help in the early diagnosis of the disease.

PRIMARY IMMUNODEFICIENCY

Complement deficiency is extremely rare but can affect the classical or alternative pathway of complement activation. An exception is angioneurotic oedema which is a relatively common hereditary disease due to a deficiency of C1 esterase inhibitor. The latter normally inactivates C1 so that a deficiency of the inhibitor allows over-activity of the complement system, generating kinins which cause increased vascular permeability. The condition may start in childhood or adult life and the patient suffers from recurrent episodes of acute subcutaneous oedema, characterized by swellings in the head and neck region. The face, lips, mouth, pharynx and larynx may be involved and may lead to respiratory obstruction. An attack can be precipitated by minor trauma, pyrexia or anxiety and the oedema may persist for up to 3 days.

388

Chronic granulomatous disease is one of the most common inherited defects of phagocytosis affecting children. It is characterized by chronic suppurative and granulomatous lymphadenitis, widespread granulomata, leucocytosis, anaemia and hypergammaglobulinaemia. Recurrent oral ulceration is found in about 16% of the affected children. Eczema may affect the skin of the face or lips and cervical lymphadenopathy is usually present. Prolonged antibiotic treatment often leads to oral candidiasis.

Chediak-Higashi syndrome is an autosomal recessive disease, presenting with recurrent respiratory infection and albinism. The polymorphonuclear leucocytes are abnormal and there is a neutropenia and impaired chemotaxis. Severe periodonal disease, dental caries, oral ulceration and cervical lymphadenopathy are commonly observed.

Cyclic neutropenia is a reduction of polymorphonuclear leucocytes at 3-weekly intervals. It is a rare condition seen in children and is caused by a maturation arrest at the promyelocyte stage. Recurrent oral ulceration can be the sole feature of this disease; otherwise the patient suffers from episodic malaise and infections of the skin and upper respiratory tract.

B-CELL DEFICIENCY

Bruton's x-linked hypogammaglobulinaemia is probably a defect in B stem cell differentiation, with intact T-cell functions. B-cell precursors are found in the bone marrow but mature B-cells and plasma cells are absent from the lymphoid tissue and blood. There is atrophy of the gut associated lymphoid tissue. IgG, IgA and IgM production is deficient and IgE and IgD are virtually absent. An IgG concentration of less than 200 mg per 100 ml of blood is of diagnostic significance in this disease.

The disease affects male infants who suffer from recurrent pyogenic bacterial infection. The mouth is not frequently involved, but there is recurrent sinusitis and the tonsillar tissue is atrophied.

IgA deficiency is the most common immunodeficiency with a prevalence of 1:600 in the general population. The number of peripheral blood, membrane-bound IgA-bearing B-cells is normal and the defect appears to be in the release rather than in the synthesis of IgA. Serum and secretory IgA are deficient but there is an abundance of free secretory component in saliva. There is a striking association of selective IgA deficiency with many autoimmune diseases. A surprising feature of IgA deficiency is that some patients experience no ill effects. IgM concentration in secretions is high and may compensate for the IgA deficiency. The majority of patients with IgA deficiency suffer from recurrent respiratory infection, allergies, gastro-intestinal disease, malignancy, autoimmune disease, relapsing neuropathies or endocrinopathies.

Oral manifestations are common, with 75% of the patients suffering from recurrent oral ulcers and 50% with recurrent *herpes labialis*. Tonsilitis and pharyngitis are also common problems. The effect on dental caries is controversial, owing to difficulties in interpretation of a lack of salivary IgA with a compensating increase in IgM, the prolonged use of antibiotics and important differences in the intake of sugar. Hence, some children were reported to have an increased and others a decreased amount of dental caries. The gingival condition, however, does not appear to be affected.

T-CELL DEFICIENCY

Di George syndrome is characterized by thymic hypoplasia due to a failure of development of the 3rd and 4th pharyngeal pouches. There is depletion of T-cells in the thymus-dependent areas of lymph nodes and in peripheral blood. Delayed hypersensitivity, graft rejection and *in vitro* lymphocyte functions are impaired. B-cells and plasma cells are normal in number and function. Patients are extremely susceptible to severe respiratory tract infection, especially with viruses and fungi.

Among the congenital abnormalities are a prominent forehead, hypertelorism, micrognathia and nasal and palatal clefts. Eruption of the teeth may be delayed and enamel hypoplasia is often found due to hypoparathyroidism. Chronic oral candidiasis is a frequent feature.

Ataxia telangiectasia is a rare condition consisting of cerebellar ataxia, telangiectasia of skin and conjunctiva and sinopulmonary infections. Both T and B functions are impaired and the prominent features are depressed cell-mediated immunity, serum IgA and IgE. The tonsils are hypoplastic and telangiectasia may involve the oral mucosa.

Wiskott-Aldrich syndrome is an x-linked immunodeficiency characterized by eczema and thrombocytopenia. Mortality is very high in infancy. The antibody response to polysaccharide antigens is poor and this is associated with a low serum IgM concentration. There is also a progressive impairment of cell-mediated immunity. The platelets fail to aggregate normally and this may cause bleeding in the gastrointestinal tract. The patient suffers from intractable viral, fungal or bacterial infections, often involving the respiratory tract.

Severe *Herpes simplex, Herpes zoster* or varicella infections may occur and can be fatal. Oral candidiasis is a common manifestation. Palatal petechiae and gingival bleeding have been recorded. Tranfer factor can be effective in controlling infection.

Chronic muco-cutaneous candidiasis is associated with a variety of T-cell defects and has been considered before (pp. 383–7).

STEM CELL DEFICIENCY

Severe combined immunodeficiency is a common condition responsible for a significant proportion of post-natal deaths. It is not entirely clear if the underlying cause is a stem cell or thymic defect. Cell-mediated immune functions are depressed or absent. The serum immunoglobulin levels are low and C1q can be also depressed. The infant develops severe bacterial, viral or protozoal infections affecting the intestines, lungs or skin.

The tonsils are absent and lymph nodes are impalpable. Chronic muco-cutaneous candidiasis is invariably present and may disseminate to other tissues. Recurrent oral ulceration may involve the tongue and cheek. Bone marrow transplants have been successful in a number of infants.

COMMON VARIABLE IMMUNODEFICIENCY

This is a mixed category of the most common immune deficiency disorders which are difficult to classify. There is a variety of defects of B-cell functions. Antibody production is impaired, although a normal number of B-cells are usually found. The patient often lacks one or two immunoglobulin classes, most commonly IgG or IgA. Recurrent pulmonary infections with pyogenic bacteria and intestinal infestations are often seen.

Recurrent oral and pharyngeal ulceration is rather common and can be associated with a neutropenia. Severe pharyngitis is also common.

Severe oral manifestations can be a prominent feature in immune deficiencies secondary to drugs, neoplasms or malnutrition. Herpetic stomatitis, oral candidiasis or intractable oral ulcers are commonly seen in patients receiving cytotoxic or immunosuppressive treatment. In addition to the pain and difficulties in eating and swallowing, there is a danger of the infection spreading to other tissues. This is particularly seen in patients with renal transplants, leukaemia, lymphoma and other neoplasms. Agranulocytosis can be caused by irradiation and a variety of drugs; cytotoxic agents (e.g. Azathioprine), analgesics (e.g. phenacetin), anti-microbial (e.g. chloramphenicol), antithyroid or anticonvulsant drugs. The presenting feature can be a sore throat and associated oropharyngeal ulceration. Malnutrition due to protein deficiency (kwashiorkor) can give rise to oral gangrene, and is seen in some of the developing countries. Iron deficiency may predispose to oral candidiasis.

The management of these lesions involves eliminating the cause of the immune defect and this is usually not possible when drugs are used for life-threatening diseases. This is however, straightforward, if diagnosed in time, with some drug-induced agranulocytosis (e.g. phenacetin) or in iron deficiency anaemia. The problem of malnutrition is partly political and has lately been dealt with successfully.

Summary

Oral manifestations of both primary and secondary immunodeficiencies are commonly seen. Recurrent throat infections and oral ulceration are the most common oral features in the various hypogammaglobulinaemias and phagocytic defects. Cell-mediated immunodeficiencies favour fungal infection by *Candida* and *Herpes simplex* viral infections. Periodontal disease appears to be decreased in secondary immunodeficiencies, but the effect on dental caries cannot be confidently assessed until detailed studies of the various immunological indices become available.

Further reading

Arnold R.R., Cole M.F., Price S. & McGhee J.R. (1977) Secretory IgM antibodies to *Streptococcus mutans* in subjects with selective IgA deficiency. *Clin. Immun. Immunopath.*, **8**, 475.

Baikie A.G., Amerena V.C. & Morley A.A. (1967) Recurring ulcers of the mouth. *Lancet*, **i,** 45.

Baringer J.R. & Swoveland P. (1973) Recovery of *Herpes simplex* virus from human trigeminal ganglions. *New Eng. J. Med.*, **288,** 648.

Buckley R.H. (1975) Clinical and immunologic features of selective IgA deficiency. In *Immunodeficiency in Man and Animals.* p. 134. Sinauer, Massachusetts.

Cawson R.A. (1973) Induction of epithelial hyperplasia by *Candida albicans*. *Br. J. Derm.*, **89,** 497.

Cooper M.D., Chase H.P., Lowman J.T., Krivit W. & Good R.A. (1968) Wiskott-Aldrich syndrome: an immunologic deficiency disease involving the afferent limb of immunity. *Am. J. Med.*, **44,** 449.

Fudenberg H.H., Good R.A., Goodman H.C., Hitzig W., Kunkel H.G., Roitt I.M., Rosen F.S., Rowe D.S., Seligmann M. & Soothill J.R. (1971) Primary immunodeficiencies. *Bull. WHO*, **45,** 125.

Gorlin R. & Pindborg J.J. (1976) *Syndromes of the Head and Neck*, 2nd edn. McGraw Hill, New York.

Hayward A.R. (1977) Immunodeficiency. In *Current Topics in Immunology Series*, No. 6. Edward Arnold, London.

Hong R., Santosham M., Schulte-Wissermann H., Horowita S., Hsu S.H. & Winkelstein J.A. (1976) Reconstitution of B and T lymphocyte function in severe combined immunodeficiency disease after transplantation with thymic epithelium. *Lancet*, **ii,** 1270.

Kirkpatrick C.H., Rich R.R. & Bennett J.E. (1971) Chronic mucocutaneous candidiasis: Model buildings in cellular immunity. *Ann. Int. Med.*, **74,** 955.

Klebanoff S.J. (1967) Iodination of bacteria; a bactericidal mechanism. *J. exp. Med.*, **126,** 1063.

Lehner T. (1965) Immunofluorescent investigation of *Candida albicans* antibodies in human saliva. *Archs. oral Biol.*, **10,** 975.

Lehner T., Wilton J.M.A. & Ivanyi L. (1972) Immunodeficiencies in chronic muco-cutaneous candidosis. *Immunology*, **22,** 775

Lehner T., Wilton J.M.A. & Shillitoe E.J. (1975) Immunological basis for latency, recurrences and putative oncogenicity of *Herpes simplex* virus. *Lancet*, **ii,** 60.

Lehrer R.I. & Cline M.J. (1969) Leukocyte myeloperoxidase deficiency and disseminated candidiasis: The role of myeloperoxidase in resistance to *Candida* infection. *J. Clin. Invest.*, **48,** 1478.

Lodmell D.L., Niwa A., Hayashi K. & Notkins A.L. (1973) Prevention of cell-to-cell spread of *Herpes simplex* virus by leucocytes. *J. exp. Med.*, **137,** 706.

Louria D.B., Smith J.K., Brayton R.G. & Buse M. (1972) Anti-candida factors in serum and their inhibition. I. Clinical and laboratory observations. *J. Infect. Dis.*, **125,** 102.

Medical Research Council (1969) Summary report of Medical Research Council working party of hypogammaglobulinaemia in the UK. *Lancet*, **i,** 163.

Nahmias A.J. & Roizman B. (1973) Infection with *Herpes simplex* virus 1 and 2. *New Eng. J. Med.*, **289,** 667.

Rasmussen L.E., Jordan G.W., Stevens D.A. & Merigan T.C. (1974) Lymphocyte interferon production and transformation after *Herpes simplex* infections in humans. *J. Immunol.*, **112,** 728.

Ray T.C. & Wuepper K.D. (1975) Experimental cutaneous *Candida albicans* infections in rodents; role of complement. *Clin. Res.*, **23,** 2304.

Robertson P.B., Wright T.E., Mackler B.F., Lenertz D.M. & Levy B.M. (1978) Periodontal status of patients with abnormalities of the immune system. *J. Perio. Res.*, **13,** 37.

Rocklin R.E. (1974) Clinical application of *in vitro* lymphocyte tests. In *Progress in Clinical Immunology.* p. 21. Grune & Stratton, New York.

Rosenberg G.L., Snyderman R. & Notkins A.L. (1974) Production of chemotactic factor and lymphotoxin by human leukocytes stimulated with *Herpes simplex* virus. *Infect. Immun.*, **10,** 111.

Russell C. & Jones J.H. (1973) The effects of oral inoculation of the yeast and mycelial phases of *Candida albicans* in rats fed a normal and carbohydrate rich diets. *Arch. Oral Biol.*, **18,** 409.

Schuller P.D., Freedman H.L. & Lewis D.W. (1973) Periodontal status of renal transplant patients receiving immunosuppressive therapy. *J. Periodont.*, **44,** 167.

Scully C.M. & Lehner T. (1980) Oral manifestations of disorders of immunity. In *Oral Manifestations of Systemic Disease*, Mason D.K. & Jones J.H. (eds). W.B. Saunders, London.

Shillitoe E.J., Wilton J.M.A. & Lehner T. (1977) Sequential changes in cell-mediated immune responses to *Herpes simplex* virus following recurrent herpetic infection in man. *Infect. Immun.*, **18,** 130.

Shillitoe E.J., Wilton J.M.A. & Lehner T. (1978) Sequential changes in T and B lymphocyte responses to *Herpes simplex* virus in man. *Scand. J. Immunol.*, **7,** 357.

Sohnle P.G., Frank M.M. & Kirkpatrick C.H. (1976) Deposition of complement components in the cutaneous lesion of chronic mucocutaneous candidiasis. *Clin. Immunol. Immunopathol.*, **5,** 340.

Stevens J.G. & Cook M.L. (1971) Restriction of *Herpes simplex* virus by macrophages. An analysis of the cell–virus interaction. *J. Exp. Med.*, **133,** 19.

Stevens J.G. & Cook M.L. (1974) Maintenance of latent herpetic infection: An apparent role for anti-viral IgG. *J. Immunol.*, **113,** 1685.

Van Sooy R.E., Hill H.R., Ritts R.E. & Quie P.G. (1975) Familial neutrophil chemotaxis defect, recurrent bacterial infections, mucocutaneous candidiasis and hyperimmunoglobulinaemia E. *Ann. Int. Med.*, **82,** 766.

Wilton J.M.A., Ivanyi L. & Lehner T. (1972) Cell-mediated immunity in Herpes virus hominis infections. *Br. Med. J.*, **i,** 723.

Wilton J.M.A. & Lehner T. (1981) Immunology of candidiasis. In *Comprehensive Immunology: Immunology of Human Infections.* Good R.A. & Day S.B. (eds). Plenum Medical Book Company, New York and London.

16

Oral manifestations of autoimmunity

Recurrent oral ulcers (ROU)

ROU are the most common lesions of the oral mucosa affecting about 10% of the normal population. There are three varieties of ROU: (a) minor aphthous ulcers (MiAU), (b) major aphthous ulcers (MjAU), and (c) herpetiform ulcers (HU). ROU are found more often in females than males and may appear at any age, though most commonly during the second decade. A family history is found in 24% to 46% of patients.

A prodromal phase is recognized by most patients as a soreness or burning sensation 1 to 2 days before the onset of ulceration. With the breakdown of epithelium and associated inflammatory reactions the pain increases in severity for a few days, but then gradually disappears. MiAU are single, small, oval ulcers, usually affecting the mucosa of the lips, cheeks and sides of the tongue (figure 16.1). They last from 4 to 14 days and recur at 1- to 4-monthly intervals. MjAU are single but large ulcers often involving the oropharynx and dorsum of the tongue (figure 16.2). They may last from 10 to 30 days, heal with scarring and recur often at less than monthly intervals. HU appear as crops of numerous minute ulcers, affecting several

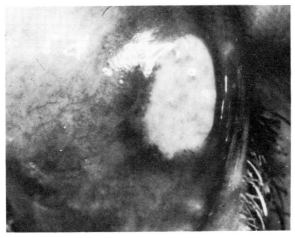

FIGURE 16.1. Minor aphthous ulcer.

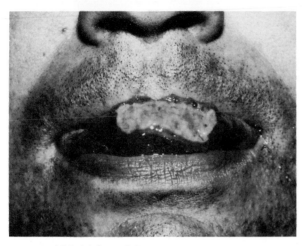

FIGURE 16.2. Major aphthous ulcer of the tip of the tongue.

sites of the oral mucosa and the crops of ulcers coalesce to single irregular lesions. HU last from 7 to 14 days and recur at intervals of less than a month. Although MjAU and HU account for less than 20% of ROU, they are the most severe types of ulcers, causing severe pain and difficulties in speaking and eating, often with loss of weight.

Behcet's syndrome (BS)

BS will be considered with ROU, as most of the aetiological and immunological features appear to be largely indistinguishable and oral ulceration is the only consistent feature in this syndrome. It should be however, noted that whilst ROU is very common BS is a rather rare disease. BS is perhaps the only disease in which oral manifestations are consistently associated with a variety of extraoral lesions. Although originally BS was defined as recurrent oral and genital ulceration with iridocyclitis, this is now extended to include cutaneous, vascular, joint, neurological and intestinal manifestations. A precise definition of this syndrome cannot be given at present, but the diagnosis is generally made when two or more major sites are involved. In order that a distinction could be drawn on clinical and prognostic grounds the syndrome can be divided into four types: (a) muco-cutaneous (M-C) type involves oral, genital and/or skin manifestations; (b) arthritic (A) type with joint involvement and two or three of the M-C manifestations; (c) neurological (N) type with brain involvement and some or all of the lesions found in the M-C and A types; (d) ocular (Oc) type with uveitis and some or all of the M-C, A and N manifestations. The presence of vascular lesions, such as thrombosis or aneurysm, can be found in any one of the four types of BS.

AETIOLOGY

Viral or bacterial agents, food allergy, hormonal disturbances, haematological abnormalities, emotional disturbance and trauma are some of the aetiological factors postulated. None of these, however, account for the majority of patients with ROU, though some of the factors may be responsible for a small proportion of ROU. Thus, about 8% of hospital out-patients with ROU may have iron, folate or B12 deficiency anaemias. Two per cent of the same population may suffer from coeliac disease, due to an allergy to dietary gluten which leads to intestinal malabsorption. About 2% develop the ulcers regularly before the onset of the menstrual period. Most of the patients, however, have some immunological abnormality, with autoimmune responses to oral mucosal antigens or some cross-reacting microbial antigens. Recently the *Herpes simplex* virus genome was found in lymphocytes of some patients with ROU and BS and this might have an effect on the pathogenesis of these diseases.

IMMUNOLOGICAL FEATURES

Some abnormalities in the immune responses have been detected in most patients with ROU and BS and these will be now described.

Immunoglobulin, complement and acute phase reactants

A slight increase in serum IgA and IgG was found especially in MjAU. Normal concentrations of C3 and C4 were found in ROU and BS. Careful sequential studies, however, have revealed that C3, C4 and C2 were markedly reduced before an attack of uveitis, suggesting complement consumption by the classical pathway. An increased concentration of C9 was found in ROU and BS but C-reactive protein (CRP) was significantly increased only in BS. An increased concentration of CRP and C9 might be a manifestation of acute phase reactants, released during epithelial inflammation. An alternative interpretation of these findings is that CRP might modulate T-cells, activate complement and promote phagocytosis, whereas C9 might play a part in cell lysis.

397

Autoantibodies

Nuclear, thyroid and gastric autoantibodies are not found in ROU or BS and the Rose-Waaler test for rheumatoid factor is also negative, even with joint involvement. However, auto-antibodies to saline homogenates of oral mucosa were found in 70% to 80% of patients with ROU and BS, as compared with 10% of controls. These antibodies belong predominantly to the IgM and, to a lesser extent, IgG classes; they are not specific to oral mucosa, as common antigenic determinants were shared between saline extracts of other epithelial tissues.

Immune complexes

The findings of some abnormalities in the complement com-ponents and the classical manifestations of BS, especially uveitis, arthritis and erythema nodosum which are commonly ascribed to immune complexes (IC), have raised the possibility that IC might be involved in BS. Circulating IC have now been detected by several assays in about 40% of patients with ROU and 60% of those with BS (figure 16.3). The amount of IC was closely associated with disease activity, so that the IC might play an important part in these diseases. The size of the IC in the ocular type of BS showed a broad range from 3×10^5 to 3×10^6 daltons (figure 16.4) and this suggested the possibility that the multifocal involvement of tissues might be associated with IC of different sizes. Electron microscopical examination of centrifuged pellets of serum revealed the presence of small membrane fragments, some of which showed complement dependent holes. These findings suggest that the soluble IC may generate C5b-9 complexes which may bind to the surface of cells and result in cell lysis.

Recent studies of phagocytosis have revealed that some patients with ROU and BS show a defect in phagocytosis by PMNL. IC in BS and in ROU might be responsible for the tissue damage in two ways: (a) direct complement dependent cell lysis; (b) the indirect effect of impairing the function of phagocytes in clearing IC as well as other substances. Increased chemotactic activity of PMNL has been found in BS but not in ROU and this appears to be due to the serum.

Immunopathology

An intense lympho-monocytic infiltration is found on histo-logical examination of the early stages of ulceration in the

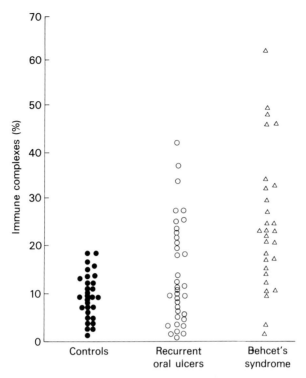

FIGURE 16.3. Immune complexes in Behcet's syndrome and recurrent oral ulcers. Complexes were assayed as a percentage inhibition of the agglutination of IgG-coated latex particles by low affinity anti-IgG. (From Levinsky R J. & Lehner T. (1978) *Clin. exp. Immunol.*, **32**, 193.)

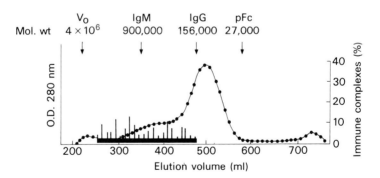

FIGURE 16.4. The broad range of size of immune complexes from a patient with Behcet's syndrome, shown by separation on a sepharose column. Complexes assayed as in figure 16.3. (From Levinsky & Lehner 1978.)

lamina propria, the adjacent epithelium (figure 16.5) and around blood vessels (figure 16.6). Later a mixed response becomes evident, with PMNL predominating and some plasma cells. The early stages are suggestive of a type IV delayed hypersensitivity reaction and this is supported by the electron-microscopical findings of intracytoplasmic phagosome-like bodies of epithelial cells adjacent to mononuclear cells and the association of phagocytosing macrophages with epithelial cells (figure 16.7).

In BS, vascular lesions are often found, initially affecting the small blood vessels, especially venules. There is an intense mononuclear, and later PMNL infiltration, with vascular endo-thelial proliferation, loss of the internal elastic lamina, fibrinoid necrosis and often obliteration of the lumen (figure 16.8). The PMNL reaction and fibrinoid necrosis are consistent with a type III Arthus reaction and this might be induced by IC. The relationship between the type IV and III immunological re-sponses is not clear and careful sequential studies will have to be carried out to clarify this. There is, however, evidence from immunopathological studies that vasculitis may be responsible for BS. Immunofluorescent studies of biopsies revealed C3 and C9 in the walls of blood vessels and sometimes in the epithelial basement membrane. However, immunoglobulin is seldom found, so that the alternative complement pathway might be involved.

In vitro cell-mediated immunity

A significant lymphoproliferative response was induced by homogenates of oral mucosa in ROU and BS but not in controls. There has been considerable support for the involve-ment of cell-mediated immunity by finding that lymphocytes from patients with ROU, but not from control subjects, induce cytotoxicity in cultures of gingival epithelial target cells. Furthermore, homogenates of oral mucosa induced significant leucocyte migration inhibition in patients with ROU but not in controls. A correlation was found in sequential studies between the clinical features of ROU and cell-mediated immunity, as assessed by DNA synthesis of lymphocytes, cytotoxicity, and leucocyte migration inhibition, but not haemagglutinating antibodies to oral mucosa.

The results of these markers of cell-mediated immunity are in agreement that the cellular responses may play an important effector part in the recurrences of oral ulcers and that this occurs in the presence of a constant level of antibodies. As the

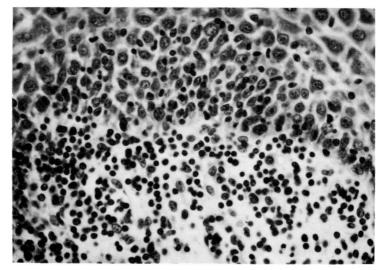

FIGURE 16.5. Lymphocytes and monocytes in the lamina propria, infiltrating through the basement membrane between the epithelial cells in a biopsy from a patient with an early minor aphthous ulcer. Haematoxylin and eosin ×375.

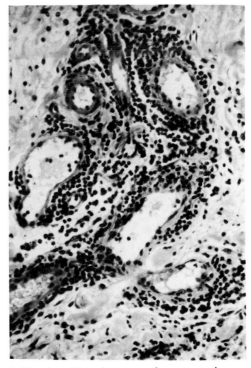

FIGURE 16.6. Perivascular infiltration of lymphocytes and monocytes in a biopsy from a patient with early minor aphthous ulceration. Haematoxylin and eosin ×315.

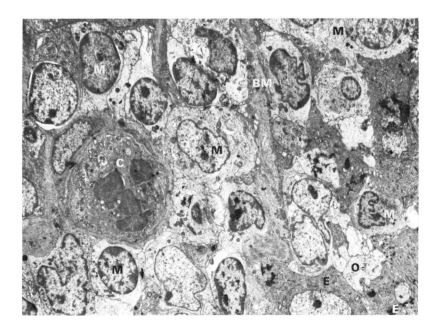

FIGURE 16.7. Electron micrograph of an early stage of aphthous ulceration showing an intense mononuclear (M) cell infiltration near the basement membrane (BM), around a capillary (C) and among epithelial cells (E) which show oedematous separation (O). Lead hydroxide ×1743.

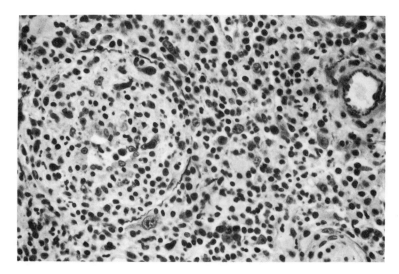

FIGURE 16.8. Intense mononuclear cell infiltration and endothelial cell proliferation, almost occluding the lumen of the blood vessel, in a biopsy from a patient with major aphthous ulceration in Behcet's syndrome. Haematoxylin-Van Gieson stain ×415.

402

cytotoxicity is antibody independent it is suggested that the antibodies may be involved in immune complex formation. The relationship between increased cellular responses and immune complexes is not clear; while immune complexes may modulate cellular immunity, they might be the principal agents in the change from focal oral ulceration to the involvement of many tissues in BS.

Histocompatibility antigens

In most of the diseases which are associated with HLA antigens in man, the immune response is thought to play an essential part in the pathogenesis of the disease. It is therefore of interest that HLA-B5 was found in 75% of Japanese patients with BS, as compared with 31% of controls, with a relative risk of 6.7. This association has been confirmed in Britain, Turkey, Israel, and France.

The studies in ROU show an association with HLA-B12. These studies suggest that the susceptibility to BS or ROU is associated with a gene near the HLA region which is in linkage disequilibrium with the HLA genes. It is possible that HLA-B12 which is significantly increased in ROU and HLA-B5 in BS might function as specific receptors for pathogens or that the antigenic determinants of some exogenous pathogens might mimic the HLA antigens.

Summary

HLA-B12 in ROU and B5 in BS offer an immunogenetic basis for the development of these diseases. Soluble IC and cell-mediated immunity to oral mucosal antigens are involved in ROU and BS. These may induce type III (complex-mediated) and type IV (cell-mediated) hypersensitivity reactions respectively, but the part that each plays in the diseases has not been clarified. Both types of reactions could be involved in the damage caused and in the recurrent nature of the diseases. The hypothesis (figure 16.9) is suggested that mononuclear cell uptake and processing of altered epithelial antigen or, more likely, cross-reacting microbial antigen may occur. This may be aided by the adjuvant effect of dental plaque and focal sepsis in the mouth or a deficiency in suppressor cells. The local lymph nodes will be induced to produce antibodies and sensitized lymphocytes which are cytotoxic to oral epithelium and can produce lymphokines. The initial epithelial damage induced by the sensitized lymphocytes will release antigen which may

403

combine with 'antibody to produce IC. The latter might be eliminated by phagocytes but the process of ingestion of IC may fail. IC will activate complement with the release of C3a and C5a and the consequent rapid infiltration of leucocytes causing damage. The generation of C5b6789 complex will lead to cell lysis. Lymphocytes may also be stimulated to produce lymphokines by immune complexes generating C3b which can interact with the corresponding receptors on lymphocytes. Thus a local pathogenic effect may result by both complex-mediated and cell-mediated hypersensitivity. Under some immunogenetic conditions, with active formation of immune complexes and a defect in phagocytic removal of immune complexes, these may spill over into the circulation and be responsible for the multifocal damage seen in BS.

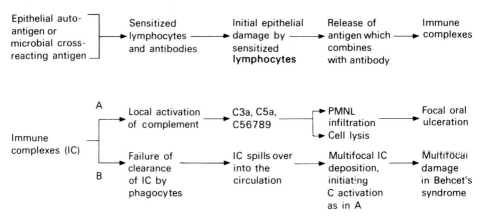

FIGURE 16.9. The immunological sequence of changes which may account for the development of oral ulceration and Behcet's syndrome.

Other autoimmune diseases with oral manifestations

PEMPHIGUS VULGARIS

This is a muco-cutaneous disorder associated with antibodies to the intercellular substance of epithelial cells. The disease shows oral manifestations in most patients. Painful vesicles or bullae may appear and burst within a few hours, resulting in shallow ulcers. These persist for weeks or months, but new lesions recur throughout the disease process. If the disease is not treated with immunosuppressive drugs the patient may die. A biopsy examination is essential and this shows epithelial bullae which are caused by a loss of the processes of prickle cells. These cells are rounded with enlarged nuclei and are termed acantholytic cells which are diagnostic on cytological examination of scrapings from the lesion. The antibodies are usually of the IgG and IgM classes and can be demonstrated by fluorescent antibody technique of diseased tissue or if the patient's serum is applied to normal epithelium; the antibodies bind to the intercellular substance.

LUPUS ERYTHEMATOSUS (see also chapter 10)

Oral manifestations in systemic and discoid lupus ery-thematosus are rarely important features of the disease, though occasionally the oral lesion may be a presenting feature. They can be recognized clinically as localized atrophic or erosive lesions surrounded by hyperkeratotic papules or striae and may involve the lips, cheeks, palate or tongue. Biopsy examin-ation shows hyperkeratosis, epithelial atrophy, liquefaction degeneration of the basal cell layer and a prominent mono-nuclear cell infiltration around the blood vessels, as well as of the lamina propria. Fibrinoid degeneration may affect the connective tissue and vessel walls.

PERNICIOUS ANAEMIA (see also chapter 10)

Soreness of the tongue, with burning and dryness of the mouth, are sometimes presenting symptoms of this disease. The tongue appears smooth, due to loss of the filliform papillae, and may also be inflamed. Recurrent oral ulcers are occasionally found in pernicious anaemia. They mimic minor aphthous ulcers but they are usually shallow and two to three in number; the ulcers last only 2 to 4 days before they heal and a new crop develops. The oral manifestations disappear when the anaemia is treated with vitamin B12.

SJÖGREN'S SYNDROME

Dryness of the mouth is a prominent feature of Sjögren's syndrome. The patient may complain of a burning sensation of the tongue, lips and cheeks, and of considerable discomfort on eating and speaking. Recurrent swelling of the parotid glands occurs commonly. The mucosa is atrophic and devoid of saliva and this makes movements between the mucosal surfaces rather difficult. Candida infection of the chronic atrophic variety commonly affects the oral mucosa and may give rise to angular cheilitis.

The syndrome consists of dry eyes and connective tissue

disease, in addition to the dry mouth. Rheumatoid arthritis is the most common but lupus erythematosus and other connective tissue diseases are often associated.

The diagnosis of Sjögren's syndrome is aided by a raised ESR, increased concentration of immunoglobulins, positive rheumatoid factor and Rose-Waaler test, presence of antinuclear factor, organ specific autoantibodies and salivary duct antibodies. An abnormal sialogram and histological evidence of sialadenitis in a lip biopsy may be more significant in the diagnosis of Sjögren's syndrome.

RHEUMATOID ARTHRITIS (see also chapter 10)

The temporomandibular joint may also be affected among the many joints involved in rheumatoid arthritis. The joints may be painful, swollen and show stiffness and crepitus. A variety of anti-inflammatory drugs used in the treatment of rheumatoid arthritis may induce lichen planus of the mouth.

Summary

Most, if not all, autoimmune diseases may have oral manifestations and some of these may be the presenting features of the disease. This is particularly common with pemphigus vulgaris which is a life-threatening disease and the presenting feature in the mouth, with the immunopathological findings in biopsies, are of some importance. Dryness of the mouth is one of the most common presenting manifestations of Sjögren's syndrome and whilst it can be a symptom of a variety of conditions, especially secondary to some drugs, the association with a connective tissue disorder and a variety of autoantibodies needs to be emphasized. A sore, smooth tongue is often found in pernicious anaemia which is due to a defect in absorption of vitamin B12, probably secondary to an autoimmune reaction to parietal cells in the stomach. It is worth noting that the temporomandibular joint in rheumatoid arthritis, oral mucosa in lupus erythematosus, muscles of mastication in myasthenia gravis and bleeding from the gingiva in autoimmune purpura should be recognized as significant oro-facial manifestations of autoimmune disorders.

Further reading

Adinolfi M. & Lehner T. (1976) Acute phase proteins and C9 in patients with Behcet's syndrome and aphthous ulcers. *Clin. exp. Immunol.*, **25**, 36.

Challacombe S.J., Barkhan P. & Lehner T. (1977) Haematological features and differentiation of recurrent oral ulceration. *Br. J. Oral Surg.*, **15**, 37.

Challacombe S.J., Batchelor J.R., Kennedy L. & Lehner T. (1977) HLA-antigens in patients with recurrent oral ulceration. *Archs. Derm.*, **113**, 1717.

Dolby A.E. (1969) Recurrent aphthous ulceration: effect of sera and peripheral blood upon epithelial tissue culture cells. *Immunology*, **17**, 709.

Donatsky O. (1976) Comparison of cellular and humoral immunity against streptococcal and adult human oral mucosa antigens in relation to exacerbation of recurrent aphthous stomatitis. *Acta Path. Micro. Scand. Sec. C*, **84**, 270.

Eglin R.P., Lehner T. & Subak-Sharpe J.H. (1982) Detection of RNA complementary to *Herpes simplex* virus in mononuclear cells from patients with Behcet's syndrome and recurrent oral ulcers. *Lancet*, **ii**, 1356.

Ferguson R., Basu M.K., Asquith P. & Cooke W.T. (1976) Jejunal mucosal abnormalities in patients with recurrent aphthous ulceration. *Brit. Med. J.*, **i**, 11.

Graykowski E.A., Barile M.F., Lee W.B. & Stanley H.R. (1966) Recurrent aphthous stomatitis. Clinical, therapeutic, histopathologic and hypersensitivity aspects. *J. Am. Med. Ass.*, **196**, 637.

Lehner T. (1969) Pathology of recurrent oral ulceration and oral ulceration in Behcet's syndrome: light, electron and fluorescence microscopy. *J. Path.*, **97**, 481.

Lehner T. (1977) Progress report: Oral ulceration and Behcet's syndrome. *Gut*, **18**, 491.

Lehner T., Almeida J. & Levinsky R. (1978) Damaged membrane fragments and immune complexes in the blood of patients with Behcet's syndrome. *Clin. exp. Immunol.*, **34**, 206.

Levinsky R.J. & Lehner T. (1978) Circulating soluble immune complexes in recurrent oral ulceration and Behcet's syndrome. *Clin. exp. Immunol.*, **32**, 193.

Ohno S., Nakayama E., Sugiura S., Itakura K., Aoki K. & Aizawa M. (1975) Specific histocompatibility antigens associated with Behcet's disease. *Am. J. Ophthalmol.*, **80**, 636.

Rogers R.S., Sams W.M. & Shorter R.G. (1974) Lymphocytotoxicity in recurrent aphthous stomatitis. *Archs. Derm.*, **109**, 361.

Shimada K., Kogure M., Kawashima T. & Nishioka K. (1974) Reduction of complement in Behcet's disease and drug allergy. *Med. Biol.*, **52**, 234.

Shimizu T., Kagami T., Matsumoto T. & Matsumura N. (1963) Clinical studies of Behcet's syndrome. Analysis of epidemiology and attack-inducing factor of the disease. *Medicine (Japan)*, **12**, 526.

Ship I.I., Morris A.L., Durocher R.T. & Burket L.W. (1961) Recurrent aphthous ulcerations and recurrent herpes labialis in a professional school student population. *Oral Surg. Med. Path.*, **13**, 1438.

Sircus W., Church R. & Kelleher J. (1957) Recurrent aphthous ulceration of the mouth. A study of the natural history, aetiology and treatment. *Qly. J. Med.*, **26**, 235.

Sobel J.D., Haim S., Obedeanu N., Meshulam T. & Merzbach D. (1977) Polymorphonuclear leucocyte function in Behcet's disease. *J. Clin. Path.*, **30**, 250.

Wray D., Ferguson M.M., Mason D.K., Hutcheon A.W. & Dagg J.H. (1975) Recurrent aphthae: treatment with vitamin B12, folic acid and iron. *Brit. Med. J.*, **ii**, 490.

407

17 Oral neoplasia

Oral cancer is an extremely distressing disease, commonly resulting in the death of the afflicted patient. In this country only about 1% of all carcinomas occur in the mouth, but in other countries, particularly in some parts of India, up to half of all cancers may be present in the mouth.

There is little that is known specifically about the immunological aspects of oral carcinoma. However, a significant association has long been recognized between some leukoplakias and carcinoma. The term leukoplakia is defined here as a white plaque that from the clinical and histological features cannot be assigned to any other disease entity. The aetiology of most oral leukoplakias is unknown, but among the variety of agents suggested, smoking, friction, use of betel nut, syphilis, chronic candidiasis and possibly latent *Herpes simplex* type 1 infection have been supported by clinical, epidemiological, pathological or immunological evidence. An important point to have evolved is that some leukoplakias can be caused by microbial, fungal, and probably viral agents, so that the immune responses might play some part in the development of leukoplakia and its transformation to carcinoma. Furthermore, smoking is also associated with immunological changes, suggesting that both chemical and microbial agents related to leukoplakia might induce their effects, to some extent, by means of the immunological response.

MONONUCLEAR CELL INFILTRATION IN LEUKOPLAKIA AND CARCINOMA

A chronic inflammatory cell infiltrate, consisting of a variable proportion of lymphocytes, monocytes and plasma cells, can usually be observed in the lamina propria of leukoplakia and carcinoma. Differential counts of the mononuclear cell infiltration in biopsies of different histological stages of leukoplakia revealed significant differences between them. Hyperkeratotic (or parakeratotic) lesions without acanthosis (epithelial hyperplasia) showed a significantly smaller number of non-pyroninophilic mononuclear cells (mostly lymphocytes) and

409

plasma cells than any of the other lesions. There was a significant increase in the number of lymphocytes and plasma cells with the development of acanthosis, epithelial atypia and carcinoma *in situ* until a maximum was reached in carcinoma. The histological grading, lymphocyte and plasma-cell counts were correlated with the risk of carcinomatous transformation in leukoplakia. It is significant that an increased number of Russell bodies has also been observed in lesions that subsequently changed to carcinomas.

CELL-MEDIATED IMMUNE RESPONSE TO TISSUE HOMOGENATES

The correlation between the mononuclear cell infiltration, and the different stages of leukoplakia and carcinoma, suggests that immunological factors might be involved in the development and progress of this disease. Homogenates of leukoplakic tissues were used to study the response of lymphocytes from these patients. This revealed a significant negative correlation between transformation of lymphocytes stimulated with autologous homogenates of leukoplakia and the lymphocyte infiltration in biopsies. Hyperkeratotic tissue without acanthosis appeared to be associated with the highest rate of lymphocyte transformation and the lowest intensity of mononuclear cell infiltration, and there was a decrease in the former and an increase in the latter as the histological grading changed to acanthosis, epithelial atypia and carcinoma. The results suggest that a new or altered antigen is detected in leukoplakia and that carcinomatous transformation is accompanied, either by a loss of or change in antigenicity, or by a specific depression in cell-mediated immunity to these antigens.

A factor is also released by sensitized lymphocytes from patients with carcinoma or leukoplakia in the presence of tumour antigen and this inhibits migration of guinea-pig macrophages in an electrical field. A serum factor depressing the lymphocytes has been detected and the titre in sera from patients with leukoplakia is intermediate between those from carcinoma and normal controls. Leucocyte migration can also be inhibited by homogenates of leukoplakia but not by normal mucosa in patients with leukoplakia. These findings are consistent with the concept that cell-mediated immune responses may play a part in the development and progress of leukoplakia.

410

Syphilis. Leukoplakia is found in tertiary syphilis and may develop 4 to 20 years after the primary and secondary stages of the disease. Carcinomatous transformation is said to occur more often in syphilitic than other types of leukoplakia. Cell-mediated immunity to treponemal antigens in primary and, particularly, early secondary syphilis is impaired, but in some patients in late secondary and especially latent syphilis the cell-mediated responses are intact. Leukoplakia becomes clinically detectable in tertiary syphilis and the cell-mediated immune responses at that stage are probably intact.

Chronic hyperplastic candidiasis. The association of a specific type of leukoplakia with Candida has been appreciated for some years and might be due to a direct effect of Candida on epithelium in subjects with some cellular immunodeficiency. However, the oral carrier rate of Candida is about 30% and the presence of hyphae of Candida in leukoplakia could result from secondary infection by Candida of a suitably altered tissue. The clinical and pathological diagnosis of chronic hyperplastic candidiasis has been discussed elsewhere (pp. 302–7).

Although the evidence for Candida causing a specific type of leukoplakia is not in doubt, there is little firm evidence, as yet, to suggest that Candida can induce carcinomatous transformation. This view arose from the increased frequency of association of Candida hyphae with epithelial atypia, as compared with other types of leukoplakia. As Candida thrives particularly well in altered tissues, its presence might indicate a secondary infection. An alternative interpretation of the presence of Candida in leukoplakia is that an impaired immune response to Candida in patients with epithelial atypia and carcinoma enables the fungus to proliferate.

Latent Herpes simplex virus type 1 infection. The oro-facial strain, *Herpes simplex* virus type 1 (HSV1), has been implicated in cancer of the head and neck. A relationship between recurrent herpetic infection and carcinoma of the lip has been suggested on clinical grounds. Oncogenic properties of HSV1 have been shown in mice by the ability of HSV1 to enhance papilloma formation when administered with methylcholanthrene and by enhancing carcinomatous transformation of papilloma. The oncogenic properties of HSV1 could be related to a non-virion antigen and can be differentiated immunologically from virion

411

antigen which is associated with infective and cytopathic functions of the virus. Significant complement fixing antibody titres to the non-virion antigen were found in patients with cancer of the head and neck, as compared with controls. Furthermore, soluble membrane antigens from carcinoma of the lip reacted specifically with an antiserum to non-virion antigen of HSV1, suggesting that a cross-reacting antigen, or the non-virion antigen is present in the tumour.

Inactivated HSV1 can impart genetic information to cells, as has been shown by transferring thymidine kinase to cells lacking this enzyme. It can be readily seen that transfer of genetic information of HSV1 might occasionally lead to neoplastic conversion. Indeed, ultraviolet light inactivated HSV1 can cause transformation of hamster embryo fibroblasts and when these cells are injected into newborn Syrian hamsters they induce metastasizing fibrosarcomas. The epidemiological relationship between sunlight and carcinoma of the lips and face in some patients, as well as sunlight and activation of HSV1 lesions of the lips and face in others might therefore be relevant.

Cell-mediated and humoral immune responses to HSV1 were also studied in patients with leukoplakia, showing a histological spectrum of changes from epithelial keratosis to acanthosis and atypia, and in patients with carcinoma. The results showed that patients with epithelial atypia had the highest indices of lymphocyte transformation and migration inhibition to HSV1. It has been postulated that HSV1 might cause neoplastic transformation of epithelial cells, for the cell-mediated immune responses could inactivate HSV1 in such a way as to prevent replication but induce oncogenic properties of the virus, as has been shown with ultraviolet light. However, as with other carcinomas, some co-factor might be required, for only a very small proportion of subjects with HSV1 infection develop leukoplakia and carcinoma.

Cell-mediated immune responses to oral carcinoma. A progressive impairment of the capacity of lymphocytes to respond to antigens and mitogens has been evident only in sequential studies of patients with early carcinoma and leukoplakia. This is best illustrated by phytohaemagglutinin, for a response to lymphocytes under 50% of normal was found in only a few patients with keratosis and/or acanthosis, but in most patients with epithelial atypia or carcinoma. A progressive decrease in the phytohaemagglutinin-responding, and therefore predominantly T-lymphocyte population of pre-cancerous patients suggests that some impairment of T-lymphocytes may occur during carcinomatous transformation.

Summary

A working hypothesis has evolved from the immunopathological investigations of leukoplakia towards a unified concept of the pathogenesis of leukoplakia and carcinomatous transformation. The initial development of leukoplakia and subsequent transformation to carcinoma is induced by microbial and/or chemical agents. The induction phase usually has a long latent period, a matter of years, during which time prolonged exposure to the chemical agent (e.g. smoking), chronic infection (*T. pallidum*, *C. albicans*), or a latent viral infection (*Herpes simplex* type 1), may initiate a local epithelial reaction as well as local and systemic immune reactions. The epithelial changes of keratosis, acanthosis, atypia and carcinoma may develop sequentially in some but may appear at any one stage and remain unchanged in others. This might be associated with a newly acquired or altered epithelial antigen. The initiation and development of any stage of leukoplakia and carcinoma might be dependent on cell-mediated immune responses, with modulating activity of antibodies. A cell-mediated immunodeficiency may play a part in chronic candidiasis, syphilis and *Herpes simplex* virus infection at the initiating stage and during carcinomatous transformation.

Further reading

Dabelsteen E. (1980) Cytological and immunological approaches to prognosis of oral premalignant lesions. In *Oral Premalignancy*. Mackenzia I.C., Dabelsteen R. & Squire C.A. (eds). University of Iowa Press, Iowa.

Hollinshead A.C. & Tarro G. (1973) Soluble membrane antigens of lip and cervical carcinomas: reactivity with antibody for Herpes virus nonvirion antigens. *Science*, **179**, 698.

Kramer I.R.H., Lucas R.B., El-Laban N. & Lister L. (1970) A computer-aided study on the tissue changes in oral keratoses and lichen planus, and an analysis of case groupings by subjective and objective criteria *Br. J. Cancer*, **24**, 407.

Lehner T. & Shillitoe E.J. (1976) Immunological aspects of cancer. In *Scientific Foundations of Dentistry*. p. 163. Cohen B. & Kramer I.R.H. (eds). Heinemann, London.

Lehner T., Wilton J.M.A., Shillitoe E.J. & Ivanyi L. (1973) Cell-mediated immunity and antibodies to Herpes virus hominis type 1 in oral leukoplakia and carcinoma. *Br. J. Cancer*, **27**, 351.

Pindborg J.J., Renstrup G., Jolst O. & Roed-Petersen B. (1968) Studies in oral leukoplakia. *J. Am. dent. Ass.*, **76**, 767.

Tarro G. & Sabin A.B. (1973) Non-virion antigens produced by *Herpes simplex* viruses 1 and 2. *Proc. nat. Acad. Sci. (Wash.)*, **70**, 1032.

18

Other aspects of oral immunology

Immune responses in dental pulp and periapical tissues

The normal pulp of a tooth is free of inflammatory cells. With the development of caries, the bactria or some soluble bacterial antigens can induce a classical inflammatory response in the pulp (figure 18.1). Some micro-organisms or their products are capable of diffusing through the dentine into the pulp and induce attraction of polymorphs into the pulp. This ability to elicit chemotaxis of polymorphs differs among the oral micro-organisms. For instance, *Actinomyces viscosus* is more potent than *Strep. mitis* in eliciting chemotaxis. It is not entirely clear whether this reaction is complement independent, but if this were to be confirmed then the chemotaxis might be a direct effect of some microbial breakdown product.

There is vasodilatation, increased vascular permeability and exudation of fluid and polymorphonuclear leucocytes. As the caries approaches the pulp, macrophages, lymphocytes and

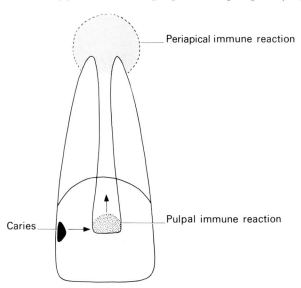

FIGURE 18.1. Pulpal and periapical immune responses to dental caries. Microbial antigenic agents diffuse to the pulp and invoke a pulpal immune reaction. If the lesion is not contained, both microbial antigen and pulpal degeneration products may induce a periapical reaction.

415

plasma cells become evident. There is extravascular immuno-globulin, predominantly IgG, and the plasma cells also belong mostly to the IgG class, though IgA, IgE and occasionally IgM containing cells are also found.

As the pulp is enclosed within the rigid structure of dentine, there is hardly any room for expansion of the inflammatory exudate. The pulp in the root canal soon becomes involved and the inflammation spreads to the periapical tissues (figure 18.1). Here it may give rise to an acute periapical abscess or if the process is chronic three types of periapical lesions may develop: chronic abscess, granuloma or a dental cyst. It can be argued that since the usual outcome of caries is death of the pulp and the development of some periapical lesion, that the protective effect of any host immune reaction is inadequate. This may be so and perhaps the most important contributing feature is the special anatomy of the dental pulp, the blood vessels of which are compressed against the rigid wall of the tooth with any inflammatory exudate. Nevertheless, the immune response might prevent acute pulpal damage in slow caries and arrested caries and might be responsible for chronic pulpitis. If the host response fails in the pulp of the tooth, it might be modified at the periapical site, where the spread of the inflammatory process may be localized to give rise to a chronic abscess, granuloma or cyst. Dental cysts show a prominent plasma cell infiltration in the cyst wall and the concentrations of IgG, IgM and IgA in the cyst fluid can be two to three times greater than those in serum. The conditions that are necessary for the development of different pulpal and periapical lesions are ill-understood and will be discussed in terms of the three immunological reactions.

A type III immune complex mediated reaction is likely to be involved, as plasma cells are found in the pulp and later in periapical tissues. These cells may produce antibodies against some of the bacterial plaque antigens, although this has not been formally demonstrated. The putative immune complex formed may activate the complement pathway and contribute to the chemotactic attraction of polymorphonuclear leucocytes into the pulp, engorgement and thrombosis of the pulpal blood vessels, leading to abscess formation.

A type IV cell-mediated reaction might also be involved, as there is some evidence for the presence of T- and B-lymphocytes and macrophages in periapical lesions. It is again likely that the cellular responses, by localizing the microbial and damaged tissue antigens, are responsible for the local damage.

416

A type I anaphylactic sensitivity: all the components necessary for this reaction have been found in the inflamed pulp. Thus, there are mast cells, IgE producing plasma cells, and histamine can be produced by the pulp. It is therefore probable that the interaction between an antigen and IgE antibody may release histamine from the mast cells and contribute to the overall inflammatory reaction.

There is very little evidence in favour of one or the other of the three types of immune responses. However, there can be little doubt that some of these reactions play an important part in the pathogenesis of pulpal and periapical lesions. Another point to appreciate is that the root canal may act as another route of immunization. Thus, serum antibodies have been elicited by introducing streptococci or non-microbial antigens into the pulp chambers or root canals of teeth. This possibility should be kept in mind when considering the potential effect of focal dental sepsis on other diseases.

The treatment of pulps and root canal therapy may involve a variety of drugs and filling materials. These may induce any of the drug hypersensitivities (see pp. 419–21), as has been found with iodine, chloramphenicol and others. Foreign body reactions of course should not be confused with hypersensitivity, as these can develop with some filling materials which are not inert.

Summary

The dental pulp and periapical tissues possess the cellular components necessary to mount three types of hypersensitivity reactions: immune complex, cell-mediated and anaphylactic types. Chemotaxis of polymorphs can be elicited as a direct effect of some bacterial product. Some or all of these mechanisms may be involved in modulating the immune responses to dental caries and especially in the development of chronic pulpitis and periapical granulomas. The root canal can function as a route of immunization to microbial antigen or as a means of sensitization to materials used in root canal therapy.

Transplantation of teeth

It is perhaps surprising to learn that transplantation of teeth between different individuals has been practised in ancient times and the tooth may well have been the first tissue to be transplanted. The basis for this apparent success is that whereas allogenic skin grafts are rejected within 8 to 12 days,

417

allogenic tooth transplants survive for about 4 years. It was therefore argued by some clinicians that the teeth are 'inert' and do not possess transplantation antigens. This is, of course, an entirely erroneous view, for transplantation antigens are present on the surface membrane of all nucleated cells. However, what has become evident is that different tissues have transplantation antigens of varying antigenic strength. Comparative studies of the immune reaction between tooth autografts and allografts placed subcutaneously in mice have shown significantly more inflammation around allografts than autografts. The leucocyte infiltration was maximal in the periapical area and this suggested that the tissues of the pulp and periodontal ligament possess the strongest antigenic determinants. Furthermore, tooth allografts are capable of inducing an accelerated rejection of skin grafts taken from the donor animal of the tooth, though this reaction is variable. Much of the experimental data suggest that the immune reaction to a tooth is weaker than that elicited by a skin graft. Tooth germs behave in the same way as other tissues but seem to have lower histocompatibility requirements. Furthermore, using a variety of strain combinations of inbred mice it was shown that tooth germs transplanted across single non-H-2 barriers (i.e. weak antigenic differences) behaved as syngeneic grafts but transplantation across multiple non-H-2 barriers showed a strong immune reaction.

Comparative studies between tooth autograft and allograft in rhesus monkeys have established the essential differences in the histopathological reactions. The pulp and periodontal ligament of the tooth autograft soon return to normal structure and the tooth becomes reattached to the bone by the periodontal ligament. The allogeneic pulp and periodontal ligament, however, never assume a normal structure or function. Within 3 weeks both the pulp and the periodontal ligament are infiltrated by lymphoid cells followed by necrosis and a persistent periapical and periodontal inflammatory reaction surrounding the entire tooth. The root undergoes resorption and periodontal reattachment does not take place. However, within a month the tooth allograft may become as firm as an autograft and this is clearly due to the root and adjacent bone undergoing resorption and bone apposition, leading to ankylosis or fusion of the root to bone. This process of tooth resorption and bony replacement eventually involves much of the tooth and results in the rejection of the allograft. The process is somewhat similar to that seen in exfoliation of deciduous teeth.

418

Tooth allograft survival can be prolonged by matching for histocompatibility and by using immunosuppressive drugs. These procedures, particularly the latter, are clearly not practicable or justifiable. However, treatment of the tooth itself can prolong graft survival. Removal of the pulp and sealing the root canal has minimized or eliminated the periapical inflammatory response and inhibited root resorption. Similarly enzymatic removal of the periodontal ligament, using collagenase or hyaluronidase was also associated with decreased inflammation and resorption and a net prolongation of a tooth graft survival. These procedures may prolong the survival of allogenic tooth transplants to about 8 years.

Summary

Allografts of teeth are antigenic and they elicit an accelerated skin graft rejection. The major sources of antigenicity of a tooth reside in the pulp and periodontal ligament, but even dentine can elicit transplantation immunity. However, a tooth allograft may survive for years without any attempt at matching for histocompatible antigens between donor and recipient and without using immunosuppressive agents. There are a number of factors which may account for the prolonged survival of tooth allografts. The teeth are antigenically weak and do not need to remain alive to continue to function (unlike, of course, kidneys). Although the pulp and periodontal ligament necrose, the rest of the tooth structure is difficult to resorb. Normal reattachment does not take place and the tooth is retained in the bone by bony replacement of the resorbed root. The tooth transplant can function in spite of attachment by ankylosis, though eventually so much of the root is resorbed that the tooth is exfoliated.

Allergies

DRUG ALLERGIES

Drug allergies are mediated by immunological reactions, they have no relation to known pharmacological properties of the drugs and there is no linear relationship to drug dosage. The reaction is often similar to that of classical protein allergy; it ceases on discontinuation of therapy, only to reappear after a further dose, and occurs only in a minority of patients. Any of the four classical immune mechanisms may be involved in the allergic reaction.

Type I immediate or anaphylactic reactions are mediated mainly by IgE antibodies which bind to receptors on mast cells and basophil leucocytes. The anaphylactic reaction is acute and has a potentially fatal outcome. Most cases are due to penicillin but streptomycin, diazepam, local anaesthetics and radio-opaque iodides may also be responsible. Anaphylaxis develops within a few minutes of administration of the responsible drug. Anaphylactic shock presents as peripheral circulatory collapse, but may be accompanied by bronchospasm, urticaria, rhinitis or angioneurotic oedema which can be lethal. Angioneurotic oedema manifests mainly as oedema of the face, eyelids, lips and tongue. The onset is rapid and often there is associated pruritis. Urticaria may be caused by the above drugs and also by codeine, salicylates, meprobamate or imipramine. Hypersensitivity to local anaesthetics is extremely uncommon in relation to the numbers being administered by dental surgeons; procaine and lignocaine have been implicated.

Testing for hypersensitivity of local anaesthetics is rather unsatisfactory but can be carried out *in vivo* by applying the test substance to the nasal mucosa, by intradermal administration or *in vitro* by assaying the lymphoproliferative response to the local anaesthetics.

Type II autoimmune or cytolytic reactions occur when a drug acting as a haptene combines with a cell surface constituent leading to auto-antibody production. These antibodies are directed at the complex of drug haptene and surface component, and result in destructions of the cells involved. Examples of type II hypersensitivity reactions include thrombocytopenia induced by quinidine and sedormid.

Type III Arthus type reactions may commence within 36 hours but more commonly occur 7 to 12 days after the onset of drug therapy. The administration of serum products, usually tetanus antitoxin, or drugs such as penicillin may be responsible. Fever, arthralgia, urticaria and maculo-papular rashes are common, while lymphadenopathy, wheezing and angioedema are less frequently seen.

Type IV or delayed hypersensitivity reactions occur with contact allergy which results from a combination of the drug, acting as a haptene, with proteins of the epidermal or epithelial cells. Contact dermatitis is characterized by the appearance of pruritis at the site of the lesion, followed by erythema and vesiculation. The allergen may be an active ingredient of a

420

preparation, often neomycin or benzocaine, or may be a base such as lanolin, or a preservative such as p-aminobenzoic acid. Contact dermatitis can be a serious problem for medical or dental personnel; the latter may become sensitized to amethocaine or mercury. Contact allergy may occasionally affect the oral mucosa or the lips, when it is due to dentifrices, cosmetics or various foods. The mucosa becomes erythematous and oedematous, sometimes with small vesicles which rupture to leave painful erosions. Allergens responsible for contact stomatitis include antibiotics, mercury, vulcanite, flavouring agents such as cinnamon in toothpaste, essential oils, epoxy resins, acrylic and walnuts.

Hypersensitivity to mercury used in the amalgam of dental fillings can be difficult to diagnose and it is rather a rare occurrence. It is often confused with hypersensitivity to local anaesthetic as the filling is inserted under local anaesthesia. Hypersensitivity to acrylic material used in dentures is even less common, though often blamed for ill-fitting dentures or difficulties in getting used to them. In spite of the rarity of true hypersensitivity to mercury and acrylic they are frequent problems referred to hospital and should be dealt with by taking a careful history and, if necessary, following this up by patch-testing with solubilized mercury and the monomer and polymer of acrylic suspended in olive oil.

Contact cheilitis may be caused by the fluorescein stain in some lipsticks or other constituents such as carmine and by some fruits.

Erythema multiforme. This deserves special attention as not infrequently it affects the oral mucosa of young men. Extensive ulcers which are preceded by bullae affect the oral mucosa. These may or may not be associated with a variety of skin lesions, genital ulcers and conjunctivitis. The aetiology of erythema multiforme is extremely varied and a large number of drugs (e.g. barbiturates, sulphonamides) and microbial agents (*Herpes simplex*, mycoplasma) have been implicated. The lesions may appear within 48 hours of the precipitating agent and the condition usually recurs.

Summary

In spite of the variety of dietary and chemical substances which make contact with the oral mucosa, the development of true allergic manifestations in the mouth is somewhat rare. Allergy to dietary constituents, drugs and materials used in dental hygiene, conservative and prosthetic dentistry are ill-understood. The material which is most often blamed for allergic reactions in the mouth is the acrylic used in dentures, although allergy to acrylic is extremely rare. Local anaesthetics employed in conservative dentistry are commonly blamed by patients who faint after an injection, usually for psychogenic reasons. Although rather rare, well authenticated histories of allergic reactions should be examined by the appropriate immunological tests.

Amyloidosis

Amyloid is a fibrillar protein deposited in between the cells of a variety of tissues and in blood vessel walls. There are three major types of amyloidosis: (a) primary amyloidosis in which there is no evidence of a predisposing disease, (b) amyloidosis associated with multiple myelomatosis, and (c) secondary amyloidosis which is associated with a variety of chronic inflammatory diseases, such as tuberculosis, rheumatoid arthritis and chronic suppurative conditions.

Light chains of immunoglobulin are found in amyloid associated with myeloma and in primary amyloid. Amyloid A protein is not part of any known fragment of immunoglobulin and is found predominantly in secondary amyloidosis. Both these types of amyloid are related to disorders of immune function.

Infiltration of tissues by amyloid arises either as a result of excessive stimulation of the reticulo-endothelial system, as in chronic infections or long-standing inflammatory disease such as rheumatoid arthritis (secondary amyloid), or because of primary derangement of immunoglobulin synthesis (primary amyloid). The concentration of normal serum immunoglobulins may be depressed and Bence Jones proteinuria may be found. Paraproteins are not found in secondary amyloidosis but they are present in a high proportion of cases of primary amyloidosis.

Enlarged tongue (macroglosia) is found in about half of the patients with primary amyloidosis and is an important, though late, manifestation of the disease. The tongue is infiltrated with amyloid which renders it large, firm and immobile.

Further reading

Benditt E.P. & Erikson N. (1971) Chemical classes of amyloid substances. *Am. J. Pathol.*, **65**, 231.

Bergenholtz G. & Lindhe J. (1975) Effect of soluble plaque factors on inflammatory reactions in the dental pulp. *Scand. J. Dent. Res.*, **83**, 153.

Calnan C.D. & Sarkanyi I. (1960) Studies in contact dermatitis. XII. Sensitivity in oleyl alcohol. *Trans. St. John's Hosp. Derm. Soc.*, **44**, 47.

Calnan C.D. & Stevenson C.J. (1963) Studies in contact dermatitis. XV. Dental materials. *Trans. St. John's Hosp. Derm. Soc.*, **49**, 9.

Cameron A.J., Baron J.H. & Priestly B.L. (1966) Erythema multiforme, drugs and ulcerative colitis. *Br. Med. J.*, **ii**, 1174.

Cronin E., Bandmann H.J., Calnan C.D., Fregert S., Hjorth N., Magnusson B., Maibach H.I., Malten K., Meneghini C.L., Pirala V. & Wilkinson D.S. (1970) Contact dermatitis in the atopic. *Acta Derm. Ven.*, **50**, 183.

Dockrill T.E. (1961) Tissue mast cells in the oral cavity. *Aus. dent. J.*, **6**, 210.

Engelman M.A. (1963) Mercury allergy resulting from amalgam restorations. *J. Am. Dent. Ass.*, **66**, 122.

Farber P.A. (1975) Scanning electron microscopy of cells from periapical lesions. *J. Endodont.*, **1**, 291.

Fisher A.A. (1954) Allergic sensitization of skin and oral mucosa to acrylic denture materials. *J. Am. Med. Assoc.*, **156**, 238.

Fong C.C., Berger J. & Morris M. (1967) Experimental allogeneic tooth transplantation in the rhesus monkey. *J. dent. Res.*, **47**, 351.

Franklin E.C., Rosenthal C.J., Pras M. & Levin M. (1976) Recent progress in amyloid. In *The Role of Immunological Factors in Infections, Allergic and Autoimmune Processes.* p. 163. Beers R.F. & Bassett E.G. (eds). Raven Press, New York.

Glenner G.G., Terry W.D. & Isersky C. (1973) Amyloidosis: Its nature and pathogenesis. *Semin. Haematol.*, **10**, 65.

Gorlin R. & Pindberg J.J. (1964) *Syndromes of the Head and Neck.* McGraw Hill, New York.

Ivanyi D. (1966) Comparison of the histocompatibility requirements of skin and tooth germ grafts. *Transplantation*, **4**, 639.

Kennedy D.R., Hamilton T.R. & Syverton J.T. (1957) Effects on monkeys of introduction of haemolytic streptococci in root canals. *J. Dent. Res.*, **36**, 494.

Klein J. (1971) Tooth transplantation in the mouth. III. The role of minor (non H-2) histocompatibility loci in tooth germ transplantation. *Transplantation*, **12**, 500.

Morgan J.K. (1968) Iatrogenic epidermal sensitivity. *Br. J. Clin. Prac.*, **22**, 261.

Okada H., Aono M., Yashida M., Munemtok K., Nishida D. & Yokomizo I. (1967) Experimental study on focal infection in rabbits by prolonged sensitization through dental pulp canals. *Archs. oral Biol.*, **12**, 1017.

Pindborg J.J. (1972) Disorders of the oral cavity and lips. In *Textbook of Dermatology.* p. 1672. Rook A., Wilkinson D.S., & Ebling F.J.G. (eds). Blackwell Scientific Publications, Oxford.

Pulver W.H., Taubman M.A. & Smith D.J. (1978) Immune components in normal and inflamed human dental pulp. *Archs. oral Biol.*, **23**, 435.

Rook A., Wilkinson D.S. & Ebling F.J.G. (1972) *Textbook of Dermatology.* Blackwell Scientific Publications, Oxford.

Scully C.M. & Lehner T. (1980) Oral manifestations of disorders of immunity. In *Oral Manifestations of Systemic Disease.* Mason D.K. & Jones J.H. (eds). W.B. Saunders, London.

Shulman L.B. (1973) The immunology of allogeneic tooth transplantation. In *Comparative Immunology of the Oral Cavity.* p. 159. DHEW Publication No. (NIH) 73–438.

423

Toller P.A. & Holborow E.J. (1969) Immunoglobulins and immunoglobulin-containing cells in cysts of the jaws. *Lancet*, **ii,** 178.

Turrell A.J.W. (1966) Allergy to denture base materials; fallacy or reality. *N.Y. State Dent. J.,* **120,** 415.

Waldman H.B. & Binkley G. (1967) Lidocaine hypersensitivity. *J. Am. Dent. Ass.,* **74,** 747.

Zachrisson B.U. (1971) Mast cells in human dental pulp. *Archs. oral Biol.,* **16,** 555.

Appendix

TABLE 1. Recommended schedule for active routine immunization of normal individuals in the United Kingdom[1]

Age	Vaccine	Interval	Notes
During the first year of life	Dip/tet/pert and oral polio vaccine (first dose)		The earliest age at which the first dose should be given is three months, but a better general immunological response can be expected if the first dose is delayed to six months of age
	Dip/tet/pert and oral polio vaccine (second dose)	Preferably after an interval of six to eight weeks	
	Dip/tet/pert and oral polio vaccine (third dose)	Preferably after an interval of four to six months	
During the second year of life	Measles vaccine	After an interval of not less than three weeks	Although measles vaccination can be given in the second year of life, delay until three years of age or more will reduce the risk of occasional severe reactions to the vaccine which occur mainly in children under the age of three years
At five years of age or school entry	Dip/tet and oral polio vaccine or dip/tet/polio vaccine		These may be given, if desired, at three years of age to children entering nursery schools, attending day nurseries or living in children's homes
Between 10 and 13 years of age	BCG vaccine		
All girls aged 11 to 13 years	Rubella vaccine	There should be an interval of not less than three weeks between BCG and rubella vaccination	All girls of this age should be offered rubella vaccine whether or not there is a past history of an attack of rubella
At 15 to 19 years of age or on leaving school	Polio vaccine (oral or inactivated) and tetanus toxoid		

[1] Data from *Immunisation Against Infectious Diseases* (1972), DHSS, London. (Reproduced from 'Immunisation', G. Dick, Update Books with permission of author and publishers.)

TABLE 2. Recommended schedule for active routine immunization of normal individuals in the USA[1]

Age	Vaccine	Notes
2 months	Dip/tet/pert and oral polio vaccine	Suitable for breast-fed as well as bottle-fed babies
4 months	Dip/tet/pert and oral polio vaccine	
6 months	Dip/tet/pert and oral polio vaccine	
1 year	Measles, rubella, mumps, tuberculin test	May be given at 1 year as combined measles–rubella or measles–mumps–rubella vaccines Measles vaccine may be given at 6 months in places where measles frequent in first year of life. In such circumstances a repeat dose should be given at 1 year. Frequency of repeated tuberculin tests depends on risk of exposure and prevalence of tuberculosis. Initial test should be at time of, or preceding, measles immunization
1½ years	Dip/tet/pert and oral polio vaccine	
4 to 6 years	Dip/tet/pert and oral polio vaccine	
14 to 16 years	Tet	And every 10 years thereafter

[1] Data from *Report of the Committee on Infectious Diseases* (1974), 17th edition, American Academy of Pediatrics, Evanston, Illinois. (Reproduced from 'Immunisation' by G. Dick, Update Books with permission of author and publisher.)

428

Index

430

438